# RESEARCH TOPICS ON BRAIN MAPPING

# RESEARCH TOPICS ON BRAIN MAPPING

YUANZHU LIÁNG
EDITOR

**Nova Science Publishers, Inc.**
New York

For permission to use material from this book please contact us:
Telephone 631-231-7269; Fax 631-231-8175
Web Site: http://www.novapublishers.com



**Library of Congress Cataloging-in-Publication Data**

Research topics on brain mapping / Yuanzhu Liang (editor).
p. ; cm.
Includes bibliographical references and index.
ISBN 978-1-60456-001-5 (hardcover)
1. Brain mapping. I. Liang, Yuanzhu.
[DNLM: 1. Brain Mapping. WL 335 R429 2007]
RC386.6.B7R47 2007
612.8'2--dc22

2007035863

*Published by Nova Science Publishers, Inc. ≃ New York*

# Contents

# Preface

This new and significant book concentrates on brain mapping which is a set of neuroscience techniques predicated on the mapping of (biological) quantities or properties onto spatial representations of the (human or non-human) brain resulting in maps. All neuroimaging can be considered part of brain mapping. Brain mapping can be conceived as a higher form of neuroimaging, producing brain images supplemented by the result of additional (imaging or non-imaging) data processing or analysis, such as maps projecting (measures of) behaviour onto brain regions (see fMRI). Brain Mapping techniques are constantly evolving, and rely on the development and refinement of image acquisition, representation, analysis, visualization and interpretation techniques. Functional and structural neuroimaging are at the core of the mapping aspect of Brain Mapping.

Short Communication - As it is known, urinary incontinence is defined as any involuntary leakage of urine, and has long been acknowledged to be a major health problem in the elderly. The authors aimed to find the brain areas, which control the bladder storage and how they work by SPECT with Neurological Statistical Image Analysis Software (NEUROSTAT).

Methods: SPECT scans were performed on forty male and right-handed subjects including fifteen healthy volunteers (Group A) and twenty-five patients with some storage symptoms of lower urinary tract. Among the twenty-five patients, nineteen patients were with DO (Group B) and six patients were with normal detrusor function (Group C). SPECT scan was performed on each subject in two states: resting state and urine withholding state with full bladder. The image of urine withholding was obtained by subtracting the resting state data from the urine withholding. NEUROSTAT was adopted to analyze the difference in rCBF between groups in resting state and to analyze the change in rCBF between urine withholding and resting states in each group. The results were displayed on Z-score images at a significance threshold of $P < 0.05$ with correction for multiple comparisons.

Results: No region reached significant threshold in comparison of Group B and Group C in resting state. Group A and Group C showed similar results in urine withholding state as compared with resting state, significant increases in tracer activity were found in bilateral inferior frontal gyri, the right superior and middle temporal gyri. Among the regions, the right inferior frontal gyrus was distinctly prominent at both Z-score and the extent. In Group B, the regions that were activated significantly in Group A and Group C did not reach significant threshold during urine withholding as compared with resting state.

Conclusions: The study indicated that bilateral inferior frontal gyri, the right superior and middle temporal gyri were associated with the control of bladder storage. Especially, the right inferior frontal gyrus played a more important role in cerebral control of bladder storage, inhibiting the contraction of detrusor during urine withholding.

Chapter I – In the past decade, functional neuroimaging studies have significantly advanced our understanding of human cognitive functions. However, much less is known about the anatomical connections underlying higher cognitive processes in humans. One of the reasons why anatomical studies have lagged behind functional studies is that there are methodological limitations on studying anatomical connections of the human brain in vivo. There are numerous detailed anatomical studies of non-human primates that serve as the basis of our understandings of connections in the brain. However, those techniques are not feasible in humans. Diffusion imaging is a new technique based on detecting the diffusion of water molecules from magnetic resonance images. Diffusion imaging allows non-invasive mapping of anatomical connections and gives a comprehensive picture of connectivity throughout the brain, but there are still numerous technical issues to be addressed. Here, the author introduces recent studies on large-scale anatomical connections underlying episodic memory in humans. The author studied an entire network based on some episodic memory tasks, and applied several new approaches to assess the tractography results. The main finding was that encoding-related areas in the left dorsolateral prefrontal cortex and the left ventrolateral prefrontal cortex connect with another encoding-related area in the left temporal cortex. This suggests that there are two pathways between prefrontal cortex and temporal cortex related to encoding processes in episodic memory. Further, the author discusses future applications of diffusion imaging in the study of the human memory system.

Chapter II – Cannabis is the most commonly used illicit drug. Its principle psychoactive compound is delta-9-tetrahydrocannabinol, acting centrally at cannabanoid 1 (CB1) receptors which are widely distributed in the neocortex with high concentrations in frontal regions and areas of associational function. Acute intoxication results in decreased attention, memory, and psychomotor speed. The effects of chronic use remain an area of debate.

A number of studies of brain structure and function have attempted to determine the neural mechanisms underlying the effect of cannabis on the CNS, and these mechanisms remain poorly understood. Evidence from CT and MRI studies does not suggest a significant association between cannabis use and structural brain abnormalities. Functional neuroimaging (fMRI, SPECT, PET) may identify brain changes to subtle to be detected by current structural imaging techniques. Although there are wide differences in study designs and considerable variations in results among different investigations, the majority of studies have demonstrated global cortical activity increases during administration of cannabis. Differential activity in specific brain regions has also been reported. Increased frontal lobe activity has been generally reported with cannabis exposure while attenuated frontal activity has been described in recently abstinent cannabis users. Studies involving the temporal lobes are limited and somewhat conflicting. Increased anterior cingulate activity correlating with subjective intoxication has been reported with cannabis administration while decreased anterior cingulate activity has been reported during abstinence in regular cannabis users.

Increases in cerebellar activity have been shown to occur in cannabis smokers while reduced cerebellar activity occurs during abstinence in regular cannabis users. Current neuroimaging has not yet helped fully clarify the role of chronic cannabis use and cognitive deficits.

Although visual EEG analysis does not yield consistent cannabis related changes, quantitative EEG has proven more revealing. Quantitative EEG studies of acute cannabis exposure showed increased relative power of alpha, combined with decreased alpha frequency and a reduction of beta activity. EEGs of chronic heavy long term users are characterized by significant elevations of absolute alpha power, relative alpha power, and interhemispheric alpha coherence over frontal and fronto-central areas, a phenomenon referred to as hyperfrontality of alpha. Most initial evoked potentials studies suggest that P300 event related potentials are not altered by chronic cannabis use, although the P50 auditory gating response may be reduced and steady state visual evoked potentials may be altered in cannabis users. The neurophysiological effects of cannabis abuse remains only partially understood and additional research is needed in this area

Chapter III – Balanced steady-state free precession (balanced SSFP or bSSFP) has gained widespread attention due to its high efficiency and unique contrast. Recently, this technique has been adapted for functional MRI in order to provide improved SNR and reduced distortion. Two different contrast mechanisms have been investigated: transition-band SSFP fMRI, which detects the bulk frequency shift from BOLD using the frequency selectivity of the SSFP profile, and pass-band SSFP fMRI, which primarily measures $T_2$ changes from the diffusion effect. Both methods utilize efficient 3D k-space trajectories, which have been developed in recent years to enable the acquisition of full 3D volumes in 2-6 seconds with minimal off-resonance artifacts (such as blurring or warping). The strong contrast and intrinsically high SNR of transition-band SSFP fMRI enables high-resolution isotropic ($1mm^3$) fMRI experiments even at low field strengths (1.5 T), and the low SAR requirements of this method also make high field imaging possible. The pass-band SSFP method has great potential for imaging in regions near susceptibility boundaries, such as the pre-frontal cortex above the sinuses. These methods are known to suffer from sensitivity to spatial and temporal off-resonance frequencies, prompting the development of new techniques, including a real-time $B_0$ shift compensation technique and an interleaved center frequency updating. Both SSFP fMRI methods could enable a wider range of neuroscience applications by enabling high resolution and reducing image artifacts.

Chapter IV – The neural large-scale dynamics and the connectivity pathways among spatially separated neural groups are conceived as a fundamental brain mechanism to integrate and process information.

The new measures of nonlinear interdependencies applied to EEG recordings, such as phase synchronization, have been recently shown to be highly sensitive to detect the dynamical change underlying the brain functions.

In the present chapter, the patterns of interdependency among different brain regions were investigated extracting the Synchronization Index (SI) from EEG response to different emotional and non-emotional film stimuli. The three basic emotions of happiness, fear and sadness were induced with the goal to investigate the synchronization patterns at different frequencies bands specifically associated with the valence dimension (positive vs. negative) and with the distinct basic emotional systems.

The comparisons among the experimental conditions showed several significant SI changes. The results demonstrated an overall decrease of SI during emotional stimulation compared to neutral, indicating an increase of complexity in the cortical dynamics. Further differences were found among the specific emotions, involving a distinct couple of electrodes with topographical effects at the frequencies bands examined. During happiness, the authors found a large pattern of synchronization in the left frontal hemisphere, especially in delta and theta waves, while fear, compared to neutral stimuli, showed a higher right synchronization, especially in beta waves. Largely different SI patterns emerged in the comparisons between the two negative emotions of fear and sadness, suggesting that the basic emotions are mediated by specific synchronized activity. The observed emotion-related SI change supports the view that coupling-decoupling patterns among the neural networks may be a relevant neural mechanism for the emotional processing and that SI nonlinear analysis may contribute to describe how the brain generates the emotion.

Chapter V – The somatosensory information processing during its course from the peripheral to the somatosensory areas is influenced by top-down modulation (centrifugal mechanism) mediated by a network comprising brain structures, motor and higher-order brain systems. However, little is known about the property of sensori-motor integration in the somatosensory cortices during the preparatory period of voluntary movement in humans. To elucidate the mechanisms underlying sensori-motor integration in the primary (SI) and secondary somatosensory cortex (SII), the authors investigated the temporal change in somatosensory evoked magnetic fields (SEFs) using a self-initiated voluntary movement task. Electrical stimulation of the right median nerve was applied continuously, while the subjects performed a self-initiated finger extension every 5 to 7 sec. They were instructed not to pay attention to the electrical stimulation. The preparatory period of self-initiated finger extension was divided into subperiods from the onset of the electromyogram, and the magnetoencephalogram signals following stimulation in each subperiod were averaged. In SI, three equivalent current dipole (ECD) components (N20m, P30m and P60m) were recognized. Although the ECD moment for N20m and P60m was not significantly changed in the preparatory period, that for P30m was significantly smaller in the 0- to -500-ms subperiod. As for bilateral SII, the ECD moment for the SII ipsilateral to movement (SIIi) showed no significant change, while that for the contralateral SII (SIIc) was significantly larger in the same subperiod. Voluntary movement is associated with both the actual motor command and a copy of the motor command (efference copy and corollary discharge) providing information about the expected sensory consequences of the movement. The opposite effects of voluntary movement on SI and SII indicated that these cortical areas are affected differently by the centrifugal mechanism and play a different role in the function of the sensori-motor integration.

Chapter VI – BOLD (blood oxygenation level dependent) contrast based functional MRI (fMRI) has been established as a noninvasive tool for brain mapping research. For most applications of BOLD fMRI, the primary objective is simply to identify activated areas in response to a specific stimulation. The fractional BOLD signal change depends on the imaging parameters such as echo time and field strength, and only its relative magnitude to the time-course signal variation (noise) is used for a statistical inference to reveal focal area(s) of interest. While a quantitative and absolute evaluation of BOLD signal change in terms of physiological parameters usually does not need to be considered, recent theoretical and experimental studies for the quantitative use of BOLD fMRI have provided us with new opportunities: 1) mapping of hemodynamic parameters of the human brain in the baseline state, such as deoxyhemoglobin concentration, venous CBV (cerebral blood volume), OEF (oxygen extraction fraction) and oxidative energetics in terms of cerebral metabolic rate of oxygen ($CMRO_2$) 2) optimization of imaging parameters, e.g., the voxel volume and echo time for given hardware settings such as the field strength and coil sensitivity.

Chapter VII – Modern neurosurgery is an arena in which advances in technology are applied to the care of patients. Neurosurgeons have been integral to the development and application of numerous methods for understanding brain-behavior relationships. Functional magnetic resonance imaging (FMRI) has been added to the neurosurgeons armamentarium over the past decade and is rapidly moving into place as established "standard of care" for surgeries involving cortical regions critical for a variety of motor, sensory, and cognitive functions. In this chapter, the authors will describe briefly the development of the FMRI technique and the history of its application to the neurosurgical theater. Technological challenges to the integration of FMRI data with other modalities of neuroimaging in the operating room are now being overcome, and the chapter provides examples of this integration as well as describing the future promise of this endeavor. The majority of this chapter is devoted to description and illustration of imaging paradigms that are used to study specific brain functions, along with case examples.

Chapter VIII – Before we can begin to search for primate homologies, it is vital to first obtain accurate structural and functional maps of human brain areas and the related regions in nonhuman primates. Functional magnetic resonance imaging (fMRI) is an excellent tool for the balanced sampling of the brain at high resolutions, but for various technical reasons it has been less than ideal for imaging certain sensory systems in either monkeys or humans. It is only recently that developments in acquisition and analysis methods have made it possible to visualize the cortical representation of the senses in at least one of the species. In this chapter the authors pursue the question of how imaging in one of the species might be assisted by developments in another. They consider the advances that have been made in imaging the visual system to reveal the underlying functional organization of a number of different visual areas and compare their organization in humans and monkeys. As a result, more visual areas are now thought to have been evolutionarily conserved in these primates. The authors also summarize recent developments in the context of the auditory, somatosensory, vestibular, olfactory and gustatory systems. In these as well as in the visual system, numerous functional areas are thought to exist, but many more remain to be localized. In the context of this research, although most developments were done in the field of human neuroimaging, there are also areas where monkey functional mapping seems to be farther advanced. Comparative approaches will help to clarify further primate evolutionary relationships by exploiting advances made in the imaging of individual species.

Chapter IX – Functional brain imaging of the somatosensory system has become an important tool in the planning of neurosurgical procedures for patients with brain tumor or cavernoma and for the discrimination of the motor cortex from the surrounding brain tissue in order to accurately define resection boundaries. Moreover, these studies are important for the monitoring of neurorehabilitation processes and the understanding of motor recovery, e.g.

after stroke, in brain trauma, spinal cord injury, extrapyramidal diseases or extremity transplantations for the planning of individual neurorehabilitation strategies.

A close relationship of movement related cortical areas and areas related to somatosensory sensation is well documented in the literature and led to the concept of the sensorimotor cortex. Positron emission tomography (PET) and functional magnetic resonance imaging (fMRI) studies have shown that somatosensory paradigms can activate somatosensory as well as motor areas of the cerebral cortex. Moreover, somatosensory stimulation for probing the nature and function of the sensorimotor cortex does not require the collaboration of the subject under examination and is therefore feasible in patients with hemiparesis or hemiplegia, which holds promise for a wide clinical applicability.

Somatosensory paradigms in fMRI also revealed a positive correlation between the intensity of phantom limb pain in amputees and the amount of reorganization of the sensorimotor cortex and thus led to a deeper understanding of the mechanisms of phantom limb pain.

For the purpose of somatosensory stimulation for the investigation of the sensorimotor cortex several MR compatible devices have been developed. These devices are based on pneumatic approaches, piezoelectric or magneto-mechanical principles. Pneumatic systems have the disadvantage of limited vibration frequencies, have shown to cause somatosensory without motorcortex activation and are difficult to control. Piezoelectric systems provide a wide range of frequencies but only small displacement amplitudes (smaller than 0.5 mm), which limits its application to the skin receptors and elicit only somatosensory without motorcortex activation, too. Magnetomechanical devices succeeded in the combined activation of the somatosensory as well as the motorcortex and are controllable.

In the paper a review of the whole area of somatosensory stimulation in functional brain imaging the past decades, advantages and disadvantages, optimal stimulation protocols and corresponding brain maps of different approaches of somatosensory stimulation in functional brain imaging and clinical and neurophysilogical applications are discussed.

Chapter X – The study of the central nervous system requires an understanding of structural and functional relationships amongst neurons. Recent advances in optical imaging techniques and fast voltage-sensitive dyes now provide a powerful tool for understanding neuronal function in the relatively intact environment of the living brain. Optical imaging provides a means to non-invasively measure changes in membrane potential using dyes that emit fluorescent signals related to changes in membrane potential. One obvious advantage of this technology is the possibility to obtain simultaneous measurements of neuronal activity from many locations, as well as offering the ability to record from processes which are too small or fragile for typical electrophysiological approaches. Optical recording also permits monitoring spatial and temporal features of information processing in complex neural networks composed of synaptically-connected populations of neurons. One potential limitation is the rather small focal penetration depth of these systems. A variety of experimental preparations (in vitro, in situ and in vivo) have been used to optically measure activity in the living brain. In this chapter, the authors will provide an overview of the recent applications of optical imaging to investigate autonomic neural networks. Autonomic circuits in the brainstem coordinate and shape motor patterns which target and control the heart, blood vessels, diaphragm and the upper airway that regulate cardiovascular and respiratory functions. With an emphasis on brainstem circuitry, the authors will discuss how optical imaging has been applied to study centrally-generated breathing activity and how spatial and temporal resolution monitoring of neuronal network activity has provided novel insights into the functional organization of brainstem autonomic circuits that are critical to overall systems homeostasis.

Chapter XI – Aim: The aim of this study is to investigate the presence of any non-linearity in the magnetoencephalographic recordings (MEG) from the temporal lobe of epileptic, Parkinson diseased and schizophrenic patients in comparison with controls, in order to find out the differences underlying their brain waves. The authors calculated the correlation dimension, which is a measure of the complexity of the dynamic system, as well as the first Lyapunov exponent that indicates the system's unpredictability.

Methods: The epileptic group comprised with 10 patients aged 20-50 years (mean: 37.5 +/- 12.8) whereas 10 subjects within the same age range served as controls. The Parkinson diseased group comprised with 10 patients aged 50 to 80 years (mean=65.1+/-10.5), whereas the controls consisted of 10 subjects within the same age range. The schizophrenic group comprised with 10 patients aged 20-30 years (mean 23.2 +/- 2.8) whereas 10 subjects within the same age range served as controls. Biomagnetic measurements were performed using a second order gradiometer SQUID (model 601 of the Biomagnetic Technologies Inc.), which was located in an electrically shielded room of low magnetic noise. For each subject the magnetic activity was recorded from a total of 64 points of the skull (32 points from each temporal lobe) as defined by a recording reference system, which is based on the 10-20 Electrode Placement System.

Results: The non-linear analysis of the MEG activity in epileptic, Parkinson diseased and schizophrenic groups showed lower dimension complexity and lower values of the first Lyapunov exponent compared with controls.

Conclusion: The application of non-linear analysis on MEG activity may offer important perspectives to better evaluate the brain function in patients with CNS disorders.

In: Research Topics on Brain Mapping
Editor: Yuanzhu Liáng, pp. 1-10
ISBN: 978-1-60456-001-5


*Short Communication A*

# Cerebral Control of Bladder Storage: Who Guides the Urine Withholding

***Yafu Yin*[*1,2], *Noriyuki Shuke*[1], *Shigeo Kaneko*[3], *Atsutaka Okizaki*[1], *Junichi Sato*[1], *Tamio Aburano*[1], *Yaming Li*[2], *Mitsuhiro Mizunaga*[3] and *Sunao Yachiku*[3]**

[1] Department of Radiology, Asahikawa Medical College, Asahikawa, Japan;
[2] Department of Nuclear Medicine, the First Hospital of China Medical University, China Medical University, Shenyang, China; [3]Department of Urology, Asahikawa Medical College, Asahikawa, Japan

## Abstract

As it is known, urinary incontinence is defined as any involuntary leakage of urine, and has long been acknowledged to be a major health problem in the elderly. We aimed to find the brain areas, which control the bladder storage and how they work by SPECT with Neurological Statistical Image Analysis Software (NEUROSTAT).

**Methods**: SPECT scans were performed on forty male and right-handed subjects including fifteen healthy volunteers (Group A) and twenty-five patients with some storage symptoms of lower urinary tract. Among the twenty-five patients, nineteen patients were with DO (Group B) and six patients were with normal detrusor function (Group C). SPECT scan was performed on each subject in two states: resting state and urine withholding state with full bladder. The image of urine withholding was obtained by subtracting the resting state data from the urine withholding. NEUROSTAT was adopted to analyze the difference in rCBF between groups in resting state and to analyze the change in rCBF between urine withholding and resting states in each group. The results were displayed on *Z*-score images at a significance threshold of $P < 0.05$ with correction for multiple comparisons.

* For correspondence or reprints contact: Yafu Yin; Address: Department of Nuclear Medicine, the First Hospital of China Medical University, China Medical University, Nanjing North St. 155, Heping Ward, Shenyang 110001, China. Telephone: +86-024-83282611; Fax: +86-024-22703576; E-mail: yinyafu@hotmail.com

**Results**: No region reached significant threshold in comparison of Group B and Group C in resting state. Group A and Group C showed similar results in urine withholding state as compared with resting state, significant increases in tracer activity were found in bilateral inferior frontal gyri, the right superior and middle temporal gyri. Among the regions, the right inferior frontal gyrus was distinctly prominent at both Z-score and the extent. In Group B, the regions that were activated significantly in Group A and Group C did not reach significant threshold during urine withholding as compared with resting state.

**Conclusions**: The study indicated that bilateral inferior frontal gyri, the right superior and middle temporal gyri were associated with the control of bladder storage. Especially, the right inferior frontal gyrus played a more important role in cerebral control of bladder storage, inhibiting the contraction of detrusor during urine withholding.

**Keywords:** *bladder storage, detrusor overactivity, NEUROSTAT,* $^{99m}$*Tc-hexamethylpropylene amine oxime, SPECT.*

# Introduction

As it is known, urinary incontinence is defined as any involuntary leakage of urine, and it is frequently found in the elderly and the patients with stroke [31], multiple sclerosis [3], Alzheimer's disease [34], multiple system atrophy [11, 32], traumatic brain lesion [12], brain tumours[20], Parkinson's disease [25, 32] and other brain disorders. It has been well known that involuntary urinary continence center is located in the pons [7, 9, 10, 21], and some regions of the frontal cortex has been considered to be associated with urine withholding [2, 9, 13, 28, 33, 36], but the cerebral control system, who guide the urine withholding, has not been well revealed.

We aimed to find the cerebral control system that guides the urine withholding and how it works. As we know, functional brain imaging and the corresponding image analysis software were chosen in previous studies [2, 9, 17], such as SPECT, PET and fMRI, Statistical Parametric Mapping (SPM), three-dimensional stereotactic surface projection (3D-SSP). In this study, SPECT and Neurological Statistical Image Analysis Software (NEUROSTAT) were adopted.

# Materials and Methods

## Subjects

Fifteen healthy volunteers (mean age 32.67±7.30 ys, range 24-45 ys) were recruited. No subject had a reported history of urological, psychiatric or neurological disease. The fifteen volunteers were named as Group A.

Twenty-five patients (mean age 72.32 ± 9.53 ys, range 40-83 ys), who were with some storage symptoms of lower urinary tract, increased daytime frequency, nocturia, urgency or urinary incontinence, underwent urodynamic studies (UDS) including Uroflowmetry,

Cystometry and Sphincter electromyography. None had a spinal cord disorder or injury, peripheral innervation disorder, history of pelvic irradiation, current genitourinary tract infection, bladder occupying disease, or with detrusor sphincter dyssynergia (DSD). Among them, nineteen patients (mean age 74.05 ± 7.55 ys, range 59-83 ys) were with detrusor overactivity (DO) confirmed by UDS and were named as Group B. And the other six patients (mean age 66.83 ± 13.53 ys, range 40-77 ys) were with normal detrusor function and were named as Group C.

All the subjects were male and right-handed and were acknowledged the full information of the study plan.

## Data Acquisition

SPECT scan was performed on each subject in two states: resting state and urine withholding state. The later was defined as the subject sensed urge to void with full bladder after 20mg furosemide administered in a drop infusion. In resting state, 444MBq of $^{99m}$Tc-HMPAO was injected intravenously, and 555MBq of $^{99m}$Tc-HMPAO was injected in urine withholding state. After two minutes of the injection, SPECT scan was performed for 10 minutes with a 4-head gamma camera (SPECT 2000H, Hitachi Medico., Tokyo, Japan), using low-energy high-resolution parallel-hole collimators. The acquisition mode was step and the matrix was 64 × 64, energy window was 20% centered at 140 KeV. In-plane FWHM of this system was 7.4mm. The interval between the two scans was about 24 minutes.

After acquisition, the data were transferred to a dedicated data processing unit (Hitachi Gamma Vision RW-3000) and processed with a Butterworth filter (cutoff frequency: 0.55 cycles per centimeter; order: 8) and reconstructed into transaxial sections of 4.0-mm-thick images in planes parallel to the orbitomeatal line. The image of urine withholding was obtained by subtracting the resting state scan data from the urine withholding state.

## Statistical Analysis

In this study, the images of two states were analyzed by NEUROSTAT, which was developed by Minoshima et al. [29].

The images of resting state for different groups were analyzed by iSSP35_2tZ, analysis software of NEUROSTAT, which can conduct an unpaired *t* test on two non-corresponding groups. The individual SPECT data was anatomically normalized to the standard brain and the regional voxel data was compared with the normal SPECT database, then the *Z*-score [(normal mean - individual value)/normal SD] for each voxel of the cerebral surface was calculated, and was displayed at the sites voxel value statistically reduced or increased. Then the brain surface extraction data files were used to perform unpaired *t* test and create *Z*-score image by iSSP35_2tZ. The results were shown on two *Z*-score images (increase and decrease images).

The images of resting and urine withholding states for each group were analyzed by another analysis software of NEUROSTAT named Stat_1tZ, which can conduct a paired *t* test of two corresponding groups using cross-sectional images. The process of analysis included six steps: co-registration, anatomic standardization, normalize, averaging of subtraction image, paired *t* test and creating *Z*-score image. Results were shown on two *Z*-score images (increase and decrease images), and detailed information was recorded in a text file.

The statistical significance was defined as $P < 0.05$ with correction for multiple comparisons [16], since many *t* values would reach a conventional level of significance by chance for there were so many voxel-by-voxel comparisons.

## Results

Decreased tracer activity was found in bilateral superior temporal gyri (STG) [Brodmann area (BA) 22, 38], medial frontal gyri (MeFG) (BA 9, 10) and anterior cingulate (AC) (BA 24, 32), the right inferior frontal gyrus (IFG) (BA 47) and left cingulate gyrus (BA 23) (figure 1) in Group B as compared with Group A.

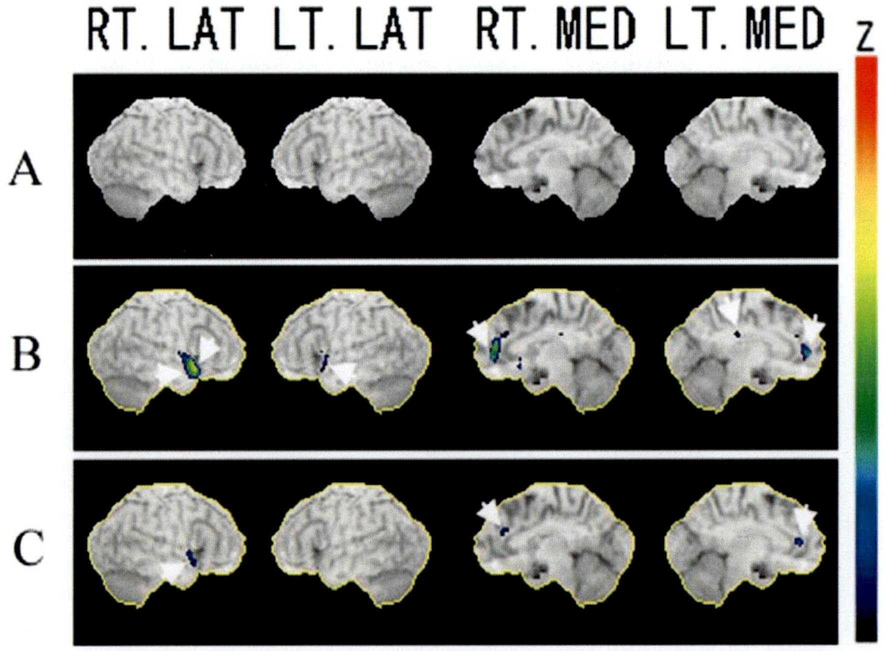


Figure 1. A: MR image of 3D-SSP; B: Z-score image (decrease image) of Group B when compared with Group A in resting state by global count; C: Z-score image (decrease image) of Group C when compared with Group A in resting state by global count.

And decreased tracer activity was found in the right STG (BA 22, 38), MeFG (BA 9) and bilateral AC (BA 32) (figure 1) in Group C as compared with Group A,

No increased or decreased activity was found in comparison of Group B and Group C.

For Group A, in urine withholding state, as compared with resting, there were significant increases in tracer activity in bilateral IFG (BA 45, 47), the right STG (BA22, 38) and middle temporal gyri (MTG) (BA21, 37) (figure 2). The cluster sizes were 219, 219, 67 and 24 voxels, respectively. Among these regions, the right IFG was distinctly prominent at both *Z*-score and the extent (cluster size).

For Group B, in urine withholding state, as compared with resting, only the left MTG and middle frontal gyrus (MFG) were activated significantly with a cluster size of 20 and 3 voxels, respectively (figure 3).

For Group C, in urine withholding state, as compared with resting, there were significant increases in tracer activity in bilateral IFG and the right MTG with a cluster size of 147, 20 and 58 voxels, respectively (figure 4).

In all of the three groups, no region with decreased activity reached significant threshold.

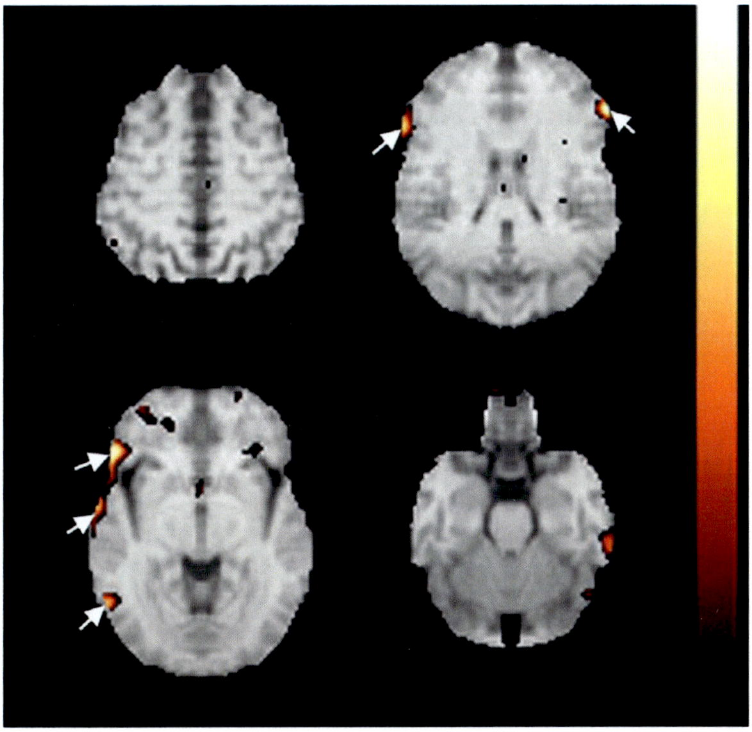

Figure 2. Results of Stat_1tZ in Group A. Increased activity in bilateral IFG and right STG and MTG as arrows indicate.

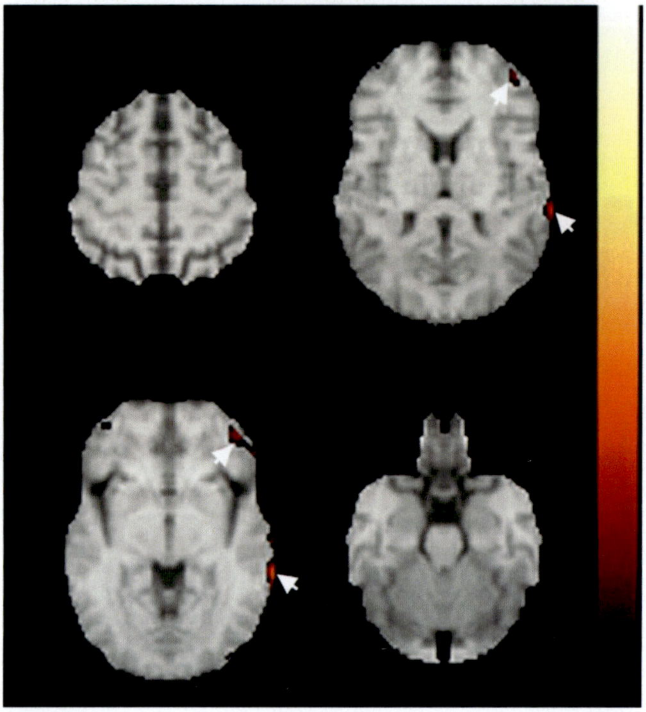

Figure 3. Results of Stat_1tZ in Group B. Increased activity in left MFG and MTG as arrows indicate.

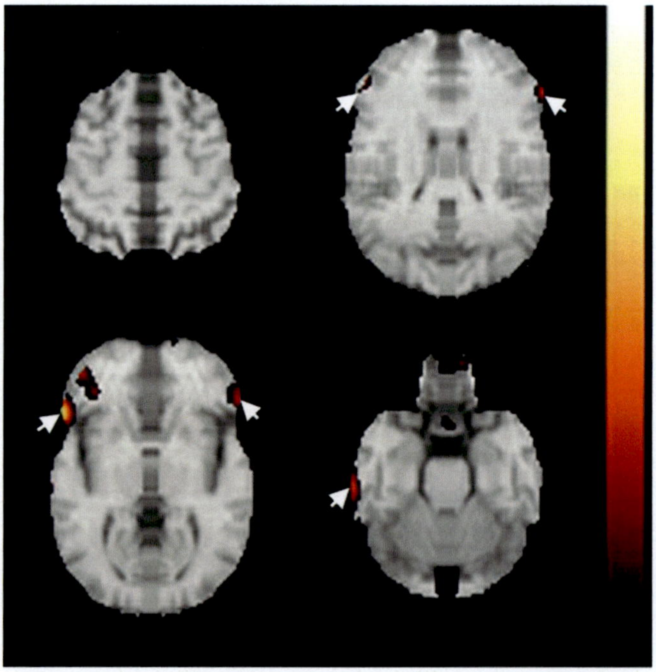

Figure 4. Results of Stat_1tZ in Group C. Increased activity in bilateral IFG and right MTG as arrows indicate.

# Discussion

As early as 1960, urinary incontinence was found in 13.2% with frontal lesions in 167 patients [36], for the first time. Later in 1964, a region in the frontal lobe was found to be important in the higher control of micturition [1]. Following that, many lesion studies in patients with cerebrovascular disorders and brain tumors all indicated that urinary incontinence was associated with the lesions in the frontal cortex[13, 28, 33, 35]. The blood flow was increased in the right frontal operculum during urine withholding in normal female subjects at a significance level with corrected $P < 0.05$ by a PET study [6]. In 2001, it was found that increasing bladder volumes resulted in increased brain activity in bilateral frontal lobes at a threshold of $P < 0.05$ without correction [2]. A clinical study of the brain and urinary tract function on 128 geriatric patients with established urinary incontinence, also confirmed that the frontal areas, especially on the right, were associated with urge incontinence by SPECT[18].

In this study, bilateral IFG, especially the right side, were distinctly activated during urine withholding at a significance threshold of $P < 0.05$ with correction for multiple comparisons in healthy men. The right IFG has been previously described to be involved in attention mechanisms [30] and the selection of response to a situation [24]. It might play a role in making the decision as to whether or not to void at the particular time and place [10] and modulation of urinary control[28]. We suggest that the frontal lobe, especially the right IFG, plays a more important role in brain control of urine withholding.

In this study, no region reached significant threshold in comparison of Group B and C in resting state, although Group B and C, as compared with Group A, showed decreases in tracer activity in STG, MeFG, IFG, AC and cingulate gyrus. According to the differences between resting and urine withholding states, similar results were found in Group A and C, bilateral IFG and the right MTG and STG were activated significantly during urine withholding, as compared with resting state. None of these regions reached significant threshold in Group B, in which the patients were with DO. The results indicated that bilateral IFG and the right STG and MTG were associated with the control of bladder storage. Among the regions, the right IFG was distinctly prominent at both *Z*-score and the extent. Additionally, Group B showed decreased activity in the right IFG, as compared with Group A, while Group C did not. We suggested that the right IFG was most correlated with the control of bladder storage.

As we know, during the urine storage phase, the detrusor is inhibited from contraction, and the striated sphincter is inhibited from relaxation. This negative feedback mechanism ensures intact continence and prevents the release of urine. In this study, bilateral IFG were activated significantly during urine withholding in both healthy subjects and the patients with normal detrusor function. While IFG were not activated significantly in Group B, in which the patients were with DO, and simultaneously, Group B showed decreased rCBF in the right IFG when compared with Group A in resting state. This was consistent with the negative feedback mechanism. Furthermore, it has been confirmed that the lesions above the pontine micturition center resulted in uninhibited bladder contractions (DO) attributed to a lack of inhibition from the cerebral cortex, while leaving relaxation of the urethral sphincter intact

[14, 15, 19]. So we could say that bilateral IFG, especially the right side, play a role in control of bladder storage, inhibiting the detrusor contraction.

In the present study, we found additional activation in the right MTG during urine withholding in Group A and C, and the right STG only in Group A. In a series of stroke patients, urinary dysfunction was found in 14% with temporal stroke[31]. Several papers [5, 23, 26] reported that the seizure of temporal lobe epilepsy patients was characterized by an aura of ictal urinary urge. Griffiths [18], who performed SPECT on 73 incontinent patients and found 10 patients with regional underperfusion in the right temporal lobe and 10 patients in the left, also gave a powerful support to our result. We suggest that the temporal lobe, especially the right STG and MTG, was associated with urine wihholding, although it was not so prominent.

As it was well known that involuntary urinary continence and micturition centers are located in the pontine tegmentum according to the results of animal studies [4, 8, 21, 27] and human studies [9, 10]. While, in this study, no significant increased or decreased activity was found in the pons in any group. We thought it might be the result from the resolution of SPECT, since the pontine urinary storage center is only a distinct group of neurons in the lateral part of the dorsolateral pontine tegmentum [7].

This is the first time that SPECT with NEUROSTAT was adopted to study the cerebral control of bladder storage in both healthy men and the patients with DO. NEUROSTAT has been reported to be useful to detect the changes in regional perfusion more easily and yield a higher accuracy than visual inspection in Alzheimer's disease [22]. The present study would be very useful for understanding the cerebral control of bladder storage and for the clinicians to determine whether the cause of bladder storage disorder, for example, urinary incontinence, is central disorder or not and to decide the treatment.

## Conclusion

The results indicated that bilateral IFG, the right STG and MTG were associated with the control of bladder storage. Especially, the right IFG played a more important role in cerebral control of bladder storage, inhibiting the contraction of detrusor during urine withholding.

## References

[1] Andrew J, Nathan PW (1964) Lesions on the Anterior Frontal Lobes and Disturbances of Micturition and Defaecation. *Brain.* 87:233-262

[2] Athwal BS, Berkley KJ, Hussain I, Brennan A, Craggs M, Sakakibara R, Frackowiak RS, Fowler CJ (2001) Brain responses to changes in bladder volume and urge to void in healthy men. *Brain.* 124:369-377

[3] Barbalias GA, Nikiforidis G, Liatsikos EN (1998) Vesicourethral dysfunction associated with multiple sclerosis: clinical and urodynamic perspectives. *J. Urol.* 160:106-111

[4] Barrington F (1921) The relation of the hind-brain to micturition. *Brain.* 44:23-53

[5] Baumgartner C, Groppel G, Leutmezer F, Aull-Watschinger S, Pataraia E, Feucht M, Trinka E, Unterberger I, Bauer G (2000) Ictal urinary urge indicates seizure onset in the nondominant temporal lobe. *Neurology.* 55:432-434

[6] Blok BF, Holstege G (1998) The central nervous system control of micturition in cats and humans. *Behav. Brain Res.* 92:119-125

[7] Blok BF, Holstege G (1999) Two pontine micturition centers in the cat are not interconnected directly: implications for the central organization of micturition. *J. Comp. Neurol.* 403:209-218

[8] Blok BF, Holstege G (1997) Ultrastructural evidence for a direct pathway from the pontine micturition center to the parasympathetic preganglionic motoneurons of the bladder of the cat. *Neurosci. Lett.* 222:195-198

[9] Blok BF, Sturms LM, Holstege G (1998) Brain activation during micturition in women. *Brain.* 121 ( Pt 11):2033-2042

[10] Blok BF, Willemsen AT, Holstege G (1997) A PET study on brain control of micturition in humans. *Brain.* 120 ( Pt 1):111-121

[11] Chandiramani VA, Palace J, Fowler CJ (1997) How to recognize patients with parkinsonism who should not have urological surgery. *Br. J. Urol.* 80:100-104

[12] Chua K, Chuo A, Kong KH (2003) Urinary incontinence after traumatic brain injury: incidence, outcomes and correlates. *Brain Inj.* 17:469-478

[13] Cummings JL (1994) Vascular subcortical dementias: clinical aspects. *Dementia.* 5:177-180

[14] de Groat WC (1997) A neurologic basis for the overactive bladder. *Urology.* 50:36-52; discussion 53-36

[15] Fall M, Ohlsson BL, Carlsson CA (1989) The neurogenic overactive bladder. Classification based on urodynamics. *Br. J. Urol.* 64:368-373

[16] Friston KJ, Frith CD, Liddle PF, Frackowiak RS (1991) Comparing functional (PET) images: the assessment of significant change. *J. Cereb. Blood Flow Metab.* 11:690-699

[17] Fukuyama H, Matsuzaki S, Ouchi Y, Yamauchi H, Nagahama Y, Kimura J, Shibasaki H (1996) Neural control of micturition in man examined with single photon emission computed tomography using 99mTc-HMPAO. *Neuroreport.* 7:3009-3012

[18] Griffiths D (1998) Clinical studies of cerebral and urinary tract function in elderly people with urinary incontinence. *Behav. Brain Res.* 92:151-155

[19] Hampel C, Wienhold D, Benken N, Eggersmann C, Thuroff JW (1997) Definition of overactive bladder and epidemiology of urinary incontinence. *Urology.* 50:4-14; discussion 15-17

[20] Hirato J (2002) Left frontal tumor in a 46-year-old man with urinary incontinence and gait disturbance. *Neuropathology.* 22:362-364

[21] Holstege G, Griffiths D, de Wall H, Dalm E (1986) Anatomical and physiological observations on supraspinal control of bladder and urethral sphincter muscles in the cat. *J. Comp. Neurol.* 250:449-461

[22] Imabayashi E, Matsuda H, Asada T, Ohnishi T, Sakamoto S, Nakano S, Inoue T (2004) Superiority of 3-dimensional stereotactic surface projection analysis over visual inspection in discrimination of patients with very early Alzheimer's disease from controls using brain perfusion SPECT. *J. Nucl. Med.* 45:1450-1457

[23] Inthaler S, Donati F, Pavlincova E, Vassella F, Staldemann C (1991) Partial complex epileptic seizures with ictal urogenital manifestation in a child. *Eur. Neurol.* 31:212-215

[24] Jenkins IH, Brooks DJ, Nixon PD, Frackowiak RS, Passingham RE (1994) Motor sequence learning: a study with positron emission tomography. *J. Neurosci.* 14:3775-3790

[25] Jost WH, Schimrigk K (1996) Urinary incontinence in patients with Parkinson syndrome. *Wien Klin. Wochenschr.* 108:296-302

[26] Loddenkemper T, Foldvary N, Raja S, Neme S, Luders HO (2003) Ictal urinary urge: further evidence for lateralization to the nondominant hemisphere. *Epilepsia.* 44:124-126

[27] Loewy AD, Saper CB, Baker RP (1979) Descending projections from the pontine micturition center. *Brain Res.* 172:533-538

[28] Maurice-Williams RS (1974) Micturition symptoms in frontal tumours. *J. Neurol. Neurosurg. Psychiatry.* 37:431-436

[29] Minoshima S, Koeppe RA, Frey KA, Kuhl DE (1994) Anatomic standardization: linear scaling and nonlinear warping of functional brain images. *J. Nucl. Med.* 35:1528-1537

[30] Pardo JV, Fox PT, Raichle ME (1991) Localization of a human system for sustained attention by positron emission tomography. *Nature.* 349:61-64

[31] Sakakibara R, Fowler CJ, Hattori T (1999) Voiding and MRI analysis of the brain. *Int. Urogynecol. J. Pelvic. Floor Dysfunct.* 10:192-199

[32] Sakakibara R, Hattori T, Uchiyama T, Yamanishi T (2001) Videourodynamic and sphincter motor unit potential analyses in Parkinson's disease and multiple system atrophy. *J. Neurol. Neurosurg. Psychiatry.* 71:600-606

[33] Sakakibara R, Hattori T, Yasuda K, Yamanishi T (1996) Micturitional disturbance after acute hemispheric stroke: analysis of the lesion site by CT and MRI. *J. Neurol. Sci.* 137:47-56

[34] Schultz-Lampel D (2003) Bladder disorders in dementia and Alzheimer's disease. Rational diagnostic and therapeutic options. *Urologe.* A 42:1579-1587

[35] Tomonaga M, Yamanouchi H, Tohgi H, Kameyama M (1982) Clinicopathologic study of progressive subcortical vascular encephalopathy (Binswanger type) in the elderly. *J. Am. Geriatr. Soc.* 30:524-529

[36] Ueki K (1960) Disturbances of micturition observed in some patients with brain tumor. *Neurol. Medico Chir.* 2:25-33

In: Research Topics on Brain Mapping
Editor: Yuanzhu Liáng, pp. 11-32
ISBN: 978-1-60456-001-5


*Chapter I*

# From Connection to Cognition: Applications of Diffusion Imaging to the Human Memory System

*Emi Takahashi*[*]
Department of Radiology; Massachusetts General Hospital;
Harvard Medical School; Boston, MA 02015, USA

## Abstract

In the past decade, functional neuroimaging studies have significantly advanced our understanding of human cognitive functions. However, much less is known about the anatomical connections underlying higher cognitive processes in humans. One of the reasons why anatomical studies have lagged behind functional studies is that there are methodological limitations on studying anatomical connections of the human brain *in vivo*. There are numerous detailed anatomical studies of non-human primates that serve as the basis of our understandings of connections in the brain. However, those techniques are not feasible in humans. Diffusion imaging is a new technique based on detecting the diffusion of water molecules from magnetic resonance images. Diffusion imaging allows non-invasive mapping of anatomical connections and gives a comprehensive picture of connectivity throughout the brain, but there are still numerous technical issues to be addressed. Here, I introduce our recent studies on large-scale anatomical connections underlying episodic memory in humans. We studied an entire network based on some episodic memory tasks, and applied several new approaches to assess our tractography results. Our main finding was that encoding-related areas in the left dorsolateral prefrontal cortex and the left ventrolateral prefrontal cortex connect with another encoding-related area in the left temporal cortex. This suggests that there are two pathways between prefrontal cortex and temporal cortex related to encoding processes in

[*] Emi Takahashi: Email: emi@nmr.mgh.harvard.edu

episodic memory. Further, I discuss future applications of diffusion imaging in the study of the human memory system.

# Introduction

## Diffusion Imaging and Tractography

Diffusion tensor imaging (DTI) is a technique that measures the diffusion properties of water molecules from diffusion-weighted magnetic resonance images (Basser et al., 1994). One promising application of diffusion images in brain research is reconstructing white matter fiber structures. Tractography algorithms are applied to DTI data to reconstruct connections between various brain regions (Mori et al., 1999; Jones et al., 1999; Conturo et al., 1999). Many studies have used DTI to show anatomical connections in the human brain (e.g. Conturo et al., 1999; Basser et al., 2000; Stieltjes et al., 2001; Xu et al., 2002; Behrens et al., 2003; Lehericy et al., 2004; Powell et al., 2004), and recent studies have used DTI to assess connectivity between functionally defined region of interest (e.g. Guye et al., 2003; Toosy et al., 2004; Dougherty et al., 2005; Kim et al., 2006; Takahashi et al., 2007). White matter occupies most of the brain, and it has been shown that disruptions of the white matter properties could cause various cognitive deficits and other kinds of variability (e.g. Catani, 2006; Sullivan and Pfefferbaum, 2003; Tuch et al., 2005). Thus, I believe that knowing white matter pathways underlying specific cognitive functions has great possibilities to contribute to our understandings of functional organization of the human brain. In this chapter, I review our recent study of anatomical connections underlying episodic memory encoding and retrieval in the human brain, along with the research trends in this field, and introduce possible future diffusion studies on the human memory system. Although results of tractography still need to be assessed for accuracy, there have been reported increasing methods to improve the technique. In our study, we used a boot-trac algorithm (Lazar and Alexander, 2005) to create probabilistic maps of DTI tractography data and several new trials to assess our results.

## A Model for Episodic Memory System

The human memory system is supported and constituted by a number of different processes (Squire and Zola-Morgan, 1991; Cabeza and Nyberg, 2000; Tulving, 2002; Habib et al., 2003). Recent functional neuroimaging studies have shown that areas in the prefrontal, parietal and temporal cortices are involved in memory encoding and retrieval (Tulving et al., 1994; Demb et al., 1995; Buckner et al., 1998; Buckner and Koutstaal, 1998; Wagner et al., 1998; Buckner et al., 1999; Lepage et al., 2000). Among these memory-related areas, prefrontal cortex (PFC) is thought to subserve cognitive control processes (Goldman-Rakic, 1987; Schacter, 1987; Shimamura, 1995; Fuster, 1997; Takahashi and Miyashita, 2002), and send top-down signals to posterior cortices (Incisa della Rocchetta, 1993; Gazzaniga, 1995; Tomita et al., 1999; Takahashi and Miyashita, 2002). Recently, a two-stage model of PFC was proposed (Petrides, 1994a, 1994b, 1996; Owen, Evans and Petrides, 1996). In this model, ventro-lateral prefrontal cortex (VLPFC) interacts with posterior cortices such as temporal cortex for active (or controlled) encoding and retrieval of information, whereas dorso-lateral prefrontal cortex (DLPFC) monitors and manipulates information maintained in VLPFC. Anatomical studies in nonhuman primates have shown direct corticocortical connections from VLPFC to temporal cortex (Petrides and Pandya, 2002), but direct connections from DLPFC to temporal cortex are still controversial (Seltzer and Pandya, 1989; Petrides and Pandya, 1994, 1999; Petrides, 2005). Based on these studies, we hypothesized two possibile models of the anatomical connections between PFC and temporal cortex in humans (figure 1A); (i) Serial Pathway Model: DLPFC connects with VLPFC, and VLPFC connects with temporal cortex, but DLPFC does not connect with temporal cortex, (ii) Parallel Pathway Model: DLPFC and VLPFC both connect with temporal cortex. In this study, we performed diffusion tensor imaging (DTI) tractography from functionally defined memory areas to test these two connectivity models.

## Functional Task

To define functional anatomy to constrain the analysis of anatomical connectivity, we used tasks that engage episodic memory. The experiment consisted of two parts, an encoding phase and a retrieval phase (figure 1B). In the encoding phase, subjects were asked to perform 4 different "encoding" tasks: 1) make a living/nonliving judgment (deep encoding), 2) detect a given letter within a non-word letter sequence (shallow encoding), 3) press a random button, and 4) fixate on a central target. Each word was presented only once throughout the encoding phase. In the retrieval phase, subjects performed randomly intermixed retrieval trials, visuo-motor control trials, and fixation trials. In the retrieval trials, subjects made yes/no recognition memory judgments for previously studied and new stimuli. Half of the words from the encoding phase were presented again, along with new words.

Activated brain areas are shown in figure 2A, B (found in the encoding phase) and figure 3A, B (found in the retrieval phase).

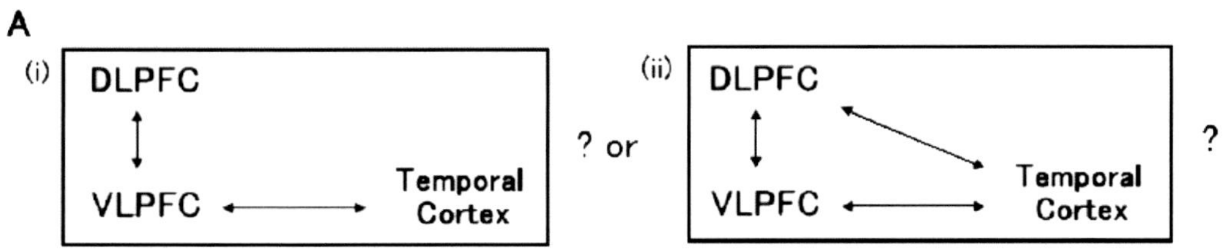


Figure 1. (Continued on next page)

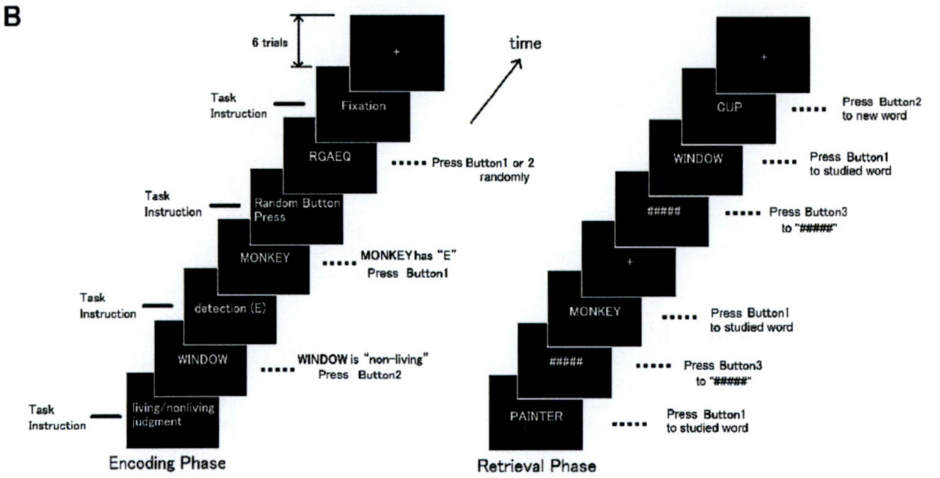


Figure 1. (A) Two possible models of connections between the prefrontal and temporal cortices. (i) Serial Pathway Model: DLPFC connects with VLPFC, but not with the temporal cortex, and VLPFC connects with the temporal cortex, (ii) Parallel Pathway Model: DLPFC and VLPFC both connect with the temporal cortex. (B) Experimental design for functional imaging in encoding (left) and retrieval (right). In encoding, there are four conditions: living/nonliving, detection, visuo-motor control, and fixation. In retrieval, there are retrieval trials and visuo-motor control trials (see text and Materials and Methods for further details).

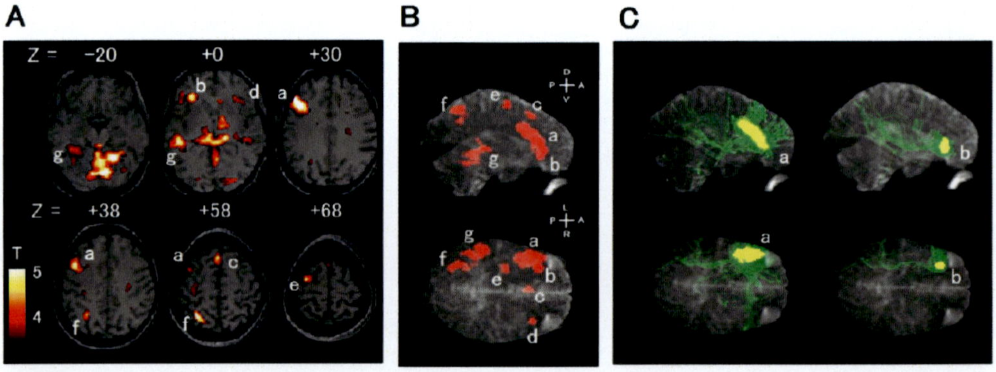


Figure 2. (A-C) Activation and fiber tracking from the activated areas in the encoding phase in the comparison "deep encoding versus visuo-motor control". (A) Activated clusters (20 subjects, random effect analysis, $p<0.001$, uncorrected; $p<0.05$ corrected for whole-brain multiple comparisons at cluster level, only cortical activation clusters are displayed) are superimposed on T1-weighted normalized brain slices. The left hemisphere of the brain corresponds to the left side of the image. A color bar for T values of activated areas is shown at the bottom of the left. Z coordinates of Talairach space are shown on the top of each slice. (a) Left DLPFC (BA9/46/45), (b) left VLPFC (BA45/47/insula), (c) medial frontal gyrus (BA6), (d) right VLPFC (BA45/46), (e) left superior frontal gyrus (BA6), (f) left intraparietal sulcus (BA7) and (g) left STS and FG (BA21/22/37). BA:Brodmann's Area. (B) Activated clusters using the same threshold as (A) are shown as red superimposed on a saggital view (top) and an axial view (bottom) of a brain. (a)-(g) represent the same areas as shown in (A). (C) All the reconstructed fibers from the left DLPFC (left) and left VLPFC (right) in single subject are shown as green in a saggital view (top) and an axial view (bottom). The activated areas are shown as yellow.

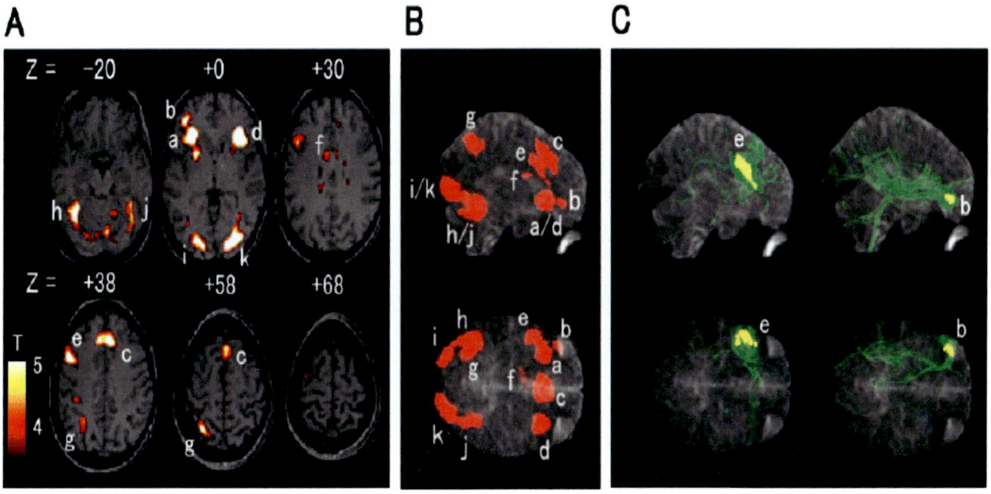


Figure 3. Activation and fiber tracking from activated areas in the retrieval phase in the comparison "all retrieval versus visuo-motor control". (A) Activated clusters (20 subjects, random effect analysis, p<0.001, uncorrected; p<0.05 corrected for whole-brain multiple comparisons at cluster level, only cortical activation clusters are displayed) are superimposed on T1-weighted normalized brain slices. The left hemisphere of the brain corresponds to the left side of the image. A color bar for T values of activated areas is shown at the bottom of the left. Z values of Talairach space are shown on the top of each slice. (a, d) bilateral VLPFC (BA47/45/insula), (b) left VLPFC (BA10/47), (c) medial frontal gyrus (BA6/8), (e) left DLPFC (BA9/8), (f) anterior cingulate cortex (BA24), (g) left intraparietal sulcus (BA7), (h, j) bilateral fusiform gyrus (BA37), and (i, k) bilateral inferior and middle occipital gyrus and cuneus (BA17/18/19). (B) Activated clusters using the same threshold as (A) are shown as red superimposed on a saggital view (top) and an axial view (bottom) of a brain. (a)-(k) represent the same areas as shown in (A). (C) All the reconstructed fibers from the left DLPFC (left) and left VLPFC (right) in single subject are shown as green in a saggital view (top) and an axial view (bottom). The activated areas are shown as yellow. (A: anterior, P: posterior, D: dorsal, V: ventral, L: left, R: right).

## Detection of Connections

We used tractography algorithms based on the method described in Basser et al. (Basser et al., 2000) and Lazar et al. (Lazar et al., 2003). At every position along the fiber trajectory, a diffusion tensor is interpolated and eigenvectors are computed. The eigenvector associated with the greatest eigenvalue indicates the principal direction of water diffusion. The fiber tract is propagated along this direction over a small distance to the next point where a new diffusion tensor is interpolated. Fiber tracking terminates when the angle between two consecutive eigenvectors is greater than a given threshold ($60^o$), or when the FA value is smaller than a given threshold (0.14). The criteria of FA < 0.14-0.15 is reported to provide the best tradeoff between fewer erroneous tracts and penetration into the white matter (Thottakara et al. 2006). This streamline approach is based on the assumption that diffusion is locally uniform and can be accurately described by a single eigenvector. Unfortunately, this approach fails to describe crossing fibers (e.g. Alexander et al., 2001). To overcome this problem, tensorline approaches (e.g. tensor deflection) have been developed that use the entire tensor information instead of reducing it to a single eigenvector (Lazar et al., 2003). In our study, both algorithms, i.e. streamline (Basser et al., 2000) and tensor deflection (Lazar et al., 2003), were used to reconstruct 3D DTI fibers (Takahashi et al, 2007).

Tractography was performed from all of the activated cortical regions (but not from cerebellum and brain stem) in 20 healthy subjects. Figure 2C and 3C show the reconstructed fibers from the left DLPFC (left) and left VLPFC (right) active in a single subject in encoding (figure 2C) and retrieval (figure 3C). The fibers from left DLPFC and VLPFC extended to other left prefrontal regions, as well as the left parietal and temporal cortices. The fibers from the region that was active in the left temporal cortex were found to be connected to the left frontal, parietal and occipital cortices.

# Design of Tractography Analyses for Cognitive Functions

## Network of Connections

By studying the pathways among all activated regions, we can see an entire network that is involved in a specific cognitive task. We examined connections between pairs of activation clusters in each subject. Fibers were obtained using any voxel in the starting cluster (as a seed) to any voxel within the end cluster, going in either direction. Examples of connections are shown in figure 4A (encoding) and 4B (retrieval). Figure 5A shows the connections found between the activated areas in the left DLPFC and the left temporal cortex for the encoding phase. Figure 5B shows the connections between the left VLPFC and the region that was active in the left temporal cortex for the encoding phase. We performed this analysis on the data obtained from all 20 subjects. The most dorsal part (BA 9) of the left DLPFC cluster connected with the dorsal part (BA21, 22) of the left temporal cortex cluster. In some subjects, there were also connections between the ventral part of the DLPFC cluster and the temporal cortex cluster. Fibers between VLPFC and STS also exhibited different pathways passing through more ventral parts. These fiber pathways were consistent across subjects.

Figure 6 summarizes the connectivity data between each pair of clusters for the entire group of subjects. The connections between the left DLPFC and the left temporal cortex, and between the left VLPFC and the left temporal cortex were found in more than 10 out of 20 subjects with both the streamline (from the left DLPFC to the left temporal cortex: 18 subjects; from the left VLPFC to the left temporal cortex: 14 subjects) and tensor deflection algorithms (from the left DLPFC to the left temporal cortex: 20 subjects; from the left VLPFC to the left temporal cortex: 18 subjects) in encoding. Fibers found in more than half of all 20 subjects with both the streamline and tensor deflection algorithms were shown as arrows in solid lines. The dotted arrow indicates the pathways found in more than 10 subjects only by tensor deflection (Some arrows are omitted).

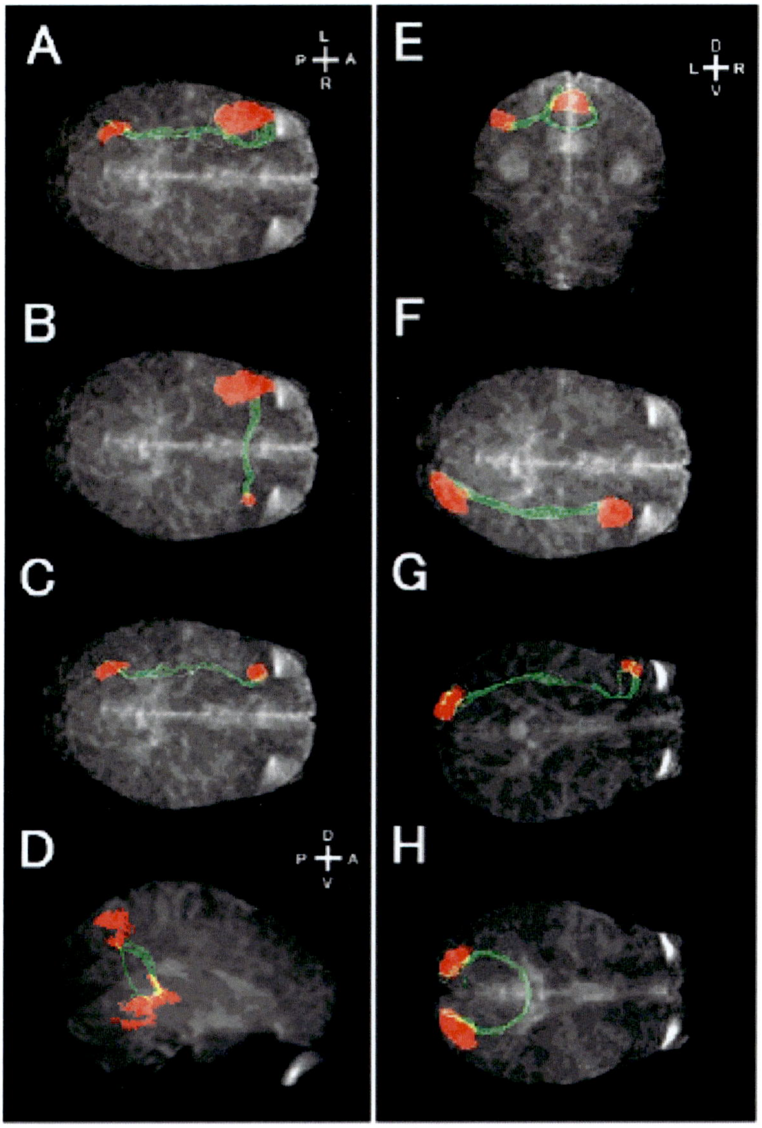


Figure 4. Examples of fiber tracking between each pair of activated areas in single subject. (A-D) "deep encoding versus control" (A) left DLPFC (BA9/8/46/45) and left middle temporal to fusiform gyrus (BA22/37), (B) left and right operculum, (C) left inferior frontal gyrus (BA47) and left intraparietal sulcus, and (D) left intraparietal gyrus (BA7/40) and left middle temporal and fusiform gyri (BA37). (E-H) "all retrieval versus control" (E) left BA9/8 and medial BA6 (SMA and pre-SMA), (F) right frontal operculum (BA47/45) and right inferior occipital gyrus (BA19), (G) left frontal operculum (BA47) and left inferior occipital gyrus (BA19), and (H) left and right inferior occipital gyrus (BA19). (A: anterior, P: posterior, D: dorsal, V: ventral, L: left, R: right).

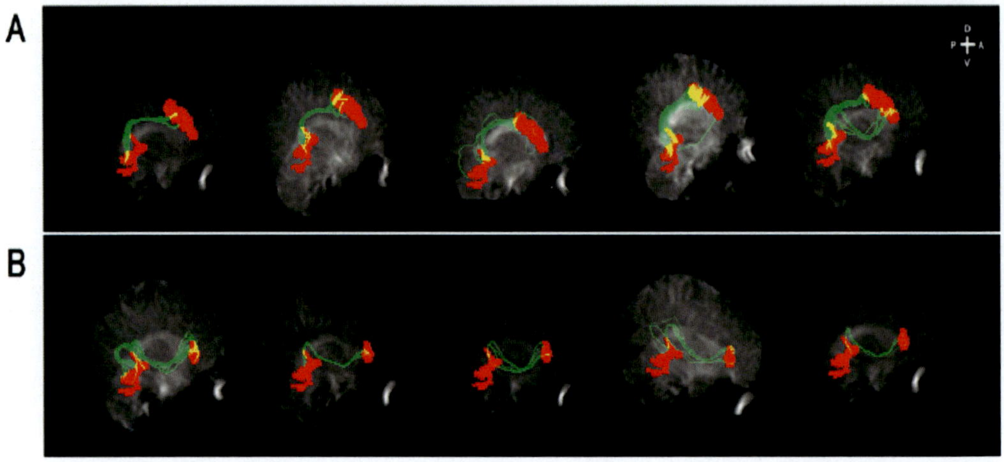


Figure 5. Fibers between two activation clusters in five different subjects. (A) Reconstructed fibers between the left DLPFC (BA9/8/46/45) and left STS to FG (BA21/22/37) in the encoding phase. (B) Reconstructed fibers between the left VLPFC and the left STS to FG (BA21/22/37) in the encoding phase. (A: Anterior, P: posterior, D: dorsal, V: ventral, L: left, R: right). Fibers were tracked in both directions.

## Specificity of Connections

If reconstructed fibers reoresented random connections between brain regions, then showing the existence of such fibers would be meaningless. Even though the connections are not entirely random, diffusely connected tracts to broad areas near the targets, are still less meaningful than they could otherwise be. To address this issue, we estimated the specificity in the connections between two activated clusters in the left DLPFC and the left temporal cortex in encoding. For this purpose, we examined the degree of connectivity between the DLPFC activation and arbitrarily defined non-activating regions. If the connection was specific, the degree of connectivity between DLPFC and arbitrary regions should be significantly lower than the connectivity between DLPFC and temporal cortex activation. However, the degree of connectivity could be affected by many factors, such as distances between regions, and shapes of regions. Thus, we restricted the arbitrary regions to those satisfying the following conditions: (1) all voxels were inside the brain, (2) there was no overlap with the activated regions, (3) the volume and shape of the region were exactly the same as the temporal cortex activation, (4) the distance from the DLPFC was exactly the same as the distance between the DLPFC and the temporal cortex activation. Following these conditions, the arbitrary regions were selected 100 times for each subject, allowing their overlap. Then, the number of the fibers between the DLPFC and these arbitrarily defined regions were obtained. The fibers between the left DLPFC and the newly placed cluster were tracked from any voxel in one cluster to any voxel in the other cluster in both directions.

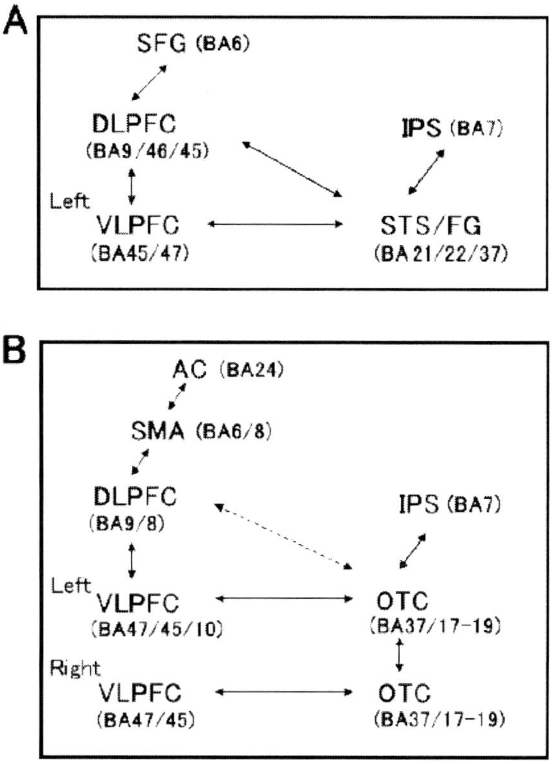


Figure 6. Summary of the fiber tracking results between the activation clusters. (A) Encoding, (B) Retrieval. The pathways found in more than 10 subjects both by streamline and tensor deflection algorithms are shown as solid arrows, while a dotted arrow indicates the pathways found in more than 10 subjects only by tensor deflection. DLPFC: dorso-lateral prefrontal cortex, VLPFC: ventro-lateral prefrontal cortex, SFG: superior frontal gyrus, STS: superior temporal sulcus, FG: fusiform gyrus, AC: anterior cingulated cortex: SMA: supplementary motor area, OTC: occipito-temporal cortex.

Arbitrary regions satisfying the selection criteria were used 100 times for each subject. Then, the number of fibers between the DLPFC and those arbitrarily defined regions were obtained. There was no connection between the DLPFC cluster and 55% of the random clusters. The median of the number of fibers between the DLPFC cluster and the random clusters was found to be 0, which is significantly different from the observed number of fibers (57 fibers). The random clusters that had more fibers than the actual number of fibers (57 fibers) were only 5%, and all of them were found in the precuneus in this particular subject.

We performed the same type of analysis on all 18 subjects who had fibers between DLPFC and temporal cortex clusters. Eleven out of 18 subjects showed a significantly larger number of actual fibers relative to fibers generated from random clusters. At the population level, the number of actual fibers and the median number of fibers from random clusters for 18 subjects were significantly different. These analyses confirmed that the connections between DLPFC and temporal cortex activation were specific. Only some restricted areas (14.0 %) located in the right PFC (BA9/46) and precuneus (BA7) showed more connections with the left DLPFC cluster.

Strength of connection is a different concept from specificity, and could be defined as the quantity of reconstructed fibers. However, one needs to be very cautious about direct comparisons of quantities because they are very sensitive to and dependent on the sampling conditions of the fibers.

## Segregation of Multiple Connections

Segregation is also a different concept from specificity, and could be contribute to our broader understanding of cognitive functions. For example, there is an unsolved relationship between the parietal cortex and temporal lobe in terms of episodic memory retrieval. The parietal cortex has traditionally been implicated in spatial attention and eye-movement processes (Hyvarinen, 1982; Corbetta, 1998; Colby and Goldberg, 1999; Mesulam, 1999). In addition, recent functional neuroimaging studies have found activation in the parietal cortex during various memory tasks, especially those related to successful recognition memory (Henson et al. 1999; Konishi et al., 2000; Donaldson et al., 2001; Cansino et al., 2002; Dobbins et al., 2003; Rugg et al., 2003; Wheeler and Buckner, 2003; Herron et al, 2004). Most studies have identified several regions in the parietal cortex that respond to "Hits" (when subjects correctly recognize previously studied old items) more than to "Correct Rejections" (when they correctly identify new items). The regions in which this effect was identified consistently include the intraparietal sulcus (IPS or Brodmann Areas (BA) 7), medial parietal cortex (the precuneus (PCu) or medial BA7, and posterior cingulate cortex or BA23/31), and several prefrontal regions. Although the roles of the prefrontal cortex in successful memory retrieval have been relatively well studied (Buckner et al., 1998a, b; Henson et al. 1999, followed by many other studies), those of the parietal cortex are still poorly understood (Shannon and Buckner, 2004; Naghavi and Nyberg, 2005; Wagner et al., 2005; Cavanna and Trimble, 2006). Since it is well known that declarative memory relies on the medial temporal lobe (MTL) and lateral temporal cortex, a key strategy for studying successful memory retrieval in the parietal cortex is to study its relationship with the temporal lobe. Given the accumulating knowledge on the functionally dissociated roles of the temporal lobe in terms of memory, studying connectivity between IPS/PCu and the temporal lobe should be fundamental to understand the roles of the parietal regions in memory.

Neuropsychological studies suggest that different types of memory depend on separated cortical structures (e.g. Squire, 1994, Takahashi and Miyashita, 2002). For example, patients with left lateral temporal lobe damage have impaired memory for semantic knowledge (De Renzi et al., 1987; Hart and Gordon, 1990; Snowden et al., 1989), but relatively preserved memory for episodic information (De Renzi et al., 1987; Snowden et al., 1994). Recent functional imaging studies also showed that lateral temporal cortex is activated by semantic memory retrieval or item-based memory, while the MTL is activated by episodic memory retrieval or relational memory (Wiggs et al., 1999; Lee et al., 2002; Konishi et al., 2006). Based on these functional dissociations between the MTL and lateral temporal cortex studies of the specific connections between these areas should provide insight into the process of memory retrieval in parietal cortex.

Another example is the dorsal and ventral information streams. When we perceive our external world, the information is divided into multiple functional streams in our brains. Especially, when we briefly hold information in working memory, "where" and "what" aspects of the percept are largely divided into dorsal and ventral pathways in the brains. However, both the functional reasons for this segregation and the underlying mechanism for recombining the information remain unsolved. Why does the brain need to separate visual information in this way to generate a percept of the world? How does the brain combine those functional streams into a perceived event or percept with distinct features? This dissociation could be based on the specific segregated anatomical connections, and our perception of complex events could be derived from the resulting specific connections from the two pathways (figure 7).

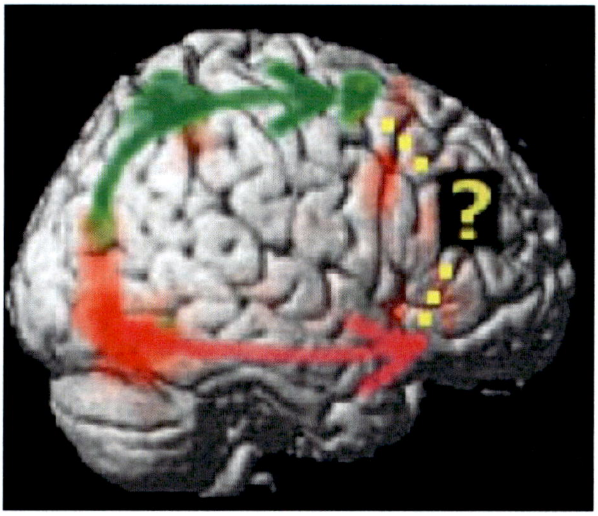


Figure 7. Dorsal and ventral streams.

## Measures of Properties on Connections

There have been increasing studies to show correlations between some measures on the connections (e.g. fractional anisotropy (FA) and apparent diffusion coefficients (ADC)) and subjects' performances (e.g. error rates and response times). These indexes reflect properties of water diffusion at each voxel. Usually, they create regions of interests (ROIs) by tractography, measure those indexes, and correlate them with performance indexes. Given that the changes of white matter properties could be related to deficits/variability of cognitive functions, those correlations would be meaningful in terms of possible detections of those relationships. However, tractography is usually done by setting a given threshold of angles and terminal conditions of the connections, which also reflect the FA values, so one needs to be very careful about determining the ROIs and seeing correlations based on the ROIs. This problem consistently arises both in studying connections between two regions and connections from one region to anywhere in the brain.

## Group Analyses

Group analysis in the tractography study has been relatively less developed compared to that in the functional study. In our study (Takahashi et al., 2007), the coordinates of the activated clusters in Talairach coordinates were reverse normalized into each subject's coordinates, and used as the basis for fiber tracking and determining the coordinates of the end points of the fibers. We then normalized the coordinates of the end points, averaged the data across all the subjects, and superimposed the resulting maps onto the normalized T1-weighted images. This approach is better than normalizing diffusion weighted images (DWIs) directly because the resolution of DWIs was reduced when we resampled DWIs during normalization.

Figure 8 shows the distribution of terminal points for reconstructed fibers in 20 subjects. The fibers were tracked from areas in the left DLPFC (top row), VLPFC (middle row) and temporal cortex (bottom row) that were activated during the encoding phase. The terminal points converged on a large number of memory-related areas also activated during the encoding phase. These areas include: left VLPFC (h), right VLPFC (k), left medial frontal (o, s), left superior frontal (t) and left temporal cortex (f). In addition, some fibers terminated in areas activated during the retrieval phase (e.g. i and p). We also found connections to the left hippocampus/parahippocampal region (c). We performed this group analysis for all the other activated areas. The results in figure 8 suggest that, consistent with our results on each subject, activated areas in the left DLPFC and VLPFC both have connections with the left temporal cortex activation.

In our study, the dispersion errors in white matter tractography were estimated by a statistical nonparametric bootstrap method (Lazar and Alexander, 2005). In each iteration, two samples were randomly selected with replacement from the pool of four independent DTI acquisitions, and were averaged. The procedure was repeated for each diffusion-encoding of the brain volume (15 directions) and for one non-diffusion weighted volume, resulting in one bootstrap DTI volume sample. The dispersion errors for the tractography were obtained by running the tractography algorithm over 100 iterations of the bootstrap DTI data set.

Thirty-three continuous seed points in the temporal cortex showed greater than 50 % probability of a connection to DLPFC. The seed cluster volume was 33 $mm^3$ (1mm sampling of seed points), corresponding to 0.7 % of the entire temporal cortex activation (4848 $mm^3$). It is clear that these seed points did not distribute diffusively across the whole activated cluster, but were rather confined in a specific region. The Talairach coordinates of these 33 voxels were located in STS (x, y, z = -54 ± 5, -40 ± 2, -1 ± 2). These results indicate that the locations in temporal cortex that had connections with DLPFC were very specific.

## Estimation of Tractography Error

We showed the results of boot-trac from a single seed point (Talairach: x, y, z = -49, -41, 0) in two ways. First, all the fibers for 100 bootstraps are shown in figure 8A. Most of the fibers (78 %) went to the DLPFC, gradually diverging by the distance from the seed point in the temporal cortex activation. To assess uncertainty of this probability, we performed boot-trac analysis 1000 times. By shuffling the orders of the 1000 boot-trac samples 1000 times, an error for each iteration was obtained. At 100 iterations of boot-trac, the error was less than 5%. Second, the boot-trac from the same seed is shown as a probabilistic map (figure 8B). This figure shows how many times, out of 100, the boot-trac fibers passed through each voxel. The probabilities were almost 100 % around the seed point in the temporal cortex activation, but soon went down less than 50 %. This is because of the divergence of the tracked fibers, which depends on the distance from the seed point, as displayed in figure 8A.

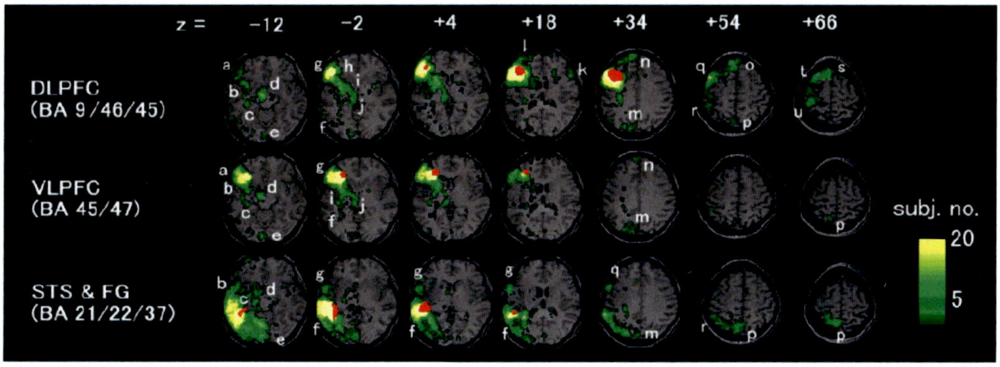


Figure 8. The average results of 20 subjects' terminal points of DTI fiber tracking. The left hemisphere of the brain corresponds to the left side of the image. The terminals of the tracked fibers are shown as yellow to green. The colors indicate the number of subjects whose fiber tracking from any seed points terminated in the voxel (see color bar). Terminal points of fibers from encoding activation in the left DLPFC (top row), left VLPFC (middle row) and the left STS (bottom row). The end points of fiber tracking converged in (a) left inferior frontal gyrus (BA47), (b) left anterior to posterior insula, (c) left hippocampus/parahippocampal formation, (d) bilateral brain stem, (e) left inferior occipital gyrus (BA18), (f) left STS and FG (BA21/22/37), (g) left inferior frontal gyrus (BA44/45), (h) left frontal operculum (BA47), (i) left striatum, (j) left thalamus, (k) right inferior frontal gyrus (BA46), (l) left superior to middle frontal gyri (BA9/10), (m) left occipital gyrus (BA19), (n) left medial frontal gyrus (BA9), (o) left supplementary motor area (BA8), (p) left precuneus (BA7), (q) left middle frontal gyrus (BA6), (r) left inferior parietal gyrus (BA40), (s) left supplementary motor area (BA6), (t) left superior frontal gyrus (BA6), and (u) left postcentral gyrus.

We obtained a probabilistic map of connections from all 33 seed points with a connection probability greater than 50% (figure 8C). These seed points are located in restricted locations, so they could compensate for the low probability of one seed point. The results indicate that the fiber tracking from those 33 seed points reached the DLPFC activation with a probability of more than 80 %. The terminal location was the posterior end of the DLPFC cluster (around x, y, z = -49, 3, 36 in the Talairach coordinate), around the precentral sulcus to the middle frontal gyrus. This result indicates that not only the seed points, but also the terminal points were in very restricted locations within the activation. Figure 8C shows the probabilities of fibers from 33 voxels in the temporal cortex to anywhere in the whole brain. Although we did not selectively show the fibers that reached the DLPFC activation, high probabilities were found only along the pathway from the temporal cortex to DLPFC. Thus, the specificity of this pathway was remarkable. We also obtained probabilistic maps (figure 9, upper row) from all the voxels in the temporal cortex activation, similar to figure 8C. All subjects' results (n=20) were averaged after normalization (figure 9, lower row).

The boot-tracked fibers were diverging by the distance from the seed points, but in many cases, as shown in figure 8A, most of the fibers reached the DLPFC activation. To see this observation quantitatively, we examined the probability of connections between any voxel in the temporal cortex and any voxel in the DLPFC. We found the connection with a probability of 100% in this subject. We performed this latter analysis for 18 subjects who showed connections between these regions. The existence of this pathway was crucial to distinguishing between the two models (the Serial and Parallel Pathway Models) mentioned above. Ten subjects out of the 18 subjects showed more than 50% probabilities for the connections between the left DLPFC and the left temporal cortex. The probability for the existence of this connection was very high in these 10 subjects (86.3 ± 18.0%, n=10). This result validates our major finding on the direct pathway between DLPFC and the temporal cortex activation.

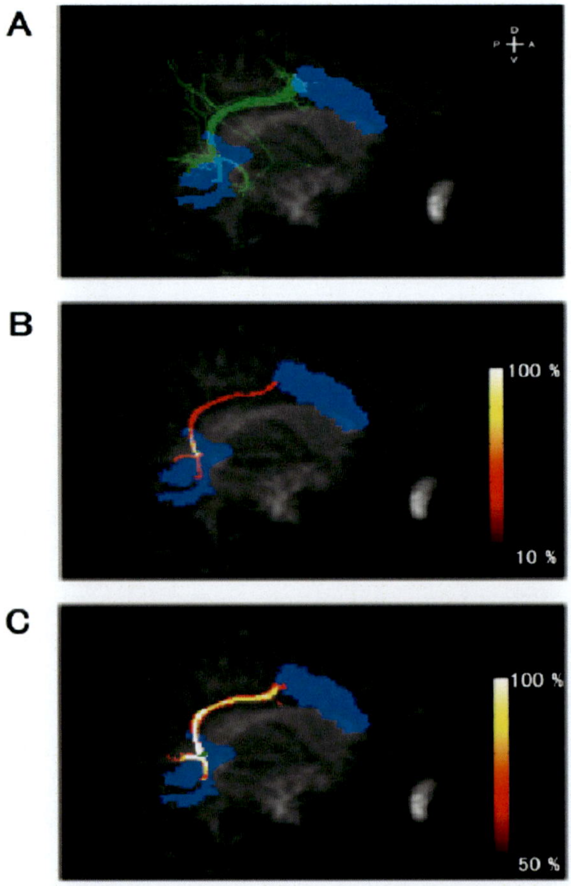


Figure 9. (A) All the fibers for 100 bootstraps from a single seed point at (-49, -41, 0). A: anterior, P: posterior, D: dorsal, V: ventral. (B) A probabilitistic map of the connection from a single seed point (Talairach: x, y, z = -49, -41, 0). The voxels with more than 10 % probabilities were color-coded. (C) A probabilitistic map of the connection from the 33 seed points of high probabilities in the temporal cortex (green). Voxels that showed more than 50 % were color-coded.

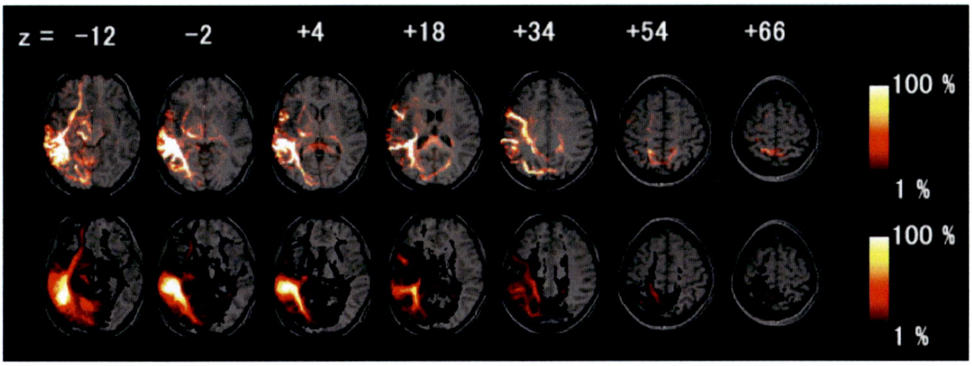


Figure 10. Probabilistic maps of the connections from all the seed points in the temporal cortex activation in a single subject (upper row) and all the 20 subjects (lower row).

# Interpretations of Tractography Results in Cognitive Functions

Although tractography provides information about anatomical pathways *in vivo*, it does not offer any functional interpretations of the reconstructed fibers. One solution to that problem is using functionally activated areas to constrain the analysis of anatomical connectivity, which I have introduced in this chapter. With knowledge of the functional roles of activated areas, outcomes of tractography (i.e. connectivity/disconnectivity of a network, probability, specificity, segregation, numbers of fibers, diffusion properties on the fibers etc.) can help us understand anatomical networks underlying specific cognitive processes. Correlations between the results of tractography, and the strength of functional activation or performance measures of subjects are an additional help. Another possible approach is to see functional correlations among areas that have anatomical connections. There have been an increasing number of studies on functional connectivity. Parallel findings of anatomical connections and functional connectivity provide another source of convergent functional evidence to explain the reconstructed fiber tracts.

# Future Directions for Tractography Studies

## Technical Improvements

One major challenge facing tractography is the crossing-fiber problem. Algorithms for tractography fail or produce errors when they encounter a voxel where neural fibers cross each other. Basically, at that point, a reconstructed fiber stops or goes in the wrong direction. There have been two approaches to solving this problem thus far: one is to assess tractography errors using a probabilistic approach, and the other is to pursue higher-resolution imaging to improve the accuracy of tractography results.

A number of studies have assessed tractography results using the probabilistic approach (e.g. Upadhyay et al., 2006; Takahashi et al., 2007). Although anatomical connections are conceptually incompatible with probability, this is one emerging trend in the study of connections *in vivo*. There are numbers of suggested methods to obtain probabilities of tracts (Behrens et al., 2003; Chung et al., 2006; Jbabdi et al., 2007). However, we currently do not have a way to directly compare the results of different implementations of the probabilistic approach. For example, the probabilities using repetition and wild bootstrap have different meanings, and it is not appropriate to compare them directly. This means that the same anatomical pathway can have different probabilities depending on the method used, even in the same brain. I believe that this problem needs to be addressed in the course of future tractography studies, in order to form a solid basis for comparative studies on large samples, similar to what has been done in tracer studies of connectivity of non-human primates. Another issue is that probability reflects both connections between the areas we are interested in, and the quality of the dataset (more precisely, various artifacts/noise on the pathway). The degree of artifact/noise could vary across different brain areas, so not addressing this problem may impair our ability to see the actual course of the pathway. These issues present challenging problems to be solved as the technology progresses.

On a different front, efforts to improve accuracy of tractography will also be very important. New techniques were proposed recently that apply multiple diffusion encoding directions (Tuch et al., 2002; Wedeen et al., 2005) together with different gradient strengths (Wedeen et al., 2005). In theory, these techniques provide us with more precise ways to uncover white matter fiber structures, by reconciling the different directions of reconstructed fibers in a single voxel. These techniques are remarkably powerful especially on post-mortem brains (Schmahmann et al., 2007). Applying them to human *in vivo* imaging is a promising future direction.

## Applications: Connectivity Studies in Human Memory Research

As I discussed earlier in this chapter, there are several unanswered questions in memory research that tractography studies could help answer. One example is studying the pathways between the medial/lateral parietal cortices and medial/lateral temporal lobes involved in successful memory retrieval, and another is dissociating dorsal and ventral streams in maintaining and encoding visual information. Both anatomical pathways are unknown in humans, so directly studying the actual pathways predicted by those models will be significant for us to understand the mechanisms of long-range networks in memory systems.

Certain other pathways are known to be important in memory processes. There are two signal pathways through which the mnemonic representation in the inferior temporal cortex can be activated in memory retrieval: the frontotemporal pathway and the limbic-temporal pathway (Takahashi and Miyashita, 2002). How do these pathways cooperate during memory retrieval? Many functional neuroimaging studies have suggested that the frontotemporal pathway is involved in retrieval. For example, Lepage and colleagues (2000) refer to the 'retrieval mode' as a neurocognitive state, in which one mentally holds in the background of focal attention an episode from one's past experience. The neural substrate of such a neurocognitive set has been identified by imaging experiments in the bilateral frontal pole (Brodmann's Area 10), the bilateral frontal operculum (BA45/47), the left dorsal prefrontal cortex (BA8/9), and the left anterior cingulate (BA 32). Our study, based on functional anatomy, showed direct anatomical pathways between the two prefrontal areas and the temporal cortex. However, so far, it is unknown how these prefrontal areas process the memory encoding/retrieval signal and which part sends the final signal to the temporal cortex. How do the two pathways play roles for the temporal cortex? It is likely that the connection between the dorsal prefrontal and temporal cortices plays a more encoding-related role (e.g. detecting novel features in an event and consolidating it into the brain) while the connection between the ventral prefrontal and temporal cortices plays a more retrieval-related role, as we showed in our study. Another signal pathway for memory retrieval originates from the medial temporal lobe. This pathway may play a crucial role for memory storage and retrieval for a while until memory is stored and retrieved by the hippocampus-independent system, perhaps until neocortical areas per se establish connectivity with each other (Takahashi and Miyashita, 2000). However, the nature of this indexing system is still unknown. Obtaining direct evidence for this hypothesis in animal experimentations remains as a challenge for future work to address.

### From Connection to Cognition

The results of tractography on humans have been compared to the results of tracer studies on non-human primates. The functional roles of connections in human brains have often been inferred based on those observed in the non-human primates. However, we should of course expect to see certain differences between humans and non-human primates that constitute the basis of uniquely human cognitive abilities. I believe that studying these differences in connectivity will provide us with a better understanding of human brains and higher-level cognitive functions.

Future comparisons of connectivity could also reveal subtle differences between individuals. This could potentially enable us to causally predict and explain the cognitive variability we see in individuals, allowing us to move beyond what is possible with today's correlation-based methods.

## Conclusion

Diffusion imaging enables us to study the white matter structure of the brain *in vivo*. Our experimental data demonstrates large-scale anatomical networks that serve as a basis of episodic memory in humans, especially two anatomical pathways between frontal and temporal lobes. Because of the limitations of current techniques, we should proceed with great care in the design of tractography studies. Future applications of tractography will be promising with development of more universally agreed-upon methods of estimating error, and more accurate detection of the trajectories of the fiber pathways.

## Acknowledgments

I gratefully thank Robert Levy for his very helpful editorial comments. This work was supported by the Uehara Memorial Foundation (Japan).

## References

Alexander A.L., Hasan K.M., Lazar M., Tsuruda J.S. and Parker D.L. (2001). Analysis of partial volume effects in diffusion-tensor MRI. *Mgn. Reson, Med.* 45, 770-780.

Basser, P.J., Mattiello, J. and LeBihan, D. (1994). MR diffusion tensor spectroscopy and imaging. *Biophs J.* 66, 259-267.

Basser P.J., Pajevic S., Pierpaoli C., Duda J. and Aldroubi A. (2000). In vivo fiber tractography using DT-MRI data. *Magn. Reson. Med.* 44, 625-632.

Behrens T.E., Johansen-Berg H., Woolrich M.W., Smith S.M., Wheeler-Kingshott C.A., Boulby P.A., Barker G.J., Sillery E.L., Sheehan K., Ciccarelli O., Thompson A.J., Brady J.M. and Matthews P.M. (2003). Non-invasive mapping of connections between human thalamus and cortex using diffusion imaging. *Nat. Neurosci.* 6, 750-757.

Buckner, R.L. and Koutstaal, W. (1998). Functional neuroimaging studies of encoding, priming, and explicit memory retrieval. *Proc. Natl. Acad. Sci. U.S.A.* 95, 891-898.

Buckner R.L., Koutstaal W., Schacter D.L., Wagner A.D. and Rosen B.R. (1998). Functional-anatomic study of episodic retrieval using fMRI. I. Retrieval effort versus retrieval success. *Neuroimage.* 7, 151-162.

Buckner, R.L., Koutstaal, W., Schacter, D.L., Dale, A.M., Rotte, M., Rosen, B.R. 1998b. Functional-anatomic study of episodic retrieval II. Selective averaging of event-related fMRI trials to test the retrieval success hypothesis. *NeuroImage.* 7: 163-175.

Buckner, R.L., Kelley, W.M. and Petersen, S.E. (1999). Frontal cortex contributes to human memory formation. *Nat. Neurosci.* 2, 311-314.

Cabeza, R. and Nyberg, L. (2000). Imaging cognition II: An empirical review of 275 PET and fMRI studies. *J. Cogn. Neurosci.* 12, 1-47.

Cansino, S., Maquet, P., Dolan, R.J., Rugg, M.D. 2002. Brain activity underlying encoding and retrieval of source memory. *Cereb. Cortex.* 12: 1048-1056.

Chung, S., Lu, Y., and Henry, R.G. (2006) Comparison of bootstrap approaches for estimation of uncertainties of DTI parameters. *Neuroimage ee,* 531-41.

Colby, C.L., Goldberg, M.E. 1999. Space and attention in parietal cortex. *Ann. Rev. Neurosci.* 22: 319-349.

Conturo T.E., Lori N.F., Cull T.S., Akbudak E., Snyder A.Z., Shimony J.S., McKinstry R.C., Burton H. and Raichle M.E. (1999). Tracking neuronal fiber pathways in the living human brain. *Proc. Natl. Acad. Sci. U.S.A.* 96, 10422-10427.

Corbetta, M. 1998. Frontoparietal cortical networks for directing attention and the eye to visual locations: identical, independent, or overlapping neural systems? *Proc. Natl. Acad. Sci. U.S.A.* 95: 831-838.

Catani, M. (2006). Diffusion tensor magnetic resonance imaging tractography in cognitive disorders. *Curr. Opin. Neurol.* 19, 599-606.

Cavanna, A.E., Trimble, M.R. 2006 The precuneus: a review of its functional anatomy and behavioural correlates. *Brain*. 129: 564-583.

De Renzi, E., Liotti, M., Nichelli, P. 1987. Semantic amnesia with preservation of autobiographical memory: *A case report. Cortex*. 23: 575-597.

Demb J.B., Desmond J.E., Wagner A.D., Vaidya C.J., Glover G.H. and Gabrieli J.D. (1995). Semantic encoding and retrieval in the left inferior prefrontal cortex: a functional MRI study of task difficulty and process specificity. *J. Neurosci.* 15, 5870-5878.

Dobbins, I.G., Rice, H.J., Wagner, A.D., Schacter, D.L. 2003. Memory orientation and success: separable neurocognitive components underlying episodic recognition. *Neuropsychologia*. 41: 318-333.

Donaldson, D.I., Petersen, S.E., Ollinger, J.M., Buckner, R.L. 2001. Dissociating state and item components of recognition memory using fMRI. *Neuroimage*. 13: 129-142.

Dougherty, R.F., Ben-Shachar, M., Bammer, R., Brewer, A.A. and Wandell, B.A. (2005). Functional organization of human occipito-callosal fiber tracts. *Proc. Natl. Acad. Sci. U.S.A.* 102, 7350-7355.

Fuster, J.M. (1997). The prefrontal cortex: Anatomy, physiology, and neuropsychology of the frontal lobe. (Philadelphia: Lippincott-Raven).

Gazzaniga, M.S. (1995). Principles of human brain organization derived from split-brain studies. *Neuron*. 14, 217-228.

Goldman-Rakic, P.S. (1987). Circuitry of primate prefrontal cortex and regulation of behavior by representational memory. In Plum, F. and Mountcastle, V. eds. *Handbook of physiology:* Section 1. The nervous system. Vol. 5. Higher functions of the brain. Part 1, pp. 373-417. (Bethesda, MD: American Physiological Society).

Guye M. et al. 2003. Combined functional MRI and tractography to demonstrate the connectivity of the human primary motor cortex in vivo. *NeuroImage*. 19: 1349-1360.

Habib, R., Nyberg, L. and Tulving, E. (2003). Hemispheric asymmetries of memory: the HERA model revisited. *TRENDS in Cogn. Sci.* 7, 241-245.

Hart, J. Jr, Gordon, B. 1990. Delineation of single-word semantic comprehension deficits in aphasia, with anatomical correlation. *Ann. Neurol.* 27: 226-231.

Henson, R.N.A., Rugg, M.D., Shallice, T., Josephs, O., Dolan, R.J. 1999. Recollection and familiarity in recognition memory: an event-related functional magnetic resonance imaging study. *J. Neurosci.* 19: 3962-3972.

Herron, J.E., Henson, R.N.A., Rugg, M.D. 2004. Probability effects on the neural correlates of retrieval success: an fMRI study. *NeuroImage*. 21: 302-310.

Hyvarinen, J. 1982. Posterior parietal lobe of the primate brain. *Physiol. Rev.* 62: 1060-1129.

Incisa della Rocchetta, A. and Milner, B. (1993). Strategic search and retrieval inhibition: The role of the frontal lobes. *Neuropsychologia*. 31, 503-524.

Jbabdi, S, Woolrich, M.W., Andersson, J.L., Behrens, T.E. (2007) *A bayesian framework for global tractography.* In press

Jones, D.K., Horsfield, M.A. and Simmons, A. (1999). Optimal strategies for measuring diffusion in anisotropic systems by magnetic resonance imaging. *Magn. Reson. Med.* 42, 515-525.

Kim, M., Ducros, M., Carlson, T., Ronen, I., He, S., Ugurbil, K., Kim, D-S. 2006. Anatomical correlates of the functional organization in the human occipitotemporal cortex. *Magn. Reson. Imaging.*

Konishi, S., Wheeler, M.E., Donaldson, D.I., Buckner, R.L. 2001. Neural correlates of episodic retrieval success. *NeuroImage.* 12: 276-286.

Konishi, S., Asari, T., Jimura, K., Chikazoe, J., Miyashita, Y. 2006. Activation shift from medial to lateral temporal cortex associated with recency judgements following impoverished encoding. *Cereb. Cortex.* 16: 469-474.

Lazar M., Weinstein D.M., Tsuruda J.S., Hasan K.M., Arfanakis K., Meyerand M.E., Badie B., Rowley H.A., Haughton V., Field A. and Alexander A.L. (2003). White matter tractography using diffusion tensor deflection. *Hum. Brain Mapp.* 18, 306-321.

Lazar, M. and Alexander, A.L. (2005). Bootstrap white matter tractography (BOOT-TRAC) *Neuroimage.* 24, 524-532.

Lehericy S., Ducros M., Krainik A., Francois C., Van de Moortele P.F., Ugurbil K. and Kim D.S. (2004). 3-D diffusion tensor axonal tracking shows distinct SMA and pre-SMA projections to the human striatum. *Cereb. Cortex.* 14, 1303-1309.

Lee, A.C., Robbins, T.W., Graham, K.S., Owen, A.M. 2002. "Pray or Prey?" dissociation of semantic memory retrieval from episodic memory processes using positronemission tomography and a nocel homophone task. *NeuroImage.* 16: 724-735.

Lepage, M., Ghaffar, O., Nyberg, L. and Tulving, E. (2000). Prefrontal cortex and episodic memory retrieval mode. *Proc. Natl. Acad. Sci. U.S.A.* 97, 506-511.

Mesulam, M.M. 1999. Spatial attention and neglct: parietal, frontal and cingulated contributions to the mental representation and attentional targeting of salient extrapersonal events. *Philos. Trans. R. Soc. Lond. B. Biol. Sci.* 354: 1325-1346.

Mori, S., Crain, B.J., Chacko V.P. and van Zijl, P.C.M. (1999). Three-dimensional tracking of axonal projections in the brain by magnetic resonance imaging. *Annal. Neurol.* 45, 265-269.

Naghavi H.R. and Nyberg L. 2005. Common fronto-parietal activity in attention, memory, and consciousness: Shared demands on integration? *Consci. Cogn.* 14: 390-425.

Owen, A.M., Evans, A.C. and Petrides, M. (1996). Evidence for a two-stage model of spatial working memory processing within the lateral frontal cortex: A positron emission tomography study. *Cerebral Cortex.* 6, 31-38.

Petrides, M. (1994a). Frontal lobes and behaviour. *Current Opinion in Neurobiology.* 4, 207-211.

Petrides, M. (1994b). Frontal lobes and working memory: Evidence from investigations of the effects of cortical excisions in nonhuman primates. In Boller, F. and Grafman, *J. eds. Handbook of neuropsychology.* Vol. 9 (Amsterdam: Elsevier), pp. 59-82.

Petrides, M. (1996). Specialized systems for the processing of mnemonic information within the primate frontal cortex. *Phil. Trans. R. Soc. B.,* 351, 1455-1462.

Petrides, M. (2005). Lateral prefrontal cortex: architectonic and functional organization. *Phil. Trans. R. Soc. B.,* 360, 781-795.

Petrides, M. and Pandya, D.N. (1994). Comparative architectonic analysis of the human and the macaque frontal cortex. In Boller, F. and Grafman, *J. eds. Handbook of neuropsychology.* Vol. 9 (Amsterdam: Elsevier), pp. 17-58.

Petrides, M. and Pandya, D.N. (1999). Dorsolateral prefrontal cortex: comparative cytoarchitectonic analysis in the human and the macaque brain and corticocortical connection patterns. *Eur. J. Neurosci.* 11, 1011-1036.

Petrides, M. and Pandya, D.N. (2002). Comparative cytoarchitectonic analysis of the human and the macaque ventrolateral prefrontal cortex and corticocortical connection patterns in the monkey. *Eur.J. Neurosci.* 16, 291-310.

Powell H.W., Guye M., Parker G.J., Symms M.R., Boulby P., Koepp M.J., Barker G.J. and Duncan J.S. (2004). Noninvasive in vivo demonstration of the connections of the human parahippocampal gyrus. *Neuroimage.* 22, 740-747.

Rajah, M.N., McIntosh, A.R. and Grady, C.L. (1999). Frontotemporal interactions in face encoding and recognition. *Cogn. Brain Res.* 8, 259-269.

Rugg, M.D., Henson, R.N.A., Robb, W.G. 2003. Neural correlates of retrieval processing in the prefrontal cortex during recognition and exclusion tasks. *Neuropsychologia.* 41: 40-52.

Schacter, D.L. (1987). Memory, amnesia, and frontal lobe dysfunction. *Psychophysiology.* 17, 568-576.

Schmahmann, J.D., Pandya, D.N., Wang, R., Dai, G., D'Arceuil, H.E., de Crespigny, A.J., and Wedeen, V.J. (2007). Association fibre pathways of the brain: parallel observations from diffusion spectrum imaging and autoradiography. *Brain.* 130, 630-53.

Seltzer, B. and Pandya, D.N. (1980). Converging visual and somatic sensory cortical input to the intraparietal sulcus of the rhesus monkey. *Brain Res.* 192, 339-351.

Seltzer, B. and Pandya, D.N. (1989). Frontal lobe connections of the superior temporal sulcus in the rhesus monkey. *J. Comp. Neurol.* 281, 97-113.

Shannon, B.J., Buckner, R.L. 2004. Functional-anatomic correlations of memory retriecal that suggest nontraditional processing roles for multiple distinct regions within posterior parietal cortex. *J. Neurosci.* 24: 10084-10092.

Shimamura, A.P. (1995). Memory and frontal lobe function. In Gazzaniga, M.S. ed. *The cognitive neurosciences.* (Cambridge, MA: MIT press), pp. 803-813.

Snowden, J.S., Goulding, P.J., Neary, D. 1989. Semantic dementia: A form of circumscribed cerebral atrophy. *Behav. Neurol.* 2: 167-182.

Snowden, J.S., Griffiths, H., Neary, D. 1994. Semantic dementia: Autobiographical contribution to preservation of meaning. *Cogn. Neuropsycol.* 11: 265-288.

Squire, L. (1994). Declarative and nondeclarative memory: multiple brain systems supporting learning and memory. In: *Mmoeyr systems.* (Schacter, D.L., and Tulving, E. eds), pp. 203-232. Cambridge, MA: MIT Press.

Squire, L.R. and Zola-Morgan, S. (1991). The medial temporal lobe memory system. *Science.* 253, 1380-1386.

Stieltjes B., Kaufmann W.E., van Zijl P.C., Fredericksen K., Pearlson G.D., Solaiyappan M. and Mori S. (2001). Diffusion tensor imaging and axonal tracking in the human brainstem. *Neuroimage.* 14, 723-735.

Sullivan, E.V. and Pfefferbaum, A. (2003). Diffusion tensor imaging in normal aging and neuropsychiatric disorders. *Eur. J. Radiol.* 45, 244-255.

Takahashi, E. and Miyashita, Y. in *Neuropsychology of Memory.* (eds. Squire, L.R. and Schacter, D.L.) 301-310 (The Guilford Press, New York, 2002).

Takahashi, E., Ohki, K., Kim, D-S. (2007). Diffusion tensor studies dissociated two fronto-temporal pathways in the human memory system. *NeuroImage.* 34: 827-838.

Thottakara, P., Lazar, M., Johnson, C. and Alexander, L. (2006) Application of Brodmann's area templates for ROI selection in white matter tractography studies. *Neuroimage.* 29, 868-878.

Tomita, H., Ohbayashi, M., Nakahara, K., Hasegawa, I. and Miyashita, Y. (1999). Top-down signal from prefrontal cortex in executive control of memory retrieval. *Nature.* 401, 699-703.

Toosy A.T. et al. 2004. Characterizing function-structure relationships in the human visual system with functional MRI and diffusion tensor imaging. *NeuroImage.* 21: 1452-1463.

Tuch, D.S., Rees, T.G., Wiegell, M.R., Makris, N., Belliveau, J.W., and Wedeen, V.J. (2002). High angular resolution diffusion imaging reveals intravoxel white matter fiber heterogeneity. *Magn. Reson Med.* 4, 577-82.

Tuch, D.S., Salat, D.H., Wisco, J.J., Zaleta, A.K., Hevelone, N.D., Rosas, H.D. (2005). Choice reaction time performance correlates with diffusion anisotropy in white matter pathways supporting visuospatial attention. *Proc. Natl. Acad. Sci. U S A.* 102, 12212-7.

Tulving E., Kapur S., Craik F.I., Moscovitch M. and Houle S. (1994). Hemispheric encoding/retrieval asymmetry in episodic memory: positron emission tomography findings. *Proc. Natl. Acad. Sci. U.S.A.* 91, 2016-2020.

Tulving, E (2002). Episodic memory: From mind to brain. *Annu. Rev. Psycol.* 53, 1-25.

Upadhyay, J., Ducros, M., Knaus, T.A., Lindgren, K.A., Silver, A., Tager-Flusberg, H., Kim, D-S. (2006) Function and Connectivity in Human Primary Auditory Cortex: A Combined fMRI and DTI Study at 3 tesla. Cereb. Cortex. In press

Wagner A.D., Schacter D.L., Rotte M., Koutstaal W., Maril A., Dale A.M., Rosen B.R. and Buckner R.L. (1998). Building memories: remembering and forgetting of verbal experiences as predicted by brain activity. *Science.* 281, 1188-1191.

Wagner, A.D., Shannon, B.J., Kahn, I., Buckner, R.L. (2005). Parietal lobe contributions to episodic memory retrieval. *Trends in Cogn. Sci.* 9: 445-453.

Wedeen, V.J., Hagmann, P., Tseng, W.Y., Rees, T.G., and Weisskoff, R.M. (2005) Mapping complex tissue architecture with diffusion spectrum magnetic resonance imaging. *Magn. Reson. Med.* 6, 1377-86.

Wheeler, M.E., Buckner, R.L. (2003). Functional dissociation among components of remembering: control, perceived oldness, and content. *J. Neurosci.* 23: 3869-3880.

Wiggs, C.L., Weisberg, J., Martin, A. (1999). Neural correlates of semantic and episodic memory retrieval. *Neuropsycologia.* 37: 103-118.

Xu D., Mori S., Solaiyappan M., van Zijl P.C. and Davatzikos C. (2002). A framework for callosal fiber distributon analysis. *Neuroimage.* 17, 1131-1143.

In: Research Topics on Brain Mapping
Editor: Yuanzhu Liáng, pp. 33-56
ISBN: 978-1-60456-001-5


*Chapter II*

# Cerebral Neuroimaging and Neurophysiological Brain Mapping of the Effects of Cannabis Abuse

***Roy R. Reeves[1,2], Frederick A. Struve[3] and Randy S. Burke[1,2]***
[1] Mental Health Service, G.V. (Sonny) Montgomery VA Medical Center, Jackson, MS
[2] Department of Psychiatry and Human Behavior,
University of Mississippi School of Medicine
[3] Department of Psychiatry, Yale University School of Medicine
and the VA Connecticut Health Care System (retired)

## Abstract

Cannabis is the most commonly used illicit drug. Its principle psychoactive compound is delta-9-tetrahydrocannabinol, acting centrally at cannabanoid 1 (CB1) receptors which are widely distributed in the neocortex with high concentrations in frontal regions and areas of associational function. Acute intoxication results in decreased attention, memory, and psychomotor speed. The effects of chronic use remain an area of debate.

A number of studies of brain structure and function have attempted to determine the neural mechanisms underlying the effect of cannabis on the CNS, and these mechanisms remain poorly understood. Evidence from CT and MRI studies does not suggest a significant association between cannabis use and structural brain abnormalities. Functional neuroimaging (fMRI, SPECT, PET) may identify brain changes to subtle to be detected by current structural imaging techniques. Although there are wide differences in study designs and considerable variations in results among different investigations, the majority of studies have demonstrated global cortical activity increases during administration of cannabis. Differential activity in specific brain regions has also been reported. Increased frontal lobe activity has been generally reported with cannabis exposure while attenuated frontal activity has been described in recently abstinent cannabis users. Studies involving the temporal lobes are limited and somewhat conflicting. Increased anterior cingulate activity correlating with subjective intoxication has been reported with cannabis administration while decreased anterior cingulate activity has been reported during abstinence in regular cannabis users. Increases in cerebellar activity have been shown to occur in cannabis smokers while reduced cerebellar activity occurs during abstinence in regular cannabis users. Current neuroimaging has not yet helped fully clarify the role of chronic cannabis use and cognitive deficits.

Although visual EEG analysis does not yield consistent cannabis related changes, quantitative EEG has proven more revealing. Quantitative EEG studies of acute cannabis exposure showed increased relative power of alpha, combined with decreased alpha frequency and a reduction of beta activity. EEGs of chronic heavy long term users are characterized by significant elevations of absolute alpha power, relative alpha power, and interhemispheric alpha coherence over frontal and fronto-central areas, a phenomenon referred to as hyperfrontality of alpha. Most initial evoked potentials studies suggest that P300 event related potentials are not altered by chronic cannabis use, although the P50 auditory gating response may be reduced and steady state visual evoked potentials may be altered in cannabis users. The neurophysiological effects of cannabis abuse remains only partially understood and additional research is needed in this area

## Introduction

Marijuana, the common name for the plant *Cannabis sativa*, is the most widely used illicit drug in the United States (Substance Abuse and Mental Health Services Administration, 2004). It has been used for centuries for its mood altering properties. Its use increased sharply among America's youth in the 1960s and 1970s. Use declined in the 1980s but since then has been on the rise again.

People smoke marijuana to obtain the psychophysiological effects that it produces. Acutely the drug produces an altered state of consciousness characterized by mild euphoria, relaxation, perceptual alterations including time distortion, and the enhancement of ordinary sensory experiences. Cognitive functions are impaired, including impaired short term memory, decreased attention, and decreased psychomotor skills and reaction time (Hall et al, 1994). The effects of chronic use remain an area of debate.

The principle psychoactive compound of cannabis is delta-9-tetrahydrocannabinol (hereafter referred to as THC) which acts centrally primarily at the cannabanoid 1 (CB1) receptor. CB1 receptor distribution is widespread throughout the neocortex, with particularly high concentrations in frontal regions and association and limbic areas, which contributes to a wide range of neurobehavioral and cognitive effects seen with acute and chronic cannabis use. Despite the prevalence and long history of cannabis use by man, the neural mechanisms underlying its influence on the brain are not well understood. This article will review investigations of neuroimaging of the effects of cannabis abuse using structural neuroimaging techniques, including pneumoencephalography (PEG), computerized tomography (CT), and magnetic resonance imaging (MRI); functional neuroimaging techniques such as single photon emission computerized tomography (SPECT), postron emission spectroscopy (PET), and functional MRI (fMRI); and analog and quantitative EEG. Because of the number of investigations to be considered, the details presented for each must necessarily be limited, and this article is not intended to be a comprehensive discussion of the topic.

## Structural Neuroimaging

Investigations of the effects of cannabis abuse utilizing structural neuroimaging are limited in number, probably because functional neuroimaging is more sensitive to the changes resulting from cannabis use. Ten studies have been performed with variable results (see table 1). As might be expected, all structural neuroimaging investigations have involved chronic users (the acute administration of cannabis would probably not be likely to produce acute structural changes).

The first such study (Campbell et al, 1971) employed PEG and reported the presence of enlarged ventricles in 10 chronic cannabis users compared to 13 healthy controls. Subsequent studies utilizing CT (Co et al, 1977; Keuhnle, et al, 1977; Hannerz et al, 1983; Wiesbeck & Taeschner, 1991) did not identify structural changes in chronic cannabis users. However there were several limitations in study design, including, in some studies, problems with subject and control selection and statistical methodology. An MRI study (Aasly et al, 1993) reported cerebral atrophy in cannabis users, but the study did not exclude subjects with significant histories of use of alcohol and other drugs which may have contributed to the atrophy. Volumetric MRI (v-MRI) investigation using more rigorous methodology showed conflicting results with two studies reporting no significant differences between users and control subjects (Block et al, 2000; Tzilos et al, 2005). However Matochik et al, 2005 reported that chronic cannabis users compared to nonusers had lower gray matter density in the right parahippocampal gyrus and greater density bilaterally near the precentral gyrus and the right thalamus. Cannabis users also had lower white matter density in the left parietal lobe and higher density around the parahippocampal and fusiform gyri compared to nonusers. Another study of chronic cannabis users employing both MRI and PET which stratified subjects by age of first use and gender (Wilson et al, 2000) reported a significant correlation between age of first use and decreased total brain volume (see discussion of PET studies below for additional detail).

It may be seen that findings among these studies are variable and inconsistent. Only one study (Matochik et al, 2005) using the highest resolution imaging and analytic techniques available has reported structural changes secondary to chronic cannabis use, and those findings have not been replicated. When the investigations are considered as a whole, minimal evidence has been found to suggest an association between cannabis use and structural brain abnormalities (Quickfall & Crockford, 2006).

## Functional Neuroimaging

Functional neuroimaging techniques are more sensitive to subtle changes in the brain than are structural imaging techniques. SPECT, PET, and fMRI have been used to study the impact of cannabis upon cerebral functioning, usually by measurement of cerebral blood flow (CBF). Usually such investigations have involved two basic paradigms: 1.) studies of subjects following exposure to cannabis under controlled laboratory conditions or 2.) studies of chronic cannabis users who have abstained from usage of the drug for at least a short period of time prior to the assessment of cerebral functioning (abstinent subjects). A small number of investigations have used both paradigms.

## SPECT Studies of the Effects of Cannabis Usage

Several investigations (summarized in table 2) have utilized SPECT to assess the impact of cannabis on the brain. A few of these have involved administration of cannabis to subjects under controlled laboratory conditions. Mathew et al (1989) recorded measurement of CBF with $^{133}$Xe SPECT in experienced and inexperienced cannabis smokers before and 60 minutes after smoking marijuana. Experienced users showed an increase in global cortical CBF while inexperienced users showed a decrease. The latter finding was explained as possibly being related to inexperienced user anxiety. Subsequent $^{133}$Xe SPECT studies of cannabis users exposed to the drug under laboratory conditions reported similar findings. Mathew et al (1992) showed that cannabis smoking was associated with bilateral CBF increase, which was maximal 30 minutes after smoking. Greater CBF increases were seen in the frontal areas and the right hemisphere. Mathew and Wilson (1993) found that cannabis smoking was accompanied by increase in cerebral blood velocity and bilateral increase in CBF, especially in the frontal regions. Behavioral changes showed significant correlations with CBF. The post-cannabis changes could not be explained by changes in general circulation and was unrelated to plasma levels of THC.

SPECT has also been utilized to examine cerebral changes in chronic cannabis users under conditions of temporary abstinence from the drug. Mathew and colleagues (1986) compared heavy users of marijuana (based on self report) and individuals who had never used cannabis. There was a nonsignificant trend toward decreased global CBF in cannabis users. A second study (Tunving et al, 1986) examined 9 users in various stages of abstinence and found that the regional CBF (rCBF) in cannabis users was significantly (11%) lower than that of healthy controls. Four of the subjects re-scanned at variable later dates showed significant increases of rCBF at followup, suggesting that hypometabolism may be a condition normalizing with a sufficient period of abstinence. Lundqvist et al (2001) compared 14 abstinent DSM-IV cannabis dependent subjects with 14 healthy individuals and found significantly reduced flow to the right frontal lobe (as opposed to other studies suggesting bifrontal reduction). Using three dimensional SPECT, Amen and Waugh (1998) reported decreased temporal lobe activity in heavy cannabis users with comorbid ADHD compared with subjects with ADHD who did not use cannabis. However, psychiatric comorbidities may have confounded their findings and makes definite conclusions difficult.

Virtually all SPECT investigations of THC have used inhaled $^{133}$Xe as the radiotracer. Reeves and Struve (2007) recorded quantitative EEGs and used injected technetium-99m hexamethylpropyleneamine oxime (HMPAO) to obtain SPECT scans of six long term daily cannabis users. $^{99m}$Tc-HMPAO is an agent with better image quality than $^{133}$Xe. SPECT scans revealed areas of decreased cerebral perfusion but in different areas among the six subjects, while EEGs demonstrated more predictable changes (discussed later).

**Table 1. Structural Neuroimaging Studies of Chronic Cannabis Users[a]**

| Study | Modality | Number of Subjects (Controls) | Duration of Cannabis Use | Amount of Cannabis Used | Comments | Results |
|---|---|---|---|---|---|---|
| Campbell et al, 1971 | PEG | 10 (13) | 3-11 years | Not specified | Less sensitive than CT or MRI | Ventricular enlargement in users compared to nonusers |
| Co et al, 1977 | CT | 12 (0) | 5-10 years | 5-35 joints/day | Limitations of study design | Not significant |
| Keuhnle et al, 1977 | CT | 19 (0) | Not specified | 28-62 times/ month | Limitations of study design | Not significant |
| Hannerz et al, 1983 | CT | 12 (0) | 6-20 years | Average 1.25 g/day | Limitations of study design | Not significant |
| Wiesbeck & Taeschner, 1991 | CT | 12 (10) | 0.5-15 years | Not specified | Controls were nonusing persons with schizophrenia | Not significant |
| Aasly et al, 1993 | MRI | 23 (17) | Not specified | 1-15 kg total lifetime intake | Some subjects had history of substance abuse | Cerebral and cerebellar atrophy |
| Block et al, 2000 | v-MRI | 18 (13) | Two or more years | 7 or more times weekly | Ventricular volumes were lower in users than controls | Not significant |
| Wilson et al, 2000 | v-MRI | 57(0) | 13.4-16.9 years | 120-240 joints/ year | PET also used as part of study | Significant correlation between age of first use and decreased total brain volume |
| Tzilos et al, 2005 | v-MRI | 22 (26) | Not specified | Mean of > 20,000 lifetime episodes | Designed to investigate older subjects with heavier use | Not significant |
| Matochik et al, 2005 | v-MRI | 11 (8) | Average 7.5 years | Average 34.7 joints/ week | No correlation of changes to age of onset of use | Changes in gray and white matter density in several areas (see text) |

[a]Modified from Quickfall & Crockford (2006).

**Table 2. Studies of the Effect of Cannabis Utilizing SPECT[a]**

| Study | Subject Type[b] | SPECT Isotope | Number of Subjects | Duration of Cannabis Use | Amount of Cannabis Use | Results |
|---|---|---|---|---|---|---|
| Mathew et al, 1989 | Abstinent/ acutely intoxicated chronic cannabis users | $^{133}Xe$ | 26 | >3 years | >10 joints/week | Inexperienced users showed a decrease in global cortical CBF, experienced users a global increase. |
| Mathew et al, 1992 | Acutely intoxicated chronic cannabis users | $^{133}Xe$ | 20 | Not reported | Not reported | Bilateral increase CBF in frontal areas and right hemisphere, maximal 30 minutes after smoking |
| Mathew & Wilson, 1993 | Acutely intoxicated chronic cannabis users | $^{133}Xe$ | 35 | Not reported | Not reported | Increased cerebral blood flow velocity, increased CBF, especially frontal regions |
| Mathew et al, 1986 | Chronic users, abstinent at least 12 hours | $^{133}Xe$ | 17 | >6 months | >6 joints/week | Trend toward decreased CBF in users |
| Tunving et al, 1986 | Abstinent chronic users | $^{133}Xe$ | 9 | 1- 15 years | 3-4 times/week or more | rCBF 11% lower in cannabis users than controls |
| Amen & Waugh, 1998 | Abstinent chronic users with ADHD | $^{133}Xe$ (3D) | 30 | Mean 5.5 years | "daily-weekly" | Decreased temporal lobe activity in users with ADHD versus nonusing controls with ADHD alone |
| Lundqvist et al, 2001 | Chronic users abstinent for an average of 1/6 days | $^{133}Xe$ | 12 | Mean 12.3 years | Mean 2.4 grams/day | Decrease CBF, right frontal lobe |
| Reeves & Struve, 2007 | Chronic daily users abstinent for over 1 week | $^{99m}Tc$-HMPAO | 6 | Over 5 years | Not specified | Variable areas of decreased CBF |

[a]Modified from Quickfall & Crockford (2006)

[b]"Acutely intoxicated" refers to subjects given cannabis under controlled laboratory conditions.

## PET Studies of the Effects of Cannabis Usage

PET imaging provides more detailed cerebral images than SPECT, resulting in PET being utilized in several more studies of the effects of cannabis use. PET studies of chronic cannabis users during periods of abstinence have shown that long term usage may effect several areas of the nervous system (see tble 3). Volkow et al (1996) demonstrated lower cerebellar metabolism in cannabis users relative to nonusing controls. Block et al (2000) also found substantially lower CBF in a large region of the posterior cerebellum. Block and colleagues (2002) later compared memory related CBF in frequent cannabis users and nonusing controls after 26+ hours of abstinence. In users memory related CBF showed decreases in prefrontal cortex, increases in memory relevant regions of the cerebellum, and altered lateralization in hippocampal areas, indicating altered memory related brain function in chronic cannabis users. Eldreth et al (2004) used PET and a modified version of the Stroop task to determine whether 25 day abstinent cannabis users have persistent deficits in executive cognitive functioning. Although the cannabis users had no deficits in task performance, they showed hypoactivity in the left perigenual anterior cingulate cortex and the left lateral prefrontal cortex and hyperactivity in the hippocampus bilaterally, suggesting that chronic cannabis users display persistent metabolic alterations in the brain regions responsible for executive cognitive functioning. In their PET/MRI study of brain volume measures, Wilson and colleagues (2000) found that subjects who started using cannabis before age 17, compared to those who started using later, had smaller whole brain and percent cortical gray matter and larger percent white matter volumes. Males who started using cannabis before age 17 had significantly higher CBF than other males. The researchers concluded that the age at which exposure to cannabis begins is important in terms of impact upon the central nervous system.

## PET Studies of the Effect of Laboratory Exposure to Cannabis

PET has been utilized in several investigations of the effects of cannabis administered under controlled conditions (see tble 4). Volkow et al (1991) investigated the effects of intravenous (IV) administration of 2 grams of THC on brain metabolism using 18F-2-fluro-2-deoxyglucose (FDG) PET in eight normal subjects at baseline and 30- 40 minutes after administration. Changes in global metabolism in response to THC were variable: three subjects showed an increase, three a decrease, and two showed no change. In contrast, all subjects demonstrated an increase in metabolism in the cerebellum following THC administration, corresponding with the high density of cannabanoid receptors known to be in this area. Cerebellar changes were the only significant regional metabolic changes due to THC administration. A later study by the same research group (Volkow et al, 1996) assessed brain glucose metabolism prior to and following THC in eight normal subjects and eight chronic marijuana abusers. At baseline abusers showed lower relative cerebellar metabolism than normal subjects. THC increased cerebellar metabolism in all subjects and abusers also showed increases in orbitofrontal cortex, prefrontal cortex, and basal ganglia.

## Table 3. Studies of the Effect of Cannabis (Abstinent Subjects) Utilizing PET[a]

| Study | Modality | Number of Subjects | Duration of Cannabis Use | Amount of Cannabis Used | Results |
|---|---|---|---|---|---|
| Volkow et al, 1996[b] | FDG-PET | 8 normal subjects, 8 abusers | Mean 5.5 years | 1- 5 joints/day | Lower relative cerebellar metabolism in cannabis users than normal subjects. |
| Block et al, 2000 | $^{15}O$-water PET | 17 | Mean 3.9 years | >7 times/week | Cannabis users showed substantially lower brain blood flow than controls in a large region of the posterior cerebellum |
| Wilson et al, 2000 | $^{15}O$-water PET | 57 | 13.4- 16.9 years | 120-240 joints/year | Subjects who started using cannabis before age 17 had smaller brain volumes and lower percent cortical grey matter compared to those who started later. |
| Block et al, 2002 | $^{15}O$-water PET | 18 | Mean 3.9 years | Mean 17 times /week | Relative to controls, CBF in cannabis users showed decreases in prefrontal cortex, increases in memory-relevant regions of the cerebellum, and altered lateralization in the hippocampus. |
| Eldreth et al, 2004 | $^{15}O$-water PET | 11 | >2 years | >4 times/week | While performing executive cognitive tasks, cannabis users showed hypoactivity of the left perigenual anterior cingulate cortex and the left lateral prefrontal cortex, and hyperactivity in the hypothalamus bilaterally compared to controls. |

[a]Modified from Quickfall & Crockford (2006)

[b]This study also involved acutely intoxicated subjects (see table 4).

## Table 4. Studies of the Effect of Cannabis Exposure Utilizing PET[a]

| Study | Modality | Number of Subjects | Duration of Cannabis Use | Amount of Cannabis Used | Laboratory Delivery of Cannabis | Results Following Cannabis Administration |
|---|---|---|---|---|---|---|
| Volkow et al, 1991 | FDG-PET | 8 | Not specified | Average 1 joint every two months | 2 mg IV | Variable or no cortical changes; increased cerebellar metabolism |
| Volkow et al, 1996[b] | $^{15}$O-water PET | 8 normal subjects, 8 cannabis abusers | Mean 5.5 years | 1- 5 joints/day 1- 7 days/week | 2 mg IV | Increased cerebellar metabolism in all subjects; abusers showed increases in orbitofrontal and prefrontal cortex and basal ganglia |
| Mathew et al, 1997 | $^{15}$O-water PET | 11 high dose, 10 low dose | Not specified | Not specified | 3 mg (low dose) and 5 mg (high dose) IV | Increased CBF especially in the frontal regions insula, cingulate gyrus, and subcortical regions. Significant changes at 60 min for the lower dose, at 30 and 60 min for the higher dose |
| Mathew et al, 1998 | $^{15}$O-water PET | 46 | Not specified | Mean 14.7 joints/year | 3 mg (low dose) and 5 mg (high dose) IV | Increase in cortical and cerebellar blood flow (not all subjects with same effect); those with decrease in cerebellar flow also had alteration of time sense |
| Mathew et al, 1999 | $^{15}$O-water PET | 19 high dose, 19 low dose | Not specifed | Not specified | 3 mg (low dose) and 5 mg (high dose) IV | Global CBF increase, more marked in the right hemisphere, frontal areas, and anterior cingulate |
| Mathew et al, 2002 | $^{15}$O-water PET | 47 | Not specified | Not specified | 3 mg (low dose) and 5 mg (high dose) IV | Significant increases in global CBF and frontal, insular, and anterior cingulate regions; rCBF remained increased up to 120 min and cerebellar flow was increased at 30 and 60 min after high dose infusion |
| O'Leary et al, 2000 | $^{15}$O-water PET | 5 sporadic users doing an auditory attention task while smoking cannabis | Mean 3.2 years | $<10$ times/week | 20 mg cigarette | Increased blood flow in several paralimbic regions including orbitofrontal areas, insula, and temporal poles. Large reductions in rCBF were observed in temporal lobe regions that are sensitive to auditory attention effects |

**Table 4. (Continued).**

| Study | Modality | Number of Subjects | Duration of Cannabis Use | Amount of Cannabis Used | Laboratory Delivery of Cannabis | Results Following Cannabis Administration |
|---|---|---|---|---|---|---|
| O'Leary et al, 2002 | $^{15}O$-water PET | 12 sporadic users doing an auditory attention task while smoking cannabis | Not specified | Mean 2.7 times/month | 20 mg cigarette | Mean global CBF did not change significantly; increased rCBF in orbital and mesial frontal lobes, insula, temporal poles, anterior cingulate, and cerebellum |
| O'Leary et al, 2003 | $^{15}O$-water PET | 12 once weekly users, 12 daily smokers performing self paced counting task during testing | Mean 5.4 years | Mean 1.8 times/day | 20 mg cigarette | Increased rCBF in the ventral forebrain and cerebellar cortex in both groups, but significantly less frontal lobe activation in chronic users |

[a]Modified from Quickfall & Crockford (2006)

[b]This study also involved abstinent subjects (see table 3).

Mathew and colleagues conducted a series of investigations of the effects of acute exposure to cannabis under laboratory conditions using $^{15}$O-water PET. In 32 subjects with a history of exposure to cannabis, scans were performed before and after IV infusion of 3 or 5 grams of THC. THC increased CBF, especially in the frontal regions bilaterally, insula, and cingulate gyrus, and subcortical regions with greater effects in the right hemisphere. Significant increases in frontal CBF occurred. While most regions showed significant change at 60 minutes for the lower dose group, the higher dose group had significant change at 30 and 60 minutes (Mathew et al, 1997). Another study (Mathew et al, 1998) of 46 volunteers confirmed significant increases in cortical and cerebellar blood flow following THC administration, but not all subjects showed this effect. Those who showed a decrease in cerebellar blood flow also had a significant alteration of time sense. An investigation (Mathew et al, 1999) of the relationship between CBF and depersonalization induced by THC following IV infusion in 59 volunteers showed a global increase in CBF which was more marked in the right hemisphere, frontal lobes, and anterior cingulate. Regression analysis showed positive correlations between right frontal and anterior cingulate blood flow and depersonalization. To assess the effect of administered THC over a two hour period, another investigation (Mathew et al, 2002) measured indices of CBF at baseline and 30, 60, 90, and 120 minutes following a 20 minute infusion of 0.15 or 0.25 mg/min of THC in 47 subjects. Intoxication peaked at 30 minutes and remained elevated at 120 minutes. rCBF remained increased up to 120 minutes after the high dose THC infusion. Significant increases were seen in global perfusion and in the frontal, insular, and anterior cingulate regions. Changes were greater in the right hemisphere. After the high dose of THC, cerebellar flow was increased at 30 and 60 minutes. Feeling intoxicated accounted for changes in rCBF better than the plasma level of THC.

O'Leary and colleagues used $^{15}$O-water PET to perform three investigations of the effects of smoked cigarettes containing 20 mg of THC. In one (O'Leary et al, 2000) rCBF was measured before and after five recreational users smoked a marijuana cigarette while they repeatedly performed an auditory attention task. Blood flow increased following smoking in a number of paralimbic regions (including orbital frontal lobes, insula, and temporal lobes) and in anterior cingulate and cerebellum. Large reductions on rCBF were observed in temporal lobe regions that are sensitive to auditory attention effects. The researchers concluded that reduction of task related CBF in temporal lobe cortices may account for the impaired cognitive functions associated with acute intoxication. In a subsequent study of 12 recreational users repeatedly performing an auditory attention task before and after smoking THC (O'Leary et al, 2002), mean global CBF did not change significantly. Increased rCBF was observed in orbital and mesial frontal lobes, insula, temporal poles, anterior cingulate, and cerebellum. Reduced rCBF was observed in temporal lobe auditory regions, in visual cortex, and in brain regions that may be a part of an attentional network (parietal and frontal lobes and thalamus). An investigation of the effects of cannabis on brain perfusion and internal timing (O'Leary et al, 2003) assessed 12 recreational users and 12 daily users performing a self paced counting task during PET imaging before and after smoking cannabis. Smoking cannabis increased rCBF in the ventral forebrain and cerebellar cortex in both groups, but resulted in significantly less frontal lobe activation in chronic users. Counting rates increased in both groups after smoking as did a behavioral measure of self paced tapping. Both increases correlated with rCBF in the cerebellum leading to the conclusion that smoking cannabis appears to accelerate a cerebellar clock altering self paced behaviors.

## fMRI Studies of the Effects of Cannabis Usage

fMRI has been used in two studies to assess the effect of chronic cannabis use on selected cerebral functions. Kanayama et al (2004) assessed brain activity in 12 long term heavy cannabis users 6 to 36 hours after last use, and in 10 control subjects while they performed a spatial working memory task. Cannabis users exhibited increased activation of brain regions typically used for spatial memory tasks, and also recruited additional regions (such as parts of the basal ganglia) not typically used for spatial working memory. Thus cannabis users displayed more widespread brain activation to perform the tasks, suggesting that they may compensate for deficits by "working harder", calling upon additional brain regions to meet the demands of the tasks.

Pillay et al (2004) used fMRI to investigate attentional areas related to motor function as well as primary and supplemental motor cortices in 9 recently abstinent cannabis smokers and 10 controls. The cannabis smokers produced reduced activation in motor cortical areas in response to finger sequencing compared to controls, suggesting that functioning in these areas may be impaired by chronic cannabis usage.

## Discrepancies in Results among Functional Imaging Studies

As may be seen from the above discussion certain findings tend to occur frequently in functional imaging studies of cannabis users, including decreased metabolism in the frontal and cerebellar areas in chronic users, and increased metabolism in the cerebellar, frontal, anterior cingulate, and paralimbic areas during cannabis intoxication. However, there is variability in reported findings in several studies with many failing to show some or all of the typical findings. Why such variations have occurred among different studies is unclear. Obviously the studies are not uniform in design, leading to some difficulty in comparing them. For studies of the effect of chronic cannabis use, it is difficult to quantitate the amount of cannabis subjects have actually used because purchased marijuana may vary significantly in quality. Other factors which may affect CBF, including abuse of other drugs, are difficult to control investigators may in some cases have to depend solely on the subjects' stated history for some information, and this may not always be reliable. Certain factors involving the process of recording scans may also come into play, for example, the subject's state of mind at the time of the procedure. Anxiety negatively effects CBF, as also do fatigue, depression, time from last drug exposure, and usage of caffeine and nicotine. Particular brain areas are activated by cognitive and emotional states and it is not always clear that these factors can be completely controlled (Gatley & Volkow, 1998).

# Neurophysiological Brain Mapping of Effects of Cannabis Abuse

Neurophysiological brain mapping of the effects of cannabis abuse has been accomplished primarily by the use of quantitative topographic EEG. Several characteristics of visual EEG (sometimes referred to as analog EEG) wave forms (e.g., frequency, voltage, or coherence) may be digitized using computer methods. The resulting numerical data may then be used to produce maps or pictures of the activity of the selected EEG characteristic. This technique has proven to be of benefit in researchers' attempts to understand the impact of cannabis use upon the functioning of the cerebral cortex. Prior to discussion of such maps, the historical applications of visual EEG in the investigation of the effects of cannabis on the brain will be reviewed. It was from these visual EEG studies that the later quantitative topographic mapping studies of the effect of cannabis later developed.

## Cannabis Exposure Studies Using Visual EEG Analysis

Many pharmacological compounds produce alterations in the human EEG, often minor and within "normal limits" for a clinical recording. An obvious strategy thus involves securing some type of EEG measure before and after exposure to cannabis and then assessing the changes induced. Table 5 summarizes selected features and results from investigations of this type that have relied on visual inspection of the raw EEG to detect changes occurring with exposure to cannabis.

A cursory inspection reveals considerable lack of comparability among the studies because of methodological differences (including differences in subject selection and variability in historical subject cannabis consumption), and in some cases, less than optimal study designs. All but a single study (Jones & Stone, 1970) employed open, nonblind methodology. It is not surprising, then, that studies of cannabis exposure using visual EEG analysis have produced, as a group, a variety of conflicting minor EEG alterations with no truly salient cannabis induced EEG effect emerging into view. Of note, however, half of the studies reported a decrease in alpha frequency following THC in from 12% to 83% of tested subjects.

## Quantitative EEG Investigations of Cannabis Exposure

Quantitative EEG has the ability to detect subtle changes in voltage, frequency, or amounts of electrical activity within user selected bandwidths. Typically recordings are made from electrodes pasted to the scalp at locations determined by the International 10-20 System (Jasper, 1958) with the data stored on optical discs. Two to five second samples or "epochs" of raw EEG activity free of contaminating artifact are selected. A computerized analog to digital conversion is used to digitize each epoch into individual data points. Data from multiple epochs may be averaged together. Spectral subdivision into basic EEG bandwidths (Delta 1.5- 3.5 Hz; Theta 3.5- 7.5 Hz; Alpha 7.5- 12.5 Hz; Beta 12.5- 20 Hz) is accomplished with a Fast Fourier Transform. Based on the collected data and averaged epochs for each subject, numerical values may be calculate at each electrode site and descriptions or maps of selected quantitative EEG parameters may be created. Absolute power, which is analogous to amplitude or signal strength, is the average amount of power in picowatts found within each EEG frequency band. Relative power involves a computation of the percentage total overall power distributed within each frequency band and is analogous to the "abundance" or relative amount of each type of activity found at each electrode site. Coherence is essentially a measure, expressed in percentage terms, of the degree of timing and phase agreement between two homologous electrodes.

Because of their increased ability to detect subtle change, quantitative EEG methods have been more useful than visual EEG methods in cannabis research. A series of studies were performed in the 1970s; this was followed by several years in which the area had virtually no investigations. Then in the late 1980s and later there was a revived interest and another series of investigations were performed. Table 6 summarizes some of the major features and results of studies of this type prior to 1980. Most of these investigations involved single or double blind placebo controlled procedures with subjects who had prior experience using marijuana, and involve more adequate methodology than did previous EEG cannabis studies.

Taken as a whole, the quantitative EEG studies presented in table 6 suggest that cannabis exposure produces transient EEG effects represented primarily by an increase in the amount of alpha activity (percentage relative power), a decrease in alpha frequency, a decrease in the relative amount of beta activity, and possibly decreased theta activity. Among these quantitative EEG studies, the work of Volvaka and colleagues (Volvaka et al, 1971, 1973, 1977) is viewed as important because if the methodological soundness of the study designs. Their findings suggest that observed cannabis EEG effects are dose dependent (higher doses producing greater effects), rapid in onset following inhalation, and transient with a decay within 30 to 70 minutes depending on other variables. Their studies also suggest that cannabis induced alpha changes are positively related to the subjective experience of feeling "high".

A review of the work of Volvaka and associates suggests that cannabis doses capable of eliciting a clear EEG effect among infrequent marijuana users produced little response when given to users with chronic and heavy habitual use patterns. Dose-finding trials for the latter group indicated that chronic cannabis users required doses at least four times higher than amounts given to occasional users in order for the expected EEG effects to occur. This finding may be compatible with the development of tolerance, or may also be consistent with a presumed persistence of EEG effects from chronic use that could obscure any transient acute effects based on low dose amounts. It is of interest that two studies that showed either limited or no post cannabis alpha changes involved subjects who were very heavy users (six joints per day or more) and laboratory exposure to low or moderate cannabis dosages (Roth et al, 1973; Bachman et al, 1979).

## Table 5. Visual EEG Studies of Exposure to Cannabis[a]

| Study | Subjects | Cannabis use history | Design[b] | Cannabis given | Results |
|---|---|---|---|---|---|
| Wikler & Lloyd, 1945 | 18 patients | Not specified | Pre vs. post cannabis exposure | 2- 3 marijuana cigarettes | Variable changes in alpha frequency and percentage |
| Williams et al, 1946 | 18 patients | Chronic, heavy use | Pre vs. post cannabis exposure | 1-4 marijuana cigarettes | Variable changes in alpha frequency and percentage |
| Ames, 1958 | 10 medical interns | None | Pre vs. post cannabis exposure | 4- 7 grains THC extract orally | Variable changes in alpha frequency and percentage |
| Daliyannakis et al, 1970 | 27 patients | "Hashish addicts" | Post cannabis EEG vs. noncannabis user EEG | Not specified | Variable changes in alpha frequency and percentage |
| Rodin et al, 1970 | 10 medical student | "Light to moderate" | Pre vs. post cannabis exposure | 2-3 300 mg marijuana cigarettes | Pre and post cannabis EEGs could not be distinguished by visual analysis |
| Jones & Stone, 1970 | 10 students | Heavy, daily use | Single blind, placebo controlled | Oral dose 10 grams; smoked dose 0.5- 1 grams | Both dose forms increased low voltage beta and decreased alpha amount; slight alpha slowing |
| Hollister et al, 1970 | 16 students | Not specified | Pre vs. post cannabis exposure | 400- 500 µg/kg THC given orally | Slowing of alpha to 7 Hz during maximal drug effect |
| Heath, 1972 | 1 patient | Chronic, heavy | Pre vs. post cannabis exposure | One 1.25 g marijuana cigarette | High voltage delta in implanted septal leads; no change in scalp EEG |
| Tassarini et al, 1973 | 10 normal volunteers | Not specified | Pre vs. post cannabis exposure | 30- 40 mg oral THC or smoked equivalent | No EEG change with oral THC, slightly higher alpha voltage with smoked THC |
| Tassarini et al, 1974 | 7 normal volunteers | Not specified | Pre vs. post cannabis exposure | 0.7- 1 mg oral THC/kg | Slight increase in alpha amplitude |
| Tassarini et al, 1976 | 11 students | Naive | Pre vs. post cannabis exposure | 0.7- 1 mg oral THC/kg | Alpha amplitude increase and frequency decrease |
| Ramani & Kanakis, 1976 | 10 normal volunteers | Light users | Pre vs. post cannabis exposure | 25 µg/kg THC IV | No EEG change noted |

[a]Modified from Stuve and Straumanis (1990).
[b]All studies were nonblinded unless otherwise noted.

**Table 6. Quantitative EEG Studies of Exposure to Cannabis Performed before 1980[a]**

| Study | Sample Size | Cannabis given | Design | Results |
|---|---|---|---|---|
| Rodin et al, 1970 | 10 | 2- 3 300 mg marijuana cigarettes | Pre vs. post THC EEG, nonblind | Increased alpha power, decreased alpha frequency |
| Hollister et al, 1970 | 8 | Oral THC, 400- 500 μg/kg | Pre vs. post THC EEG, single blind | Increased synchronization of alpha, posterior leads |
| Volvaka et al, 1971 | 10 | 7.5 and 22.5 mg marijuana cigarette | Pre vs. post THC EEG, multiple dose level placebo controlled double blind | Dose dependent increase in percentage alpha, decrease percentage beta |
| Volvaka et al, 1973 | 14 | 3 different preparations of marijuana | Pre vs. post THC EEG, placebo controlled double blind | Increase percentage alpha, decrease percentage beta, decrease alpha frequency |
| Roth et al, 1973 | 12 | 10 mg marijuana cigarette | Pre vs. post THC EEG, placebo controlled double blind | Increase in alpha power |
| Low et al, 1970 | 75 | 4.8 and 9.1 mg marijuana cigarette | Pre vs. post THC EEG, multiple dose level placebo controlled double blind | Trend for increase in alpha power, decrease in alpha frequency |
| Hanley et al, 1976 | 18 | 2.2 mg THC marijuana cigarettes | Pre vs. post THC EEG, nonblind | Decrease in alpha frequency |
| Fernadez-Guardiola et al, 1976 | 10 | 250 mg/kg oral THC | Pre vs. post THC EEG, nonblind | Decrease in alpha abundance, increase in theta |
| Volvaka et al, 1977 | 20 | 4 different preparations of marijuana | Pre vs. post THC EEG, multiple dose level placebo controlled double blind | Transient increase in alpha abundance and decrease alpha frequency, decrease beta and theta abundance, |
| Bachman et al, 1979 | 4 | THC 30.0- 44.8 μg/kg IV | Pre vs. post THC EEG, nonblind | Reduction of theta power. No effect on alpha. |

[a]Modified from Stuve and Straumanis (1990).

For reasons that are unclear there was virtually no research in this area from 1977 until the late 1980s. Then a series of studies were completed by Struve and colleagues and by Lukas and associates that further explored the effects of cannabis, many of which presented quantitative topographic maps of EEG activity related to cannabis. Quantitative topographic mapping may be considered an extention of quantitative EEG in which data for a selected EEG variable is visually displayed, essentially producing a map of the activity of that variable in the cerebral cortex. In one of the first studies (Struve et al, 1989) which compared ten chronic heavy cannabis users (at least once per day for more than a year) to nonusing controls, results revealed that chronic users displayed significant increases in absolute power of alpha, relative power of alpha, and interhemispheric coherence of alpha over the bilateral frontal cortex. The researchers referred to these findings as "hyperfrontality of alpha"). Samples of visual EEG from a control and chronic cannabis users are shown in figure 1. Increased voltage is easily observable in the frontal areas in the users compared to the nonuser control. Even more impressive is topographic mapping of alpha absolute power shown in figure 2. The color maps easily highlight the difference between user and controls. A second study (Struve et al, 1994) involving 17 psychiatric inpatient chronic cannabis users compared to nonusing controls comfirmed these findings. A quantitative EEG discriminant function analysis permitted a 95% correct user versus nonuser classification. An investigation (Struve et al, 1998) of very long duration users (daily use for 15- 24 years) compared to users for shorter periods of time reported that the longer users were found to have significantly elevated absolute power of theta activity over bilateral frontal central cortex, as well as significantly increased interhemispheric coherence of theta activity across central and posterior regions compared to the shorter term users.

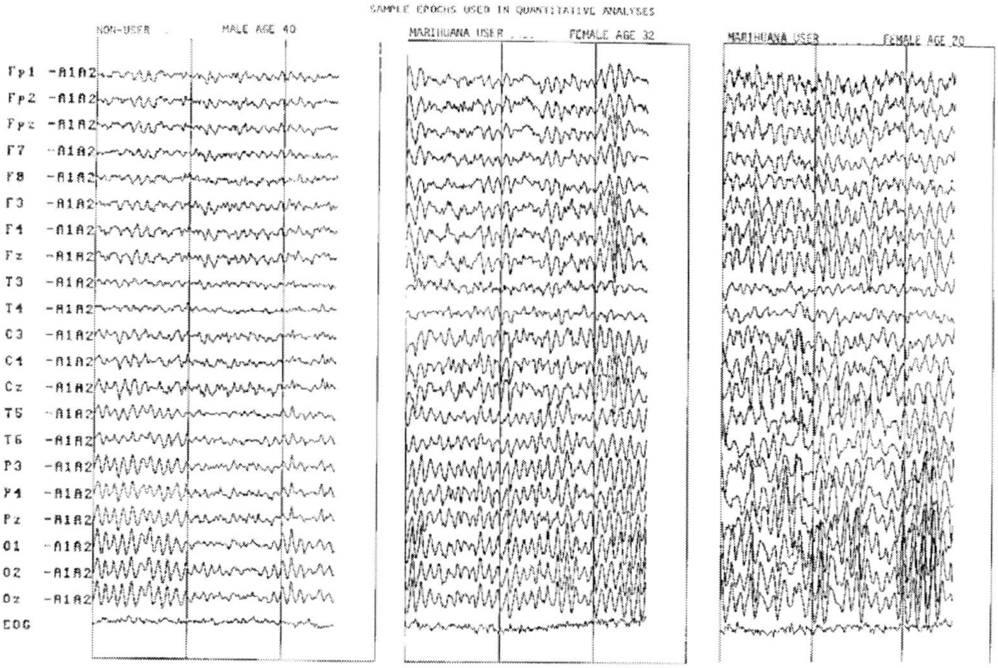


Figure 1. Representative Visual EEG Tracings from Chronic Cannabis Users and a Normal Control Subject (From Stuve et al, Clin Electroencephalogr 1989; 20:6-23. Used with permission).

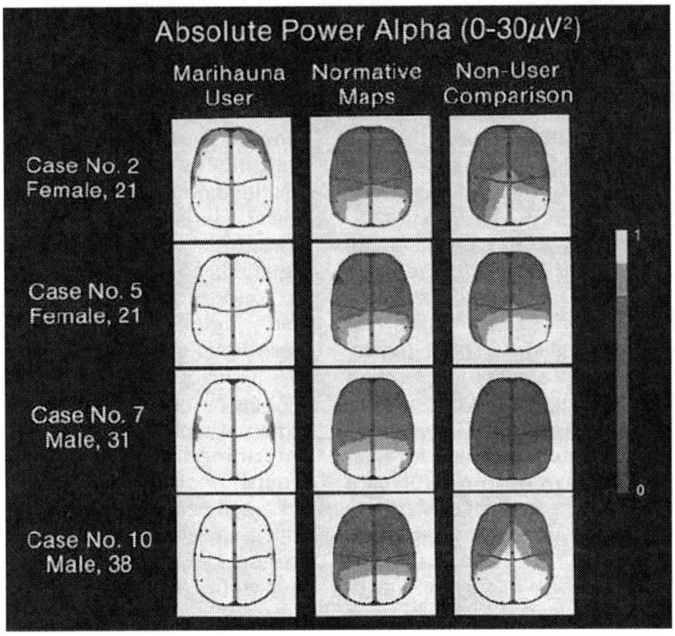


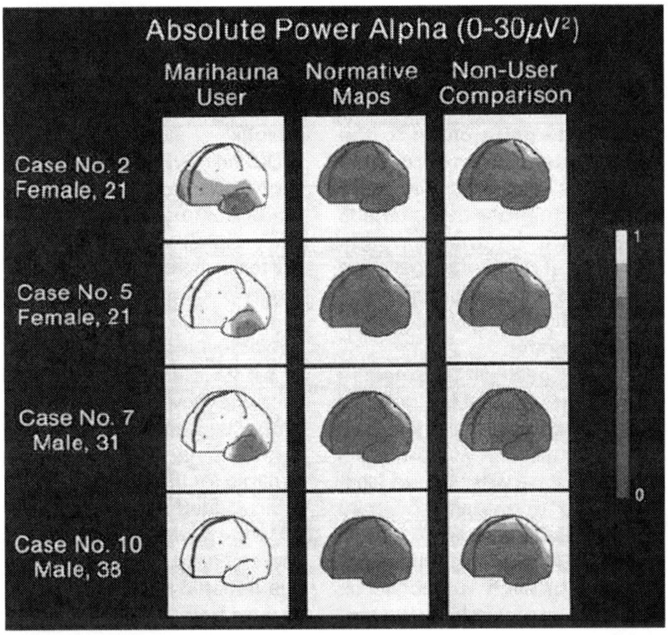


Figure 2. Examples of Topographic Quantitative EEG Mapping of Alpha Absolute Power in Chronic Cannabis Users and Normal Subjects (From Stuve et al, Clin Electroencephalogr 1989; 20:6-23. Used with permission).

Because the previous studies had used psychiatric patients as subjects, an extensive investigation (Struve et al, 1999) of chronic cannabis who had undergone a rigorous examination to insure that they were medically and psychiatrically healthy was preformed.

The results of previous studies were replicated. Summing up the conclusions of this and previous studies the researchers cited a comprehensive summary of quantitative EEG findings which occur with chronic cannabis abuse and suggested that significant statistical associations may exist between long term exposure to cannabis and: 1.) increased absolute power, relative power, and coherence of alpha over bilateral frontal cortex, i.e., hyperfrontality of alpha; 2.) generalized increase of absolute power of non alpha frequencies over widespread cortical regions; 3.) decreased relative power of delta and beta over frontal cortex; 4.) increased interhemispheric coherence of theta and delta activity over the frontal cortex; and 5.) slowing of alpha activity.

The researchers felt that there still remained the need to establish the causal influence of cannabis in the production of this characteristic EEG profile in subjects who did not display it at the beginning. The characteristic profile of elevation of absolute and relative power and coherence of alpha over bilateral frontal cortex as well as decrease in alpha frequency was clearly demonstrated using laboratory paced smoking of cannabis with high and low dose content and placebo in a counterbalanced design with double blind conditions (Struve et al, 2003). The publication of these findings was accompanied by a method or tool (the Alpha Hyperfrontality Score) to avoid the necessity of analyzing data separately for a multitude of scalp electrodes during assessment of the EEG effect of cannabis. A composite Alpha Hyperfrontality Score is generated by entering the Z-Scores (departures of measured EEG values from established normative data base means in standard deviation units) for alpha absolute power, alpha relative power, and alpha interhemispheric coherence at various electrode sites into the following expressions:

Absolute Power Component (AHA) "Alpha Hyperfrontality- Absolute"

$$AHA = \frac{\frac{[Fp1+Fp2+Fpz]}{3} + \frac{[F3+F4+Fz]}{3} + \frac{[F7+F8]}{2}}{3}$$

Relative Power Component (AHR) "Alpha Hyperfrontality- Relative

$$AHR = \frac{\frac{[Fp1+Fp2+Fpz]}{3} + \frac{F3+F4+Fz]}{3} + \frac{[F7+F8]}{2}}{3}$$

Coherence Component (AHC) "Alpha Hyperfrontality- Coherence"

$$AHC = \frac{[Fp1/Fp2] + [F3/F4] + F7/F8]}{3}$$

Total Alpha Hyperfrontality Score (AHS)

$$AHS = \frac{AHA + AHR + AHC}{3}$$

In this study total AHS scores did not differ significantly from those scores among the nonusers (nonusers mean AHS = 0.49; casual users mean AHS = 0.65, p = ns). In contrast chronic daily users had total AHS scores that were significantly elevated compared to casual users in the study (daily users mean AHS = 1.42; casual users mean AHS score = 0.65, p = 0.009).

Although other topographic quantitative EEG studies of cannabis exposure are rare, Lukas and colleagues (Lukas et al, 1986; Lukas et al, 1989; Lukas et al, 1995) have conducted detailed studies of acute cannabis administration combined with quantitative EEG and behavioral measures, which have generated results compatible with the findings discussed above. Although not using the same quantitative EEG measure as the composite measure of alpha hyperfrontality discussed above, Lukas et al have demonstrated that EEG alpha activity significantly increases and spreads to anterior cortical regions following cannabis inhalation. In an attempt to demonstrate a relationship between SPECT neuroimaging of chronic cannabis use and quantitative EEG findings, Reeves and Struve (2007) recorded quantitative EEGs and employed injected $^{99m}$Tc-HMPAO to obtain SPECT scans of six long term daily cannabis users. Although EEG results were compatible with the alpha hyperfrontality pattern discussed above, SPECT scans revealed areas of decreased cerebral perfusion but in different areas among the subjects.

## Evoked Potentials and Cannabis Exposure

Evoked potentials (EP) studies of the effects of cannabis on the human brain have overall yielded inconsistent results, particularly earlier studies which may have lacked methodological sophistication. In a review of studies done up to that time, Struve & Straumanis (1990) concluded that although EP, P300, and contingent negative variation (CNV) results with cannabis use had been variable, certain trends, although weak, had emerged: 1.) all of the EP studies showed either no drug effect or prolongation of latency, with none showing reduction of latency; 2.) P300 amplitude tends to be decreased and latency increased; and 3.) CNV is augmented with low dose but not with high dose cannabis. Some additional studies since then have suggested that EPs might have some promise for assessing the effects of cannabis use, but the evidence is not yet convincing. Patrick and colleagues (Patrick et al, 1997; Patrick et al, 1999; Patrick et al, 2000) performed a series of investigations on EP changes related to cannabis with the following findings: 1.) Latency and amplitude of auditory, visual, and somatosensory EPs were not effected by cannabis with the exception of an elevated P50 amplitude in daily cannabis users; 2.) reduced P50 suppression in the sensory gating paradigm was observed; 3.) The degree of sensory gating impairment among cannabis users was correlated with frequency of cannabis use per week.

Two other relatively recent studies suggest possible usefulness of EPs. An investigation of EPs elicited during a complex auditory selective attention task revealed that the latency of the greatest negative peak of EPs (200 and 300 ms) to target times was shorter in controls than in cannabis users suggesting that chronic cannabis use relates to different types of information processing under conditions of selective attention (Kempel et al, 2003). Skosnick et al (2006) conducted the first investigation demonstrating altered visual steady state visual evoked potentials (SSVEP), showing that age of onset of cannabis use positively correlated with 18 Hz spectral power values and that the transient N160 component was reduced in cannabis users. Currently, however, EPs could probably not be considered a useful tool for assessing cannabis effects, but this may change with additional investigations.

# Conclusions

There can be little doubt that cannabis use has a significant impact on the human nervous system. However the details of the precise effects are still poorly understood. Studies to date suggest that cannabis exerts prominent effects at least in the frontal, perilimbic, and anterior cingulate areas and the cerebellum. The impact of cannabis on other brain areas remain unclear. Further research is needed in this area.

# References


Amen DG, Waugh M. High resolution brain SPECT imaging of marijuana smokers with AD/HD. *J. Psychoactive Drugs.* 1998; 30:209-214.

Aasly J, Storsaeter O, Nilsen G, et al. Minor structural brain changes in young adult drug abusers. A magnetic resonance study. *Acta Neurol. Scand.* 1993; 87:210-214.

Block RI, O'Leary DS, Ehrhardt JC, et al. Effects of frequent marijuana use on brain tissue volume and composition. *Neuroreport.* 2000; 11:491-496.

Block RI, O'Leary DS, Hichwa RD, et al. Cerebellar hypoactivity in frequent marijuana users. *Neuroreport.* 2000; 11:749-753.

Block RI, O'Leary DS, Hichwa RD, et al. Effects of frequent marijuana use on memory-related regional cerebral blood flow. *Pharmacol. Biochem. Behav.* 2002; 72:237-250.

Campbell AM, Evans M, Thomson JL, Williams MJ. Cerebral atrophy in young cannabis smokers. *Lancet.* 1971 Dec 4; 2(7736):1219-1224.

Co BT, Goodwin DW, Gado M, et al. Absence of cerebral atrophy in chronic cannabis users. *JAMA.* 1977; 237:1229-1230.

Eldreth DA, Matochik JA, Cadet JL, Bolla KI. Abnormal brain activity in prefrontal brain regions in abstinent marijuana users. *Neuroimage.* 2004; 23:914-920.

Gatley SJ, Volkow ND. Addiction and imaging of the living brain. *Drug Alcohol. Depend.* 1998; 51:97-108.

Hall W, Solowij N, Lemon J. The health and psychological consequences of cannabis use. *National Drug Strategy Monograph Series* No 25, Australian Government Publication Service, Canberra, 1994.

Hannerz J, Hindmarsh T. Neurological and neuroradiological examination of chronic cannabis smokers. *Ann. Neurol.* 1983; 13:207-210.

Jasper HH. The ten-twenty electrode system of the International Federation. *Electroencephal. Clin. Neurophysiol.* 1958; 10:371-375.

Kanayama G, Rogowska J, Pope HG, et al. Spatial working memory in heavy cannabis users: a functional magnetic resonance imaging study. *Psychopharmacology.* (Berl) 2004; 176:239-247.

Kempel P, Lampe K, Parneford R, et al. Auditory-evoked potentials and selective attention: Different ways of information processing in cannabis users and controls. *Neuropsychobiol.* 2003; 48:95-101.

Kuehnle J, Mendelson JH, Davis KR, New PF. Computerized tomographic examination of heavy marijuana smokers. *JAMA.* 1977; 237:1231-1232.

Lukas SE, Mendelson JH, Amass L, Smith R. Plasma-9-tetrahydrocannabinol (THC) levels during marijuana-induced EEG and behavioral effects in human subjects. *The Pharmacologist.* 1986; 28:534.

Lukas SE, Mendelson JH, Henry J, et al. Ethanol effects on marijuana-induced intoxication and electroencephalographic activity. In: Harris LS (ed). *Problems of Drug Dependence* 1988. Washington DC: US Government Printing Office (NIDA Research Monograph No 90); 1989:62.

Lukas SE, Mendelson JH, Benedikt R. Electroencephalographic correlates of marijuana-induced euphoria. *Drug Alc. Depend.* 1995; 37:11-140.

Lundqvist T, Jonsson S, Warkentin S. Frontal lobe dysfunction in long-term cannabis users. *Neurotoxicol. Teratol.* 2001; 23:437-443.

Mathew RJ, Tant SR. Regional cerebral blood flow in marijuana smokers. *Br. J. Addict.* 1986; 81:567-571.

Mathew RJ, Wilson WH, Tant SR. Acute changes in cerebral blood flow associated with marijuana smoking. *Acta Psychiatri. Scand.* 1989; 79:118-128.

Mathew RJ, Wilson WH, Humphries DF, et al. Regional cerebral blood flow after marijuana smoking. *J. Cereb. Blood Flow Metab.* 1992; 12:750-758.

Mathew RJ, Wilson WH. Acute changes in cerebral blood flow after smoking marijuana. *Life Sci.* 1993; 52:757-767.

Mathew RJ, Wilson WH, Coleman RE. Marijuana intoxication and brain activation in marijuana smokers. *Life Sci.* 1997; 60:2075-2089.

Mathew RJ, Wilson WH, Turkington TG, Coleman RE. Cerebellar activity and disturbed time sense after THC. *Brain Res.* 1998; 797:183-189.

Mathew RJ, Wilson WH, Turkington TG, et al. Regional cerebral blood flow and depersonalization after tetrahydrocannabinol administration. *Acta Psychiatr. Scand.* 1999; 100:67-75.

Mathew RJ, Wilson WH, Turkington TG, et al. Time course of tetrahydrocannabinol-induced changes in regional cerebral blood flow measured with positron emission tomography. 2002; 116:173-185.

Matochik JA, Eldreth DA, Cadet JL, Bolla KI. Altered brain tissue composition in heavy marijuana users. *Drug Alcohol. Depend.* 2005; 77:23-30.

O'Leary DS, Block RI, Flaum M, et al. Acute marijuana effects on rCBF and cognition: a PET study. *Neuroreport.* 2000; 11:3835-3841.

O'Leary DS, Block RI, Koeppel JA, et al. Effects of smoking marijuana on brain perfusion and cognition. *Neuropsychopharmacology.* 2002; 26:802-816.

O'Leary DS, Block RI, Turner BM, et al. Marijuana alters the human cerebellar clock. *Neuroreport.* 2003; 14:1145-1151.

Patrick G, Straumanis JJ, Struve FA, et al. Early and middle latency evoked potentials in medically and psychiatrically normal daily marijuana smokers: A paucity of significant findings. *Clin. Electroencephalogr.* 1997; 28:26-31.

Patrick G, Straumanis JJ, Struve FA, et al. Reduced P0 auditory gating response in psychiatrically normal chronic marijuana users. *Biol. Psychiatry.* 1999; 45:1307-1312.

Patrick G, Struve FA. Reduction of P50 gating response in marijuana users: Further supporting data. *Clin. Electroencephalogr.* 2000; 31:88-93.

Pillay SS, Rogowska J, Kanayama G, et al. Neurophysiology of motor function following cannabis discontinuation in chronic cannabis smokers: an fMRI study. *Drug Alcohol. Depend.* 2004; 76:261-271.

Quickfall J, Crockford D. Brain neuroimaging in cannabis: A review. *J. Neuropsychiatry Clin. Neurosci.* 2006; 18:318-332.

Reeves RR, Struve FA. Technitium-99m-HMPAO SPECT cerebral blood flow alterations and quantitative EEG sequelae of daily cannabis use. *Clinical EEG and Neuroscience,* In press.

Skosnik PD, Krishnan GP, Vohs JL, O'Donnell BF. The effect of cannabis use and gender on the visual steady state evoked potential. *Clin. Neurophysiol.* 2006; 117:144-156.

Struve FA, Strumanis JJ, Patrick G, Price L. Topographic mapping of quantitative EEG variables in chronic heavy marijuana users: Empirical findings with psychiatric patients. *Clin. Electroencephalogr.* 1989; 20:6-23.

Struve FA, Strumanis JJ. Electroencephalographic and evoked potential methods in human marijuana research: Historical review and future trends. *Drug. Dev. Res.* 1990; 20:369-388.

Struve FA, Strumanis JJ, Patrick G. Persistent topographic quantitative EEG sequelae of chronic marijuana use: A replication study and initial discriminant function analysis. *Clin. Electroencephalogr.* 1994; 25:63-75.

Struve FA, Patrick G, Strumanis JJ, Fitz-Gerald MJ, Manno J. Possible EEG sequelae of very long duration marijuana use: Pilot findings from topographic quantitative EEG analysis of subjects with 15 to 24 years of cumulative daily exposure to THC. *Clin. Electroencephalogr.* 1998; 29:31-36.

Struve FA, Strumanis JJ, Patrick G, Leavitt J, Manno JE, Manno BR. Topographic quantitative EEG analysis of chronic marijuana use: A replication using medically and psychiatrically screened normal subjects. *Drug Alc. Depend.* 1999; 56:167-169.

Struve FA, Manno BR, Kemp P, Patrick G, Manno JR. Acute marijuana (THC) exposure Produces a "transient" topographic quantitative EEG profile identical to the "persistent" Profile seen in chronic heavy users. *Clin. Electroencephalogr.* 2003; 34:75-83.

Substance Abuse and Mental Health Services Administration. *Results from the 2003 National Survey on Drug Use and Health: National findings.* Rockville, MD, Office of Applied Studies, NSDUH Series H-25, DHHS Publication No. SMA-043964, 2004.

Tunving K, Thulin SO, Risberg J, Warkentin S. Regional cerebral blood flow in long-term heavy marijuana use. *Psychiatry Res.* 1986; 17:15-21.

Tzilos GK, Cintron CB, Wood JB, et al. Lack of hippocampal volume change in long-term heavy cannabis users. *Am. J. Addict.* 2005; 14:64-71.

Volkow ND, Gillespie H, Mullani N, et al. Cerebellar metabolic activation by delta-9-tetrahydro-cannabinol in human brain: a study with positron emission tomography and 18F-2-fluoro-2-deoxyglucose. *Psychiatry Res.* 1991; 40:69-78.

Volkow ND, Gillespie H, Mullani N, et al. Brain glucose metabolism in chronic marijuana users at baseline and during marijuana intoxication. *Psychiatry Res.* 1996; 67:29-38.

Wiesbeck GA, Taeschner KL. A cerebral computed tomography study of patients with drug-induced psychosis. *Eur. Arch. Psychiatry.* 1991; 241:88-90.

Wilson W, Mathew R, Turkington T, et al. Brain morphological changes and early marijuana use: a magnetic resonance and positron emission tomography study. *J. Addict. Dis.* 2000; 19:1-22.

In: Research Topics on Brain Mapping
Editor: Yuanzhu Liáng, pp. 57-85
ISBN: 978-1-60456-001-5


*Chapter III*

# Steady-State Free Precession (SSFP) Techniques for Functional MRI

***Jongho Lee*[*1], *Taek S. Kim*[1], *Jin Hyung Lee*[1] *and Karla L. Miller*[2]***
[1] Magnetic Resonance Systems Research Laboratory, Department of Electrical Engineering, Stanford University, Stanford, California
[2] Oxford Centre for Functional MRI of the Brain (FMRIB); Department of Clinical Neurology; Oxford University, Oxford, United Kingdom

## Abstract

Balanced steady-state free precession (balanced SSFP or bSSFP) has gained widespread attention due to its high efficiency and unique contrast. Recently, this technique has been adapted for functional MRI in order to provide improved SNR and reduced distortion. Two different contrast mechanisms have been investigated: transition-band SSFP fMRI, which detects the bulk frequency shift from BOLD using the frequency selectivity of the SSFP profile, and pass-band SSFP fMRI, which primarily measures $T_2$ changes from the diffusion effect. Both methods utilize efficient 3D *k*-space trajectories, which have been developed in recent years to enable the acquisition of full 3D volumes in 2-6 seconds with minimal off-resonance artifacts (such as blurring or warping). The strong contrast and intrinsically high SNR of transition-band SSFP fMRI enables high-resolution isotropic ($1mm^3$) fMRI experiments even at low field strengths (1.5 T), and the low SAR requirements of this method also make high field imaging possible. The pass-band SSFP method has great potential for imaging in regions near susceptibility boundaries, such as the pre-frontal cortex above the sinuses. These methods are known to suffer from sensitivity to spatial and temporal off-resonance frequencies, prompting the development of new techniques, including a real-time $B_0$ shift

* *Address correspondence to:* Jongho Lee; Room 208, Packard Electrical Engineering Bldg. Stanford University; Stanford, CA 94305-9510; TEL: (650) 725-5638; FAX: (650) 723-8473; E-MAIL: jonghoyi@mrsrl.stanford.edu

compensation technique and an interleaved center frequency updating. Both SSFP fMRI methods could enable a wider range of neuroscience applications by enabling high resolution and reducing image artifacts.

# Introduction

Since its first inception in the early 1990s, functional magnetic resonance imaging (fMRI) has become a primary research tool for studying human brain activity. The most popular contrast mechanism is referred to as blood oxygenation level dependency (BOLD) [1,2]. To optimize the detection of this contrast, a single shot EPI or spiral trajectory sequence with a long echo time, which is typically matched to the $T_2^*$ value of gray matter, is widely used [3,4]. Despite its popularity, the resulting images from these sequences often suffer from severe imaging artifacts such as image distortion and signal dropout in the areas with high field inhomogeneity [5]. These artifacts make it difficult to acquire functional contrast in the frontal and temporal lobes of a brain and also complicate the registration of functional images to anatomical reference images. Several methods have been suggested to mitigate these artifacts: tailored RF pulse [6], z-shimming [7], spiral in-out readouts [8], and supplementary devices [9,10]. They provide different levels of compensation with different levels of complexity, but none of these are completely satisfactory.

In addition to the image artifacts, the signal to noise ratio for the acquired functional images is low due to the high temporal sampling rate. Moreover, the signal change from BOLD contrast is only a few percent, which is comparable to that of the temporal noise fluctuation. As a result, detecting the task-correlated signal changes is a challenging task that requires a complicated statistical data analysis to extract the hidden brain activation from the noisy data. One approach to increase signal to noise ratio (SNR) and more importantly contrast to noise ratio (CNR) is using a high field system ($\geq$ 3 T). It has been shown that both SNR and CNR increase as the field strength increases [11,12]. In particular, the contrast from the parenchyma and small veins increases super-linearly with $B_0$ field strength [13], providing better spatial specificity at high field systems [14,15]. As a result, most of the functional MRI experiments currently are performed on widely available 3 T systems. A number of institutes have installed higher field systems ($\geq$ 7 T) for human brain studies [12,16]. However, 3 T systems are still SNR limited for high-resolution (~ 1 mm$^3$) studies, whereas 7 T systems have several technical difficulties such as $B_1$ inhomogeneity and increased specific absorption rate (SAR). These issues have not yet been solved, and have limited the use of 7 T scanners for routine neuroscience research [17,18].

Recently, new fMRI methods that are based on balanced steady-state free precession (bSSFP) were proposed to allow high SNR and low distortion fMRI to be possible [19-22]. These methods benefit from the intrinsic SNR efficiency of the balanced SSFP sequence and provide much improved image quality. These methods possess the potential for solving the primary limitations of conventional fMRI methods. In this chapter, two different SSFP fMRI approaches, transition-band SSFP fMRI and pass-band SSFP fMRI, are discussed as alternatives to conventional fMRI methods.

# Balanced Steady-State Free Precession

Balanced steady-state free precession (bSSFP) has a long history, along with many acronyms (refocused SSFP, FIESTA, trueFISP and balanced FFE) used in literature. It was first introduced in 1958 by Carr [23] and was rediscovered by Freeman and Hill [24], and Oppelt *et al.* [25]. The term "balanced" comes from the fact that all gradients are refocused in every TR (net zero gradient area in each axis in every TR, see figures 1a and c). In other words, the *k*-space trajectory, which starts from the origin of *k*-space, returns to the origin at the end of each TR (figures 1b and d). As a consequence, the gradients do not influence the phase of the spins, and the off-resonance frequency of the spins becomes the sole contributor to the phase accrual of the spins.

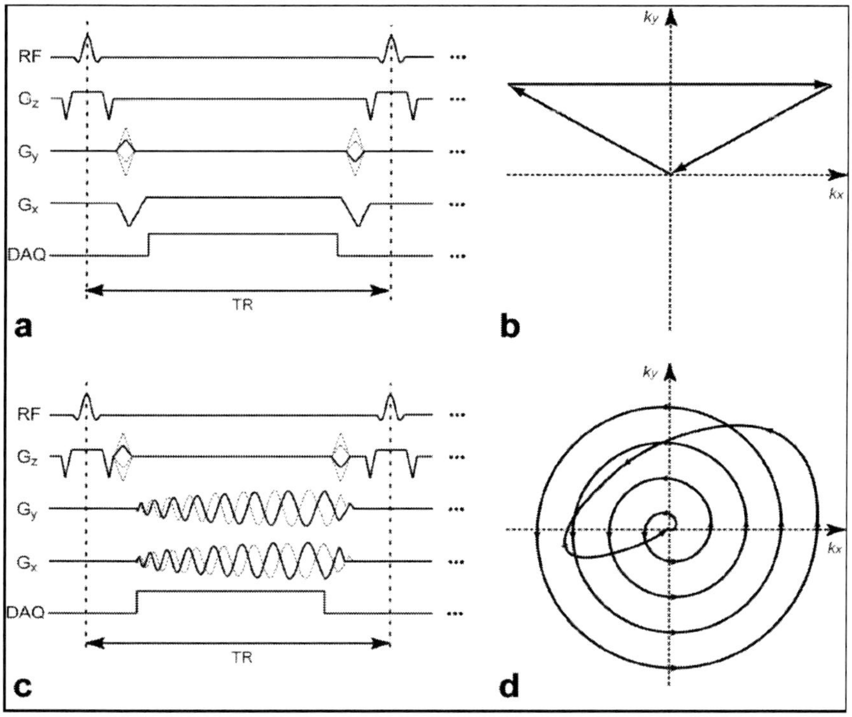


Figure 1. Balanced SSFP sequence: (a) a pulse sequence diagram for a 2D Cartesian trajectory and (b) its *k*-space. (c) a pulse sequence diagram for a 3D stack-of-spiral trajectory and (d) its *k*-space. A typical TR for bSSFP is less than 10 ms. In each RF excitation, the integration of the total gradient area at the end of a TR becomes zero in each axis. This means that the *k*-space is covered starting from the origin of the *k*-space and returns back to the origin. A short TR and fully balanced gradients make the magnetization from the previous RF excitations persists to the following readouts. This results in an increased SNR efficiency in bSSFP.

Due to these balanced gradients, the magnetization of the spins is strongly dependent upon the off-resonance frequency of the spins. This effect is illustrated in figure 2. The magnetization profile, which plots the magnitude and phase of the transverse magnetization as a function of off-resonance frequency, possesses very unique characteristics: a significant signal dip is observed near the on-resonance frequency (0 Hz), and also every *n*/TR, where *n* is an integer (figure 2a). This signal dip creates so-called dark bands or banding artifacts in the resulting images (figure 3) [26]. There is also a sharp 180° phase shift at this signal dip frequency band (figure 2b). This signal profile can be thought of as a frequency-domain filter, with some off-resonance frequencies exhibiting high signal and other frequencies being heavily attenuated. For this reason, it is useful to adopt the language of filter design: we will refer to a flat and high part of the profile as the "pass band", a flat and low part of the profile as a "stop band" and a part of the profile that has a strong dependence on resonance frequency as a "transition band". The shapes of the magnetization profile can be modified by changing scan parameters such as the flip angle (figures 2c and d) and the transmit RF and receiver phases (figures 2e and f). At high flip angle, there are pass bands centered at multiples of $\pm(2TR)^{-1}$ Hz (figure 2a), whereas these frequencies correspond to stop bands at low flip angle (figure 2c). Both high and low flip angles exhibit transition bands at 0 Hz and multiples of $\pm(TR)^{-1}$ Hz, with both the magnitude and phase of the signal exhibiting a strong dependence on resonance frequency (figures 2a-d).

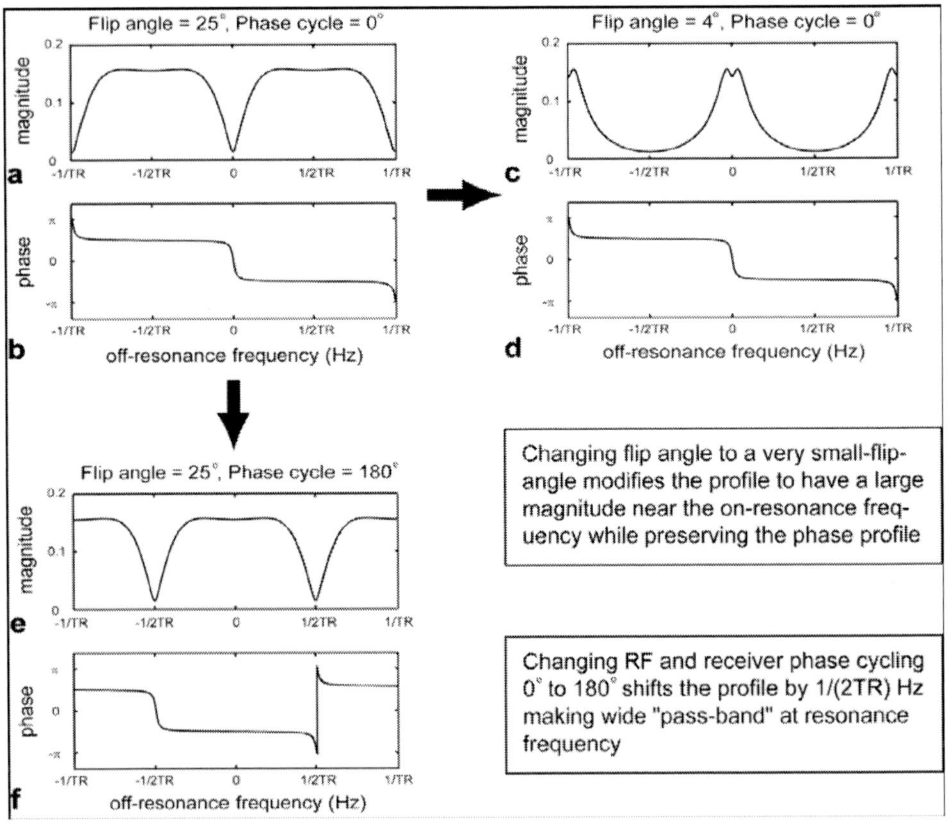


Figure 2. Balanced SSFP magnetization profiles: The balanced SSFP (a) magnitude and (b) phase profiles for a large flip angle (25°) with no phase cycling. The magnitude signal dip and 180° phase transition exist near the on-resonance frequency and every *n*/TR (*n* is an integer). These profiles are modified by changing the flip angle (c and d) and transmit RF and receiver phase cycles (e and f). The common simulation parameters are TR = 10 ms, TE = 5 ms, $T_1$ = 870 ms, and $T_2$ = 100 ms.

Because of this unique magnetization profile, particularly the banding artifacts, the bSSFP technique had been slow to be adopted as a major imaging sequence. The hardware, especially the gradient systems, had to become fast enough to support a short repetition time. A short repetition time increases the absolute frequency difference between transition bands, such that for a given range of frequencies across the brain, the relatively uniform pass band (figure 2e) is wide enough to cover the imaging volume without signal drop-out areas.

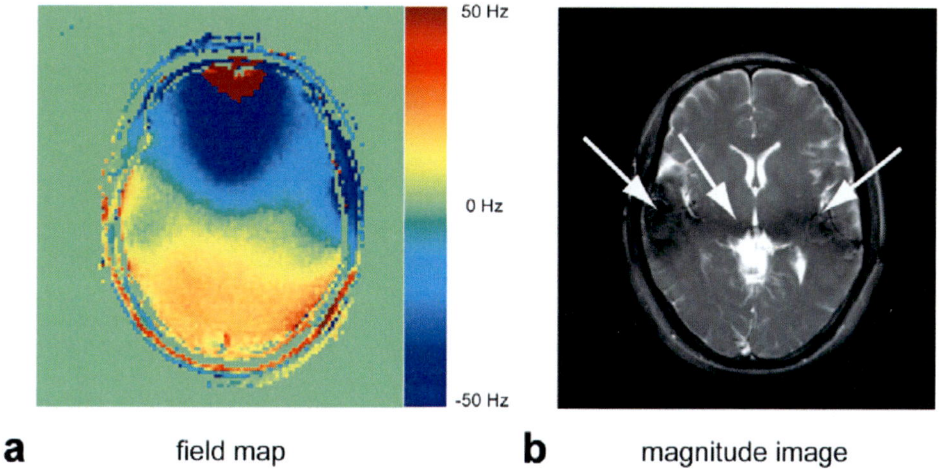


Figure 3. Banding artifacts in bSSFP: The areas near the on-resonance frequency, which are identified in field map (a), experience significant signal reductions in the magnitude image shown in (b). This artifact is called as a banding artifact (arrows).

One of the most exciting features that has attracted attention to this sequence is the high SNR efficiency (SNR normalized by the square root of the acquisition time). Balanced SSFP typically utilizes a very short TR (usually less than 10 ms) with fully balanced gradients; this allows magnetization to persist for several subsequent TRs and generates multiple echo pathways. As a result, the magnetization created by one RF excitation is "reused" in the following readouts. The persistence of the previous magnetization yields a much higher SNR efficiency compared to other sequences in which the transverse magnetization is usually spoiled (suppressed) at the end of each TR [27]. Figure 4 shows this advantage: for a short TR, the signal becomes much larger in bSSFP (in the pass band) than gradient-spoiled gradient recalled echo (GRE). The experimental SNR comparison among different sequences can be found in [27].

Another advantage of the bSSFP technique comes from its unique contrast, which is proportional to $T_2/T_1$. In certain applications, this contrast provides an improved image quality. For example, in the cardiac application, this $T_2/T_1$ contrast provides good separation between blood and myocardium because the blood has a much higher $T_2/T_1$ value compared to the surrounding tissue (see figure 6 in [28]).

With these advantages, the bSSFP technique has been widely applied in various applications such as angiography, cardiac imaging, and musculoskeletal imaging. Readers are recommended to read the review articles [26,29-31] for more detailed descriptions and applications of the technique.

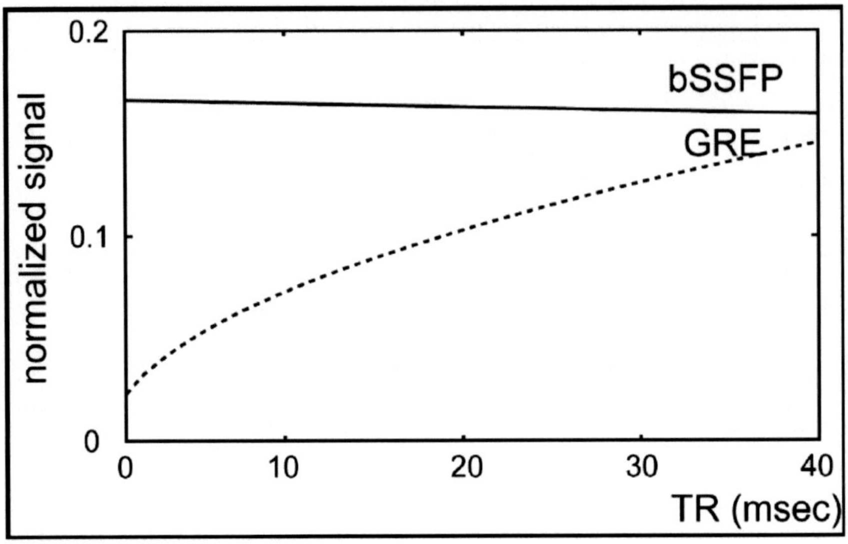


Figure 4. SNR efficiency of bSSFP vs. GRE: Due to the multi-pathway echo signals, the bSSFP signal is high even for a short TR. This results in an increased SNR efficiency ($SNR/\sqrt{t}$) for a short TR.

Recently, there have been several proposals to use this bSSFP sequence to address the fundamental limitations on fMRI image quality and SNR. The idea was first introduced by Cho *et al* [19], and later by Scheffler *et al* [20] and Miller *et al* [21]. These methods acquire data near the transition band so that the frequency shifts that accompany brain activity induce signal changes. This method is referred to as transition-band SSFP fMRI since the contrast is obtained in the transition band. Recently, another SSFP fMRI method that obtains more conventional ($T_2$-based) BOLD contrast in the pass band was introduced by Bowen *et al.* to provide wider spatial coverage [22]. This new method is different from transition-band SSFP fMRI in its contrast mechanism and is referred to as pass-band SSFP fMRI. The contrast mechanism and signal characteristics of these two SSFP fMRI methods are explained in more detail below.

## Contrast Mechanism and Signal Characteristics of SSFP fMRI

### Transition-Band SSFP fMRI

The functional contrast in transition-band SSFP fMRI comes from the frequency sensitivity of the bSSFP profile [20,21]. When oxygenation concentration changes in a blood vessel, it creates a bulk frequency shift both inside and outside of the blood vessel [32,33]. For tissue that lies in the transition band, this bulk frequency shift induces changes in the magnetization magnitude and phase because the bSSFP magnetization profile is a strong function of the off-resonance frequency of the voxel (figure 5a). The signal change in a voxel is determined by the intra- and extra-vascular frequency shifts, the fractional volume of the vessels, and the off-resonance frequency distribution. It is also strongly dependent on the details of the bSSFP magnetization profile, with large signal changes in the part of the profile with greatest sensitivity to off-resonance frequency - that is, in the transition band.

The first proposed methods were based on the presence of the large magnitude modulations in the transition band at high flip angle, and aimed to cause the signal to move in and out of the magnitude dip at 0 Hz (figure 2a) [19,20]. Later work [21] proposed another approach that avoids having to acquire data with low-signal by changing to a very small flip angle (~ 5°, figure 2c) such that the transition band has high signal and the abrupt phase change contributes to functional contrast. This profile provides higher SNR near the on-resonance frequency compared to the large-flip-angle case since the transverse magnetization is much larger near the on-resonance frequency. On the other hand, the phase profile is the same as in the large flip angle case: a 180° phase transition over a very narrow off-resonance frequency band (~ 10 Hz) exists in the high SNR frequency band. As a result, the bulk frequency shift from BOLD induces a large phase shift that comes from the sharp phase transition (figure 5a). The fraction of tissue within a voxel that exhibits a task-correlated frequency shift therefore acquires a significant phase offset relative to un-shifted tissue, creating both phase cancellation (i.e., magnitude changes) and bulk phase shifts (i.e., phase changes). Because the phase change is caused by the bSSFP profile rather than slow accumulation of phase during the echo time, the signal change can be significant for small frequency shifts even at short TE and TR. The bulk frequency shift can also modulate the magnitude signal due to variations in the magnitude profile. The phase and magnitude signal correlations that are observed therefore depend on the vessel network and the off-resonance distribution within a voxel [34].

In short, in transition-band SSFP fMRI, the bulk frequency shift induced from the BOLD effect is the major contrast mechanism for detecting the functional signal. This means that many of the well-known properties of GRE-based fMRI need to be re-considered in the context of SSFP. For example, it suggests that functional contrast is not strongly dependent upon the echo time [34], unlike GRE-based methods where the percent signal change increases approximately linearly with TE. The signal dependence of bSSFP on field strength also has somewhat unusual properties [35] compared to those found in GRE BOLD [36], as shown in figure 6. The SNR of bSSFP is higher than GRE at 1.5-3 T as expected, but the two sequences have similar SNR at 7 T. At high field, the increasing dominance of $T_2^*$ effects may cause significant loss for echo pathways from previous TRs, reducing the so-called "SSFP condition". The CNR of transition-band SSFP also has an unusual dependence on field strength, as shown in figure 6c. While the CNR of GRE increases approximately linearly with field strength, bSSFP has approximately constant CNR at 1.5-3 T and reduced CNR at 7 T. This somewhat surprising behavior is believed to reflect the combination of reduced percent signal change due loss of signal from $T_2^*$ decay and increased noise due to physiological fluctuations [35]. These data suggest that, unlike most other fMRI methods, transition-band SSFP may be well-suited to imaging at low field.

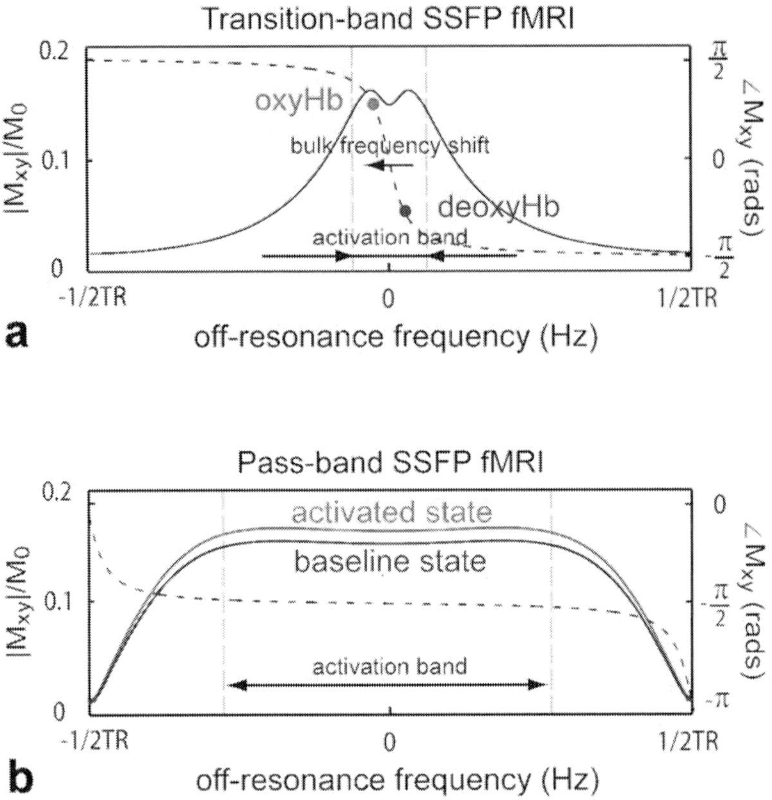


Figure 5. Magnetization profiles of the two SSFP fMRI methods: (a) In transition-band SSFP fMRI, a small flip angle (4°) provides high signal near the on-resonance frequency where the phase transition exists. When the bulk frequency shift is induced by BOLD, the large phase transition provides functional contrast. (b) In the pass-band case, the functional contrast is acquired from the $T_2$ change of BOLD effect. In the activated state, $T_2$ is increased due to the reduced deoxy-hemoglobin concentration. This results in an increased signal intensity providing positive contrast in fMRI. Since the activation band is wider in the pass band, the pass-band method will provide wider spatial coverage than transition-band SSFP fMRI.

The inherent SNR efficiency of balanced SSFP and short TR with short readout duration make this technique suitable for high-resolution fMRI studies [34,37,38]. Figure 7 shows an example. Even at 1.5 T, a high-resolution (1 x 1 x 1 $mm^3$) fMRI result was successfully obtained with a wide coverage (FOV = 16 x 16 $mm^2$, number of slices = 18, every 3 sec). This high-resolution is difficult to achieve using conventional methods due to SNR limitation. The activation is primarily localized in the gray matter regions following the sulci of the anatomical images. This good match between the activation map and the underlying anatomy indicates the high quality of the functional data in SSFP fMRI.

Unfortunately the functional contrast is a strong function of the off-resonance frequency of the voxel; the contrast is primarily concentrated in a narrow off-resonance frequency band, which is referred to as an "activation band" (4 ~ 6 Hz wide near the on-resonance frequency). As a result, the method suffers from spatial and temporal off-resonance variations. Compensation techniques that mitigate these off-resonance effects have been proposed [39,40] and will be discussed later.

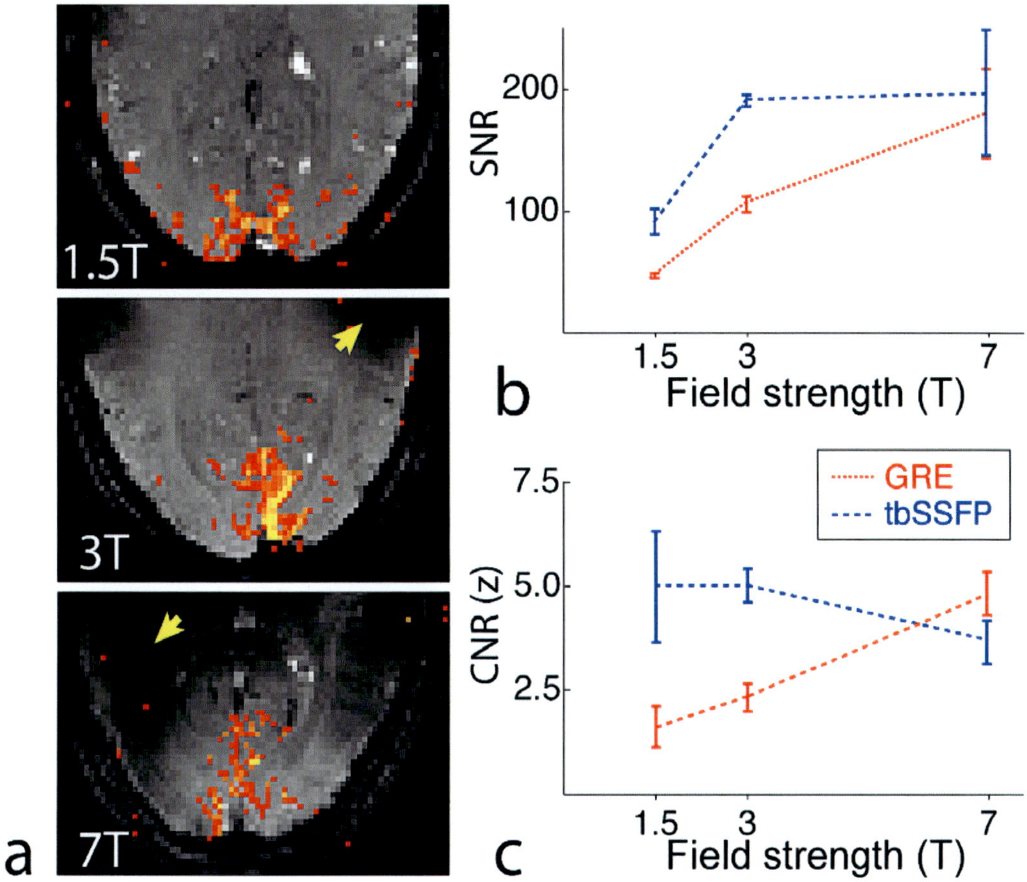


Figure 6. Effects of field strength on transition-band SSFP fMRI, using matched GRE acquisitions as a reference. All data were acquired using 3D stack-of-EPI acquisitions (2 x 2 x 2 $mm^3$ resolution, $\alpha = 4^{\circ}$, TR = 12 ms, 2.4-2.9 s/volume) with 2 minutes of visual stimulation, and acquisition was repeated at three off-resonance frequencies to cover all of visual cortex. (a) Example activation maps for representative subjects at three different field strengths, with the three different frequencies combined using a fixed-effects analysis. Similar patterns of activation are detectable, although the increased effects of banding are readily visible at higher field (arrows). (b) SNR increases with field strength for both GRE and SSFP, with higher SNR in SSFP at low field strengths. However, the SNR benefit is not significant at 7 T, which likely reflects the increasing effect of $T_2^*$ at high field, causing SSFP and GRE to have similar signal levels. (c) The contrast-to-noise ratio, which is ultimately a more important measure in fMRI, exhibits distinct properties from SNR. Most strikingly, at low field strength, transition-band SSFP has significantly higher CNR than the matched GRE data. An additional, unusual property is the dependence of the CNR on field strength: whereas the GRE CNR increases with field strength, transition-band SSFP has equivalent CNR at 1.5 and 3 T, but significantly reduced CNR at 7 T. This reduction is believed to reflect increased sensitivity to physiological noise at high field.

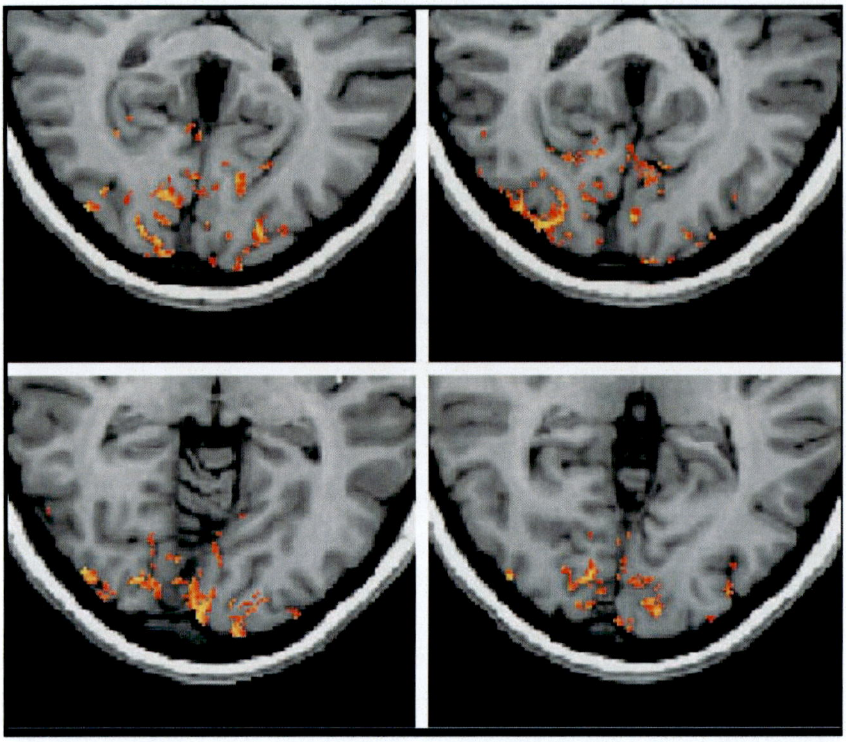

Figure 7. High-resolution transition-band SSFP fMRI: A high-resolution (1 $mm^3$) was obtained at 1.5 T using transition-band SSFP fMRI. The scan parameters were FOV = 16 x 16 $cm^2$, TR = 15 ms, flip angle = 5°, BW = ±125 kHz, and 18 slices per 3 sec. Three center frequencies ($\Delta f_{center}$ = -3, 0 and 3 Hz) were covered to increased the spatial coverage. The total scan time was 6 min 45 sec. Functional data were analyzed by a complex-data analysis method [34] and the three z-score maps were combined by maximum z-score projection.

## Pass-Band SSFP fMRI

The signal change induced from the bulk frequency shift discussed above becomes significantly smaller in the pass band since the profile is largely insensitive to frequency offsets over a wide range of frequencies (figure 5b). However, it has been demonstrated that one can still detect brain activation robustly in this pass-band off-resonance frequency band using 3–4 T scanners (figure 8a) [22,35,41,42]. This method, which is referred to as pass-band SSFP fMRI, is primarily based on the BOLD-induced $T_2$ change [35,43,44]. As mentioned earlier, in bSSFP, magnetization that is excited during a given TR may persist for multiple subsequent repetition periods, creating a signal which sums the contribution from a range of signal “pathways”. The signal contributed from pathways with several periods in the transverse plane is heavily $T_2$ weighted, resulting in an increased BOLD contrast for a short TR and TE where the GRE-type sequence shows little or no contrast [35].

The origin of the BOLD-induced $T_2$ contrast (as opposed to the $T_2^*$ BOLD effect detected with GRE) results from the diffusion of spins in the field patterns surrounding blood vessels [45,46]. Spins diffusing in these field patterns accumulate random phase offsets, leading to signal loss that cannot be refocused in a spin echo experiment; in other words, it leads to $T_2$ relaxation. Because the field patterns depend on deoxy-hemoglobin concentration, these $T_2$ changes reflect local activity in much the same way as more conventional $T_2$* BOLD [47]. In the intra-vascular space, the motion of the spins near deoxy-hemoglobin alters the $T_2$ value of blood [48,49]. Once $T_2$ changes, the magnitude of the bSSFP profile is modified, providing signal changes from the BOLD contrast (figure 5b) [44]. As deoxy-hemoglobin concentration deceases (*i.e.*, in the activation state), the $T_2$ value becomes longer, which results in an increased steady-state signal.

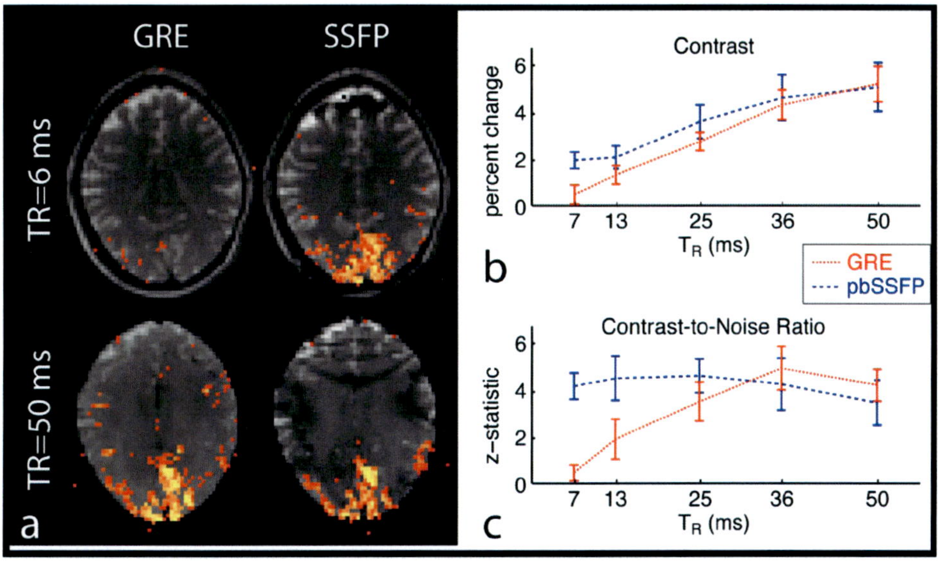


Figure 8. Pass-band SSFP fMRI example data, highlighting several key differences with matched GRE acquisitions. Pass-band SSFP and GRE data were acquired with identical 3D stack-of-EPI readouts (2.9 x 2.9 x 2.9 $mm^3$ resolution, $\alpha = 30^o$, 2.8-3.7 s/volume) at a range of TR (and with TE = TR/2) for seven subjects. (a) Example activation maps in a single subject at long and short TR. At short TR, GRE and pass-band SSFP have drastically different sensitivity to brain activity, with no activation in GRE, but robust activation with pass-band SSFP. At long TR, activation maps from the two acquisitions are essentially identical. (b) The fMRI contrast (percent signal change) demonstrates different signal from pass-band SSFP and GRE at short TR, but similar signal changes at long TR. This is in good agreement with theoretical calculations which suggest that pass-band SSFP exhibits $T_2$ BOLD contrast at short TR (where GRE has no $T_2^*$ contrast due to short TE), and that both sequences have $T_2^*$ contrast at long TR. (c) The contrast-to-noise ratio (z-statistic) in pass-band SSFP fMRI also differs from GRE in an interesting manner. Whereas the CNR of GRE rapidly drops to zero as the TR is decreased, the CNR of pass-band SSFP is relatively constant across TR. Given that the contrast in pass-band SSFP is decreasing with TR, this is indicative of lower noise variance at short TR, which reflects a decreased sensitivity to physiological noise as the TR is decreased. This property is also visible in (a) where the activation maps are highly similar at short and long TR.

These theoretical predictions have been validated by comparing pass-band SSFP and GRE fMRI data, shown in figure 8. To minimize the contribution of the transition-band effects described above, the bSSFP acquisition utilized a flip angle for which the pass band is predicted to be maximally. In this experiment, the acquisition parameters in pass-band SSFP and GRE data are matched so that the GRE sequence only differs from bSSFP by the addition of a spoiling gradient after the readout. The GRE data can thus provide an estimate of the $T_2^*$

effect in the matched pass-band SSFP. At short TR, the GRE signal tends toward zero percent signal change, whereas the pass-band SSFP signal exhibits residual signal, in agreement with theoretical predictions of $T_2$ contrast at short TE/TR (figure 8b). When TR (and TE) become relatively long, the $T_2^*$ decay from the last RF excitation becomes significant, creating GRE-like contrast. Therefore a long TR causes the signal characteristics of bSSFP to converge to GRE [35,41]. This result is in good agreement with simulations which show significant functional signal change at TE = 0 [44].

Although the percent signal change is an important aspect of functional contrast, ultimately the CNR determines the robustness (and therefore sensitivity) of the signal. As with transition-band SSFP, the CNR of pass-band SSFP fMRI has unusual properties when compared to a conventional GRE acquisition (and keeping in mind that for these acquisitions, TE = TR/2). As shown in figure 8c, the CNR of pass-band SSFP is relatively insensitive to the TR, whereas the CNR of GRE rapidly degrades as the TR (and therefore the TE) is reduced. This property has been shown to reflect reduced sensitivity to physiological noise in pass-band SSFP [35] as the sequence transitions from $T_2^*$ BOLD contrast at long TR to $T_2$ BOLD at short TR. This crucial property means that the reduced contrast at short TR does not imply a reduction in the robustness of the fMRI signal.

The extra-vascular signal change of pass-band SSFP, which was simulated by the Monte-Carlo simulation, has shown other important signal characteristics [44]: when the TR is short (< 20 ms), the contrast possesses the so-called spin-echo characteristics [50]. This means that the signal change from large veins is significantly reduced in pass-band SSFP. As a result, the method is expected to provide a better spatial specificity compared to GRE fMRI.

Compared to the transition-band case, the pass-band method is much more immune to the off-resonance effects. However, large spatial off-resonance variations in some brain regions are still an issue in pass-band SSFP fMRI. Therefore, the compensation of spatial and temporal off-resonance is an important topic for both SSFP fMRI.

## 3D Acquisitions for SSFP fMRI

One crucial difference between bSSFP and GRE or SE sequences is that, while the latter sequences perform poorly at short TR, bSSFP requires short TR. One implication of this is that the image must be acquired over multiple excitations. Further, in order to acquire multiple slices while maintaining the steady state, data must be acquired in 3D *k*-space. The use of a multi-shot 2D acquisition would require sequential excitation of each slice, causing an unacceptable increase in TR. The use of 3D acquisitions represents a significant departure from the 2D single-shot spiral or EPI acquisitions that dominate conventional fMRI.

To date, 3D extensions of spiral [38] and EPI [37] acquisitions have been developed for use with SSFP fMRI, as illustrated in figure 9. The 3D stack-of-EPI acquisition extends 2D segmented EPI scans (figure 9a) to acquire multiple planes in *k*-space (figure 9c); a similar strategy can be made to extend interleaved spiral scans to 3D (figures 9b and d). These *k*-space trajectories are readily incorporated into bSSFP by zeroing the accumulated gradient area after the readout (figures 9e and f), which returns to the center of *k*-space as discussed above. While these are the only 3D trajectories proposed to date, alternate 3D trajectories are certainly possible (for example, radial [51] or cone trajectories [52]).

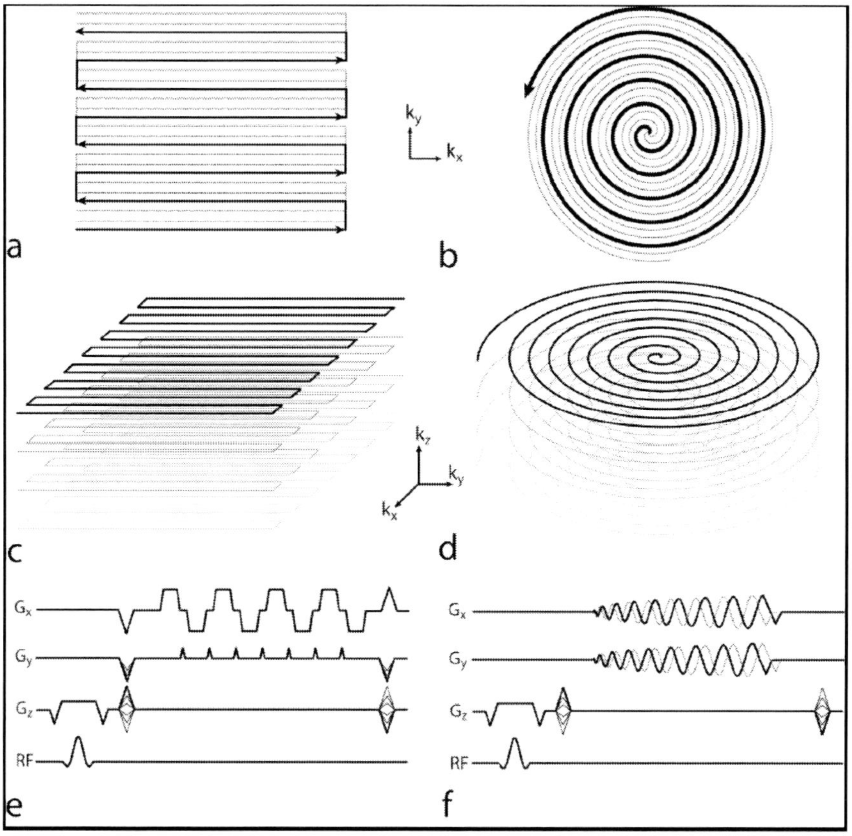


Figure 9. Example 3D acquisitions developed for use with SSFP fMRI, based on echo-planar imaging (left column) and spiral trajectories (right column). (a and b) Both EPI and spiral trajectories are based on multi-shot 2D *k*-space acquisitions where the $k_x$-$k_y$ plane is acquired over multiple excitations (in these examples, 3 interleaved acquisitions, indicated by dashed lines). (c and d) These 2D multi-shot acquisitions are then extended to cover 3D *k*-space by repeating these *k*-space planes for multiple $k_z$ locations (in these examples, 4 $k_z$ planes indicated by gray lines). (e and f) These 3D acquisitions can be incorporated into a bSSFP sequence in a straightforward manner by simply ensuring that zero total gradient area is accumulated on every gradient axis.

There are several properties of these 3D acquisitions that are advantageous for fMRI. First, 3D acquisitions tend to have high SNR because signal is received from the entire magnetization in every TR (by comparison, a 2D multi-slice acquisition with *n* slices can dedicate only 1/*n* of the total scan time to receiving signal from each slice). Second, the requirement for TR limits the duration of each 3D segment, so that off-resonance artifacts (distortion for EPI and blurring for spirals) are very low relative to conventional single-shot acquisitions. Third, the use of 3D *k*-space acquisitions avoids the problems associated with 2D slice excitations, which have fundamental limits on slice resolution (2-3 mm) and are prone to slice warping. There are also disadvantages of 3D acquisitions, such as the inability to define a specific time-point at which the data is acquired (which can be crucial for some fMRI paradigm designs) and the requirement that 3D slices be contiguous (compared with 2D acquisitions which can allow for gaps between slices). For most studies, however, these issues are not overly problematic, and recent advances in 3D trajectories for SSFP fMRI have enabled the acquisition of large 3D volumes in *k*-space [53].

## Off-Resonance Effects in SSFP fMRI and Their Compensation

One important characteristic that differentiates bSSFP from other sequences is the signal dependence on the off-resonance frequency (figure 5). Banding artifacts clearly distinguish a bSSFP image (figure 3). In the transition-band SSFP fMRI case, the signal dependence on off-resonance provides functional contrast from the bulk frequency shift change. However, there exist several other sources of frequency drift that affect the resonance frequency of a voxel and subsequently change the magnitude and phase of the voxel signal. These sources can hamper the stability of both pass-band and transition-band SSFP fMRI methods by adding unwanted variations in the data. In this section, the problems of both spatial and temporal off-resonance will be discussed as well as their compensation techniques.

### Spatial off-Resonance

When a slice or slab is selected for imaging, the first step for a modern MRI scanner is to match the precession frequencies of the imaging volume to the Larmor frequency as closely as possible so that off-resonance frequency induced imaging artifacts can be minimized. This procedure, which is referred to as "shimming", involves measuring the field distribution and correcting it by changing the shim gradient magnetic fields (x, y, z linear shim gradients and additional higher order shim systems available) [54-57]. Despite this effort, one might not be able to correct for spatial off-resonance frequencies completely. When scanning a whole brain volume, for example, a frequency distribution of a few hundred Hertz is often measured, even after shimming; these effects are more problematic at high field than low field. The sources of this spatial off-resonance include hardware imperfection [58], chemical shift [59], eddy currents [60], subject related sources [61], and other extraneous fields induced from external sources [62]. Figure 3a shows an example of a field map that represents the spatial off-resonance frequency distribution of an imaging slice.

In SSFP fMRI, this spatial off-resonance becomes a limiting factor for the spatial coverage. Figure 10 illustrates the spatial coverage of both SSFP methods. In pass-band SSFP fMRI, the banding artifacts can be observed in the areas of large off-resonance (figures 10a and d). This artifact hinders whole brain coverage in the pass-band method, even though it has better spatial coverage than conventional GRE fMRI (figures 10c and f). In the transition-band case, the area near the on-resonance frequency is where functional contrast is acquired (high signal areas in figures 10b and e). As a result, the spatial off-resonance variation poses a major limitation in the spatial coverage of transition-band SSFP fMRI.

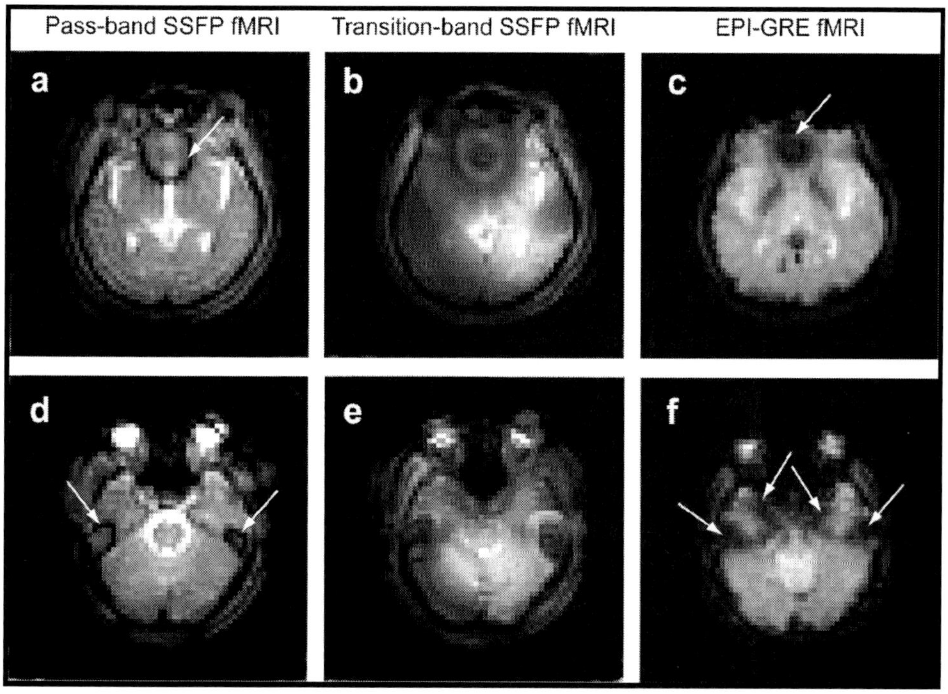


Figure 10. Comparison of the image quality. The pass-band SSFP images show the banding artifacts (arrows) in the areas of large off-resonance (a and d). However, the bands exist in narrow regions. In the transition-band SSFP case, significant signal intensity variation is observed (b and e). This variation comes from the large magnitude profile change based on the off-resonance frequency. In both pass-band and transition-band SSFP, the acquisition is optimized (primarily via the flip angle) such that the bright areas are the activation band regions where functional contrast can be acquired. Due to the off-resonance sensitivity, the spatial coverage of transition-band SSFP is significantly limited. The EPI-GRE results show signal dropout and image distortion (arrows). These artifacts limit functional studies for these regions in GRE fMRI. The images of both SSFP fMRI are acquired using the 3D stack-of-spiral trajectory whereas the GRE images are from an EPI sequence. The resolution for all the images is 3.75 x 3.75 x 5 $mm^3$. A total of 20 slices are acquired in every 1 sec for SSFP fMRI and 2 sec for GRE fMRI.

One can increase the spatial coverage of SSFP fMRI by focusing on a small ROI and shimming within the ROI such that no banding artifacts occur in this region. Another method to improve the spatial coverage is repeating the experiments with shifted center frequencies (figure 11) [21,42]. This repetition with shifted center frequencies help to increase the spatial coverage of SSFP fMRI at the expense of an increased scan time. In the pass-band case, two repetitions can provide the whole brain coverage [42]. In transition-band SSFP fMRI, three repetitions were performed to cover the visual cortex [38], whereas eleven repetitions were used to cover a whole brain area [37]. The multi-frequency acquisitions can then be combined to produce a single statistical activation map; the statistical maps from individual frequencies can be combined, for example, using maximum-intensity projections [21,42] or fixed-effects analysis [37].

Instead of repeating the acquisition, one can interleave different center frequencies in every volume acquisition time [40]. Figure 12 illustrates the concept of this interleaved center frequency method. In the pass-band method, only two different center frequencies (for example, F1 = F3 = 0 Hz, and F2 = F4 = $(2TR)^{-1}$ Hz) are enough whereas in the transition-band method, one needs to have enough center frequencies (for example, F1 = -6 Hz, F2 = -2 Hz, F3 = 2 Hz, and F4 = 6 Hz) that cover the spatial off-resonance of a ROI. This interleaved method helps to reduce unwanted complications such as the spatial coverage mismatch from scanner $B_0$ field drift or subject condition variation. This method bears some resemblance to z-shim acquisitions, in which GRE images are acquired with multiple shim settings to reduce signal dropout [7]. For transition-band SSFP fMRI, this interleaved method enabled wider spatial coverage without repeating the experiments. The location of the activation and the number of activated voxels were similar to that of the repeated method [40]. For the pass-band case, the method is still under investigation.

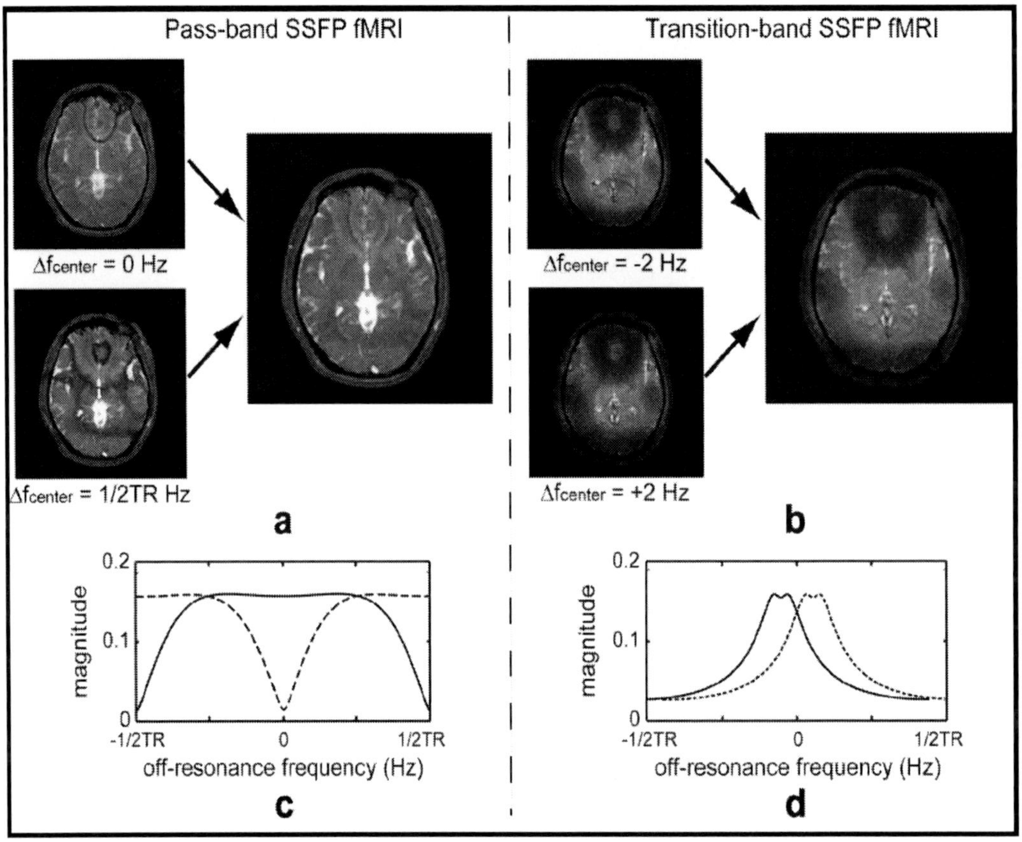


Figure 11. Increasing spatial coverage in SSFP fMRI: In both SSFP fMRI methods, the spatial coverage can be increased by multiple scans with shifted center frequencies. The composite images, the larger figures in (a) and (b), show wider spatial coverage than the single center frequency acquisition. In the pass-band case, the two center frequencies, which are separated by $(2TR)^{-1}$ Hz, can yield enough spatial coverage for the whole brain. Therefore, functional contrast can be obtained in the large susceptibility areas.

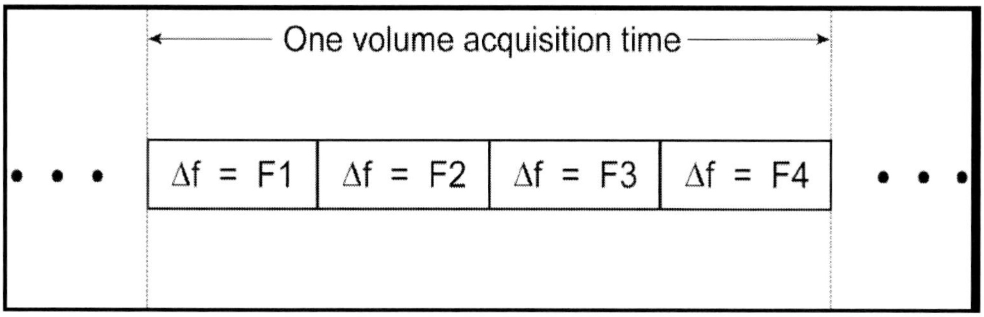


Figure 12. Interleaved center frequency model: Different center frequencies can be interleaved within one volume acquisition time (~ 3 sec) to provide wider spatial off-resonance frequency coverage without repeating the experiment. Two interleaves (F1 = F3 = 0 and F2 = F4 = $(2TR)^{-1}$) are enough for pass-band SSFP fMRI whereas multiple interleaves that cover the ROI are necessary for transition-band SSFP fMRI.

## Temporal off-Resonance

Another source of frequency instability that degrades the performance of SSFP fMRI occurs in the temporal domain. The temporal off-resonance variation, which is related to the stability of the $B_0$ field, can introduce unwanted signal variability and contrast change in SSFP fMRI. There are two major sources that are related to the $B_0$ stability: respiration induced field change and slow scanner field drift. Respiration-induced $B_0$ field change has been well investigated since it is one of the major physiological noise sources [61,63,64]. A bulk susceptibility change from the varying lung volume causes $B_0$ field fluctuations over time. A typical range of resonance offsets is between 0.15 Hz and 1 Hz in the brain at 1.5 T [61], which fluctuate in a quasi-sinusoidal manner. The effect is relatively uniform in an axial slice [65] and increases with the field strength [65]. Another source for the $B_0$ field change is the slow scanner $B_0$ resonance frequency drift. It has been investigated that the heating of passive iron shims can induce about 1 Hz/min $B_0$ field drift [58,66,67]. This source of resonance frequency drift is unidirectional, introducing a quasi-linear trend in the time series data.

In conventional fMRI, drift in $B_0$ induces a slow shift (for EPI) or blurring (for spiral). These temporal instabilities can largely be removed by post-processing methods such as filtering [68-70], navigator based methods [71-77] and other methods [78-81]. However, these methods are not effective in SSFP fMRI. The $B_0$ field change from respiration and/or scanner drift shifts the balanced SSFP magnetization profile and this shift induces time varying contrast in addition to the additive noise. In transition-band SSFP fMRI, for instance, the scanner $B_0$ field drift can gradually shift the location of the activation band over time resulting in time-varying functional contrast, and eventually, the ability to acquire the contrast for a targeted ROI is lost (figure 13a). In the pass-band case, these effects are less detrimental due to the broad activation band, but the dark band can nevertheless gradually encroach on the ROI causing similar problems (figure 13b). These effects fundamentally alter the local contrast in SSFP, and therefore cannot be removed in post-processing. As a result, compensation for temporal $B_0$ field changes in SSFP fMRI should be done in real time so that the field distribution is spatially stationary, and temporally stable.

Recently, a real-time compensation method for $B_0$ field change in SSFP fMRI has been proposed [39,82]. This method measures $B_0$ field drift from phase changes in the free induction decay (FID) and compensates for it using a real-time feedback system [83]. The real-time system updates the center frequency of the scanner (or the transmit RF and receiver phases) based on the measurement and tracks the $B_0$ field change (figure 14). As a result, the effects from the $B_0$ field change are cancelled and the bands remain spatially stable. In fMRI experiments, it has been demonstrated that this technique provides higher z-scores for the activated voxels (figure 15).

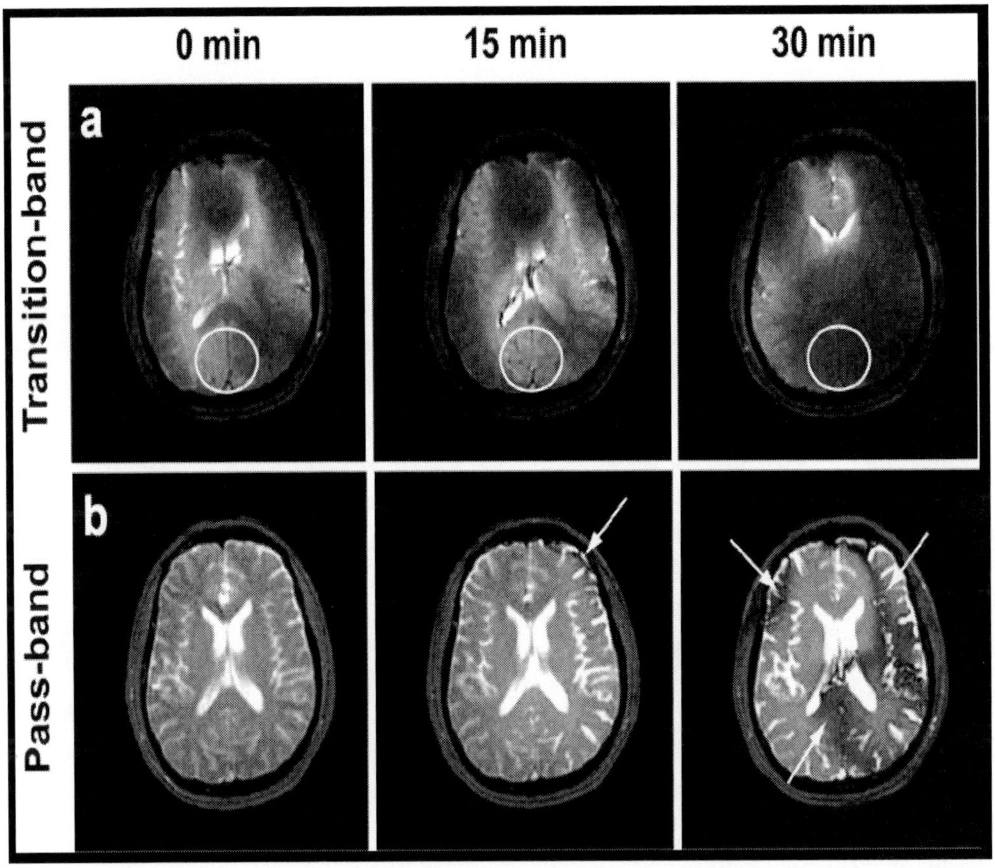


Figure 13. Temporal off-resonance in SSFP fMRI: In both SSFP methods, the $B_0$ drift of the scanner can cause severe image artifacts. In the pass-band case, the unwanted dark bands can gradually encroach into the image. In transition-band SSFP fMRI, the drift shifts the location of the activation band (bright areas) generating time varying functional contrast. After 30 min, the ability to detect functional contrast in a ROI (circled area) was lost. Once the activation band is moved out of a ROI or the dark band is located within a ROI, no activation can be restored using post-processing methods.

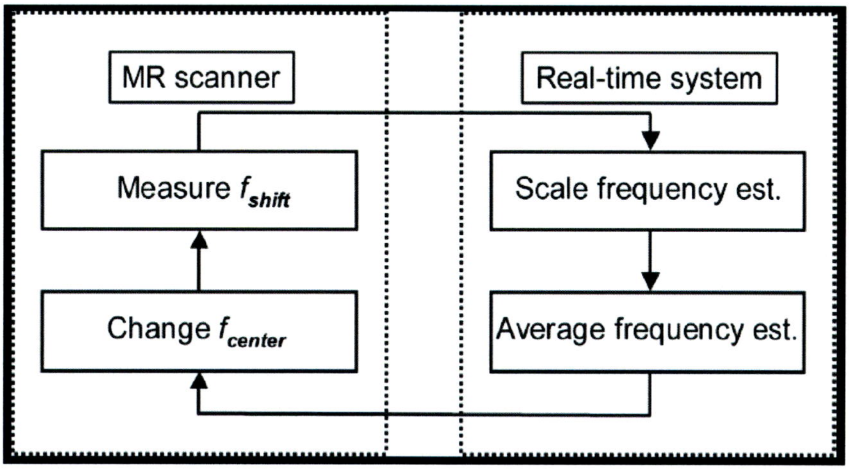


Figure 14. Conceptual model for real-time compensation: The measurement of the frequency shift is transferred to the real-time system in every TR. The real-time system processes the information and feed it back to the scanner so that the scanner can track the frequency shift by changing the center frequency of the scanner. Instead of changing the center frequency, the transmit RF and receiver phases are modified to have finer control of the center frequency change.

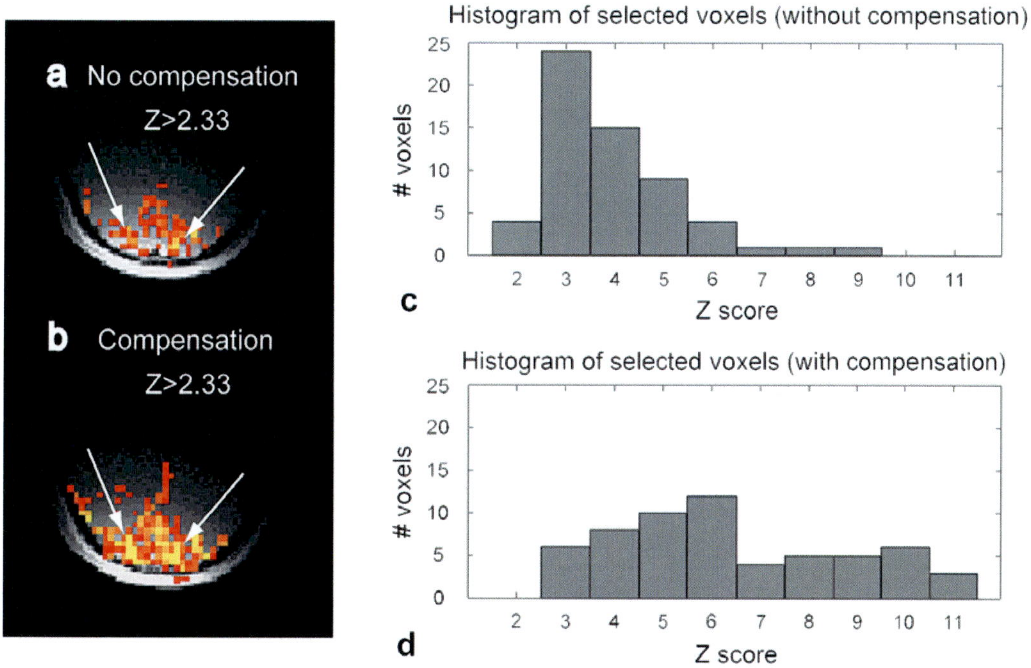


Figure 15. Temporal off-resonance compensation in SSFP fMRI: The transition-band SSFP fMRI results show significant increases both in the number of activated voxels and z-scores when the real-time temporal off-resonance compensation was used. The histograms of the commonly activated voxels show the shifts of the z-scores to higher scores (c and d).

# Advantages and Applications of SSFP fMRI

The advantages of SSFP fMRI that have been mentioned several times in this article is the high SNR efficiency and improved image quality. Figure 16 demonstrates the image quality difference between GRE and SSFP sequences for a high-resolution study (FOV = 14 x 14 $cm^2$, resolution = 1 x 1 $mm^2$, slice thickness = 4, and field strength = 3 T). The single shot EPI-GRE image shows significant artifacts compared to the SSFP image. More importantly, these artifacts reduce the true resolution of the GRE images.

Another important characteristic of bSSFP is that, in order to efficiently acquire multiple slices, data must be acquired in 3D *k*-space rather than using 2D multi-slice methods. This requirement has a few disadvantages, as discussed above. However, there are also several important advantages to 3D acquisitions. While 2D slice excitations place fundamental limits on the achievable resolution in the third dimension (typically 2-3 mm), 3D *k*-space trajectories can achieve high-resolution, isotropic voxels. As demonstrated in figure 18, this enables a much more accurate visualization of cortical structure, which is highly convoluted and rarely planar. In addition, 3D acquisitions have higher SNR for sequences with high signal at short TR such as bSSFP. It has been shown that 3D acquisitions have SNR and CNR advantages in GRE fMRI [84], particularly in conjunction with partial *k*-space acquisitions where physiological noise appears to be reduced [85]. For these reasons, although fMRI is conventionally acquired using 2D multi-slice acquisitions, the compatibility of bSSFP with 3D acquisitions is expected to be advantageous, particularly for high-resolution fMRI.

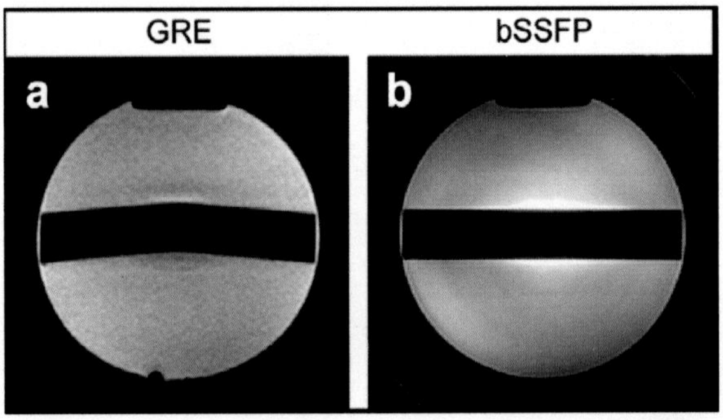


Figure 16. Comparison of the image quality at high-resolution in a water phantom: The GRE image shows significant image distortion compared to bSSFP image. This artifact comes from the long echo time and data acquisition time. For the GRE image, a single shot 2D EPI sequence was used (12 slices per 2sec). For the bSSFP image, a 3D stack-of-spiral sequence with 10 interleaves was used (22 slices per 2 sec). The time series SNR for the GRE data was only 0.59 of the bSSFP SNR. Hence, bSSFP provides more slices, higher SNR and better image quality compared to GRE.

One more advantage comes from the increased acquisition duty cycle. In GRE and SE fMRI, the data acquisition starts after a long echo time ($T_2^*$ or $T_2$) to optimize the contrast. This implies that the acquisition duty cycle is low, typically less than 25%. This reduces the SNR of the acquired images and limits the spatial coverage and temporal sampling rate of conventional fMRI. In SSFP fMRI, however, the readout duty cycle is much higher (~ 70 %) and this high duty cycle can be used to increase the spatial coverage and/or the temporal sampling rate of the data. For example, when FOV = 24 x 24 $cm^2$ and resolution = 3.75 x

3.75 $mm^2$, the GRE fMRI sequence with spiral gradients covers approximately 30 slices in every 2 seconds (single shot, TR = 66.7 ms, TE = 40 ms, BW = ± 125 kHz), whereas the SSFP fMRI sequence can cover over 60 slices in the same time (multi-shot, TR = 7.8 ms, number of interleaves = 4, BW = ± 125 kHz).

With these advantages, SSFP fMRI is applicable to several important applications. First, the pass-band method can be used for standard resolution studies. In particular, the broad activation band should enable acquisition near susceptibility boundaries where conventional GRE BOLD suffers from severe signal loss due to through-slice dephasing [42]. The ability to acquire complete coverage of these regions in two acquisitions may be crucial for imaging problematic regions such as pre-frontal cortex involved in basic cognition [86] and brainstem regions implicated in pain [87]. In addition, the improved image quality simplifies alignment with the anatomical reference images. It is expected that pass-band method will also enable improved spatial specificity due to reduced sensitivity to draining veins, giving rise to better localization of brain activity. Finally, pass-band SSFP fMRI may also enable high-resolution fMRI at moderate field strengths (3-4 T) [53]. Figure 17 demonstrates the high-resolution results of pass-band SSFP fMRI.

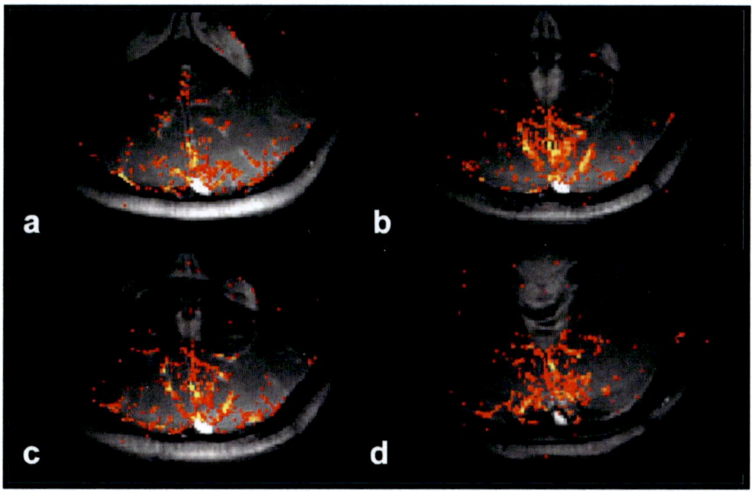


Figure 17. High-resolution (1 x 1 x 3$mm^3$) pass-band SSFP fMRI at 3T. Data was acquired using 3D stack-of-spiral (TR = 10 ms, $\alpha = 30^o$, 2 s/vol, 10 slices). The activation is well localized in the occipital lobe along the brain sulcus. No spatial smoothing was performed to preserve the original resolution.

Transition-band SSFP fMRI appears to have great potential for high-resolution fMRI across a wide range of field strengths. Most notably, it has been shown in several studies to enable high-resolution studies even on low field strength systems (1.5 T) [34,37]. Although the CNR characteristics at low resolution appear to discourage the use of transition-band SSFP at high field (see figure 6c), at high resolution the advantages of high field may be much greater. Figure 18 demonstrates dramatic improvement in the quality of activation maps with increasing field strength (1.5-7 T) for transition-band SSFP fMRI, and figure 19 demonstrates the ability to acquire even high resolution at 7 T. The use of real-time feedback to reduce sensitivity to physiological noise is expected to have even greater importance at high field, and may significantly improve the performance of transition-band SSFP fMRI in this regime. Transition-band SSFP therefore may be applicable at a broad range of field strengths, with the strong contrast being crucial at low field and the low SAR requirements combined with real-time compensation creating great potential at high field.

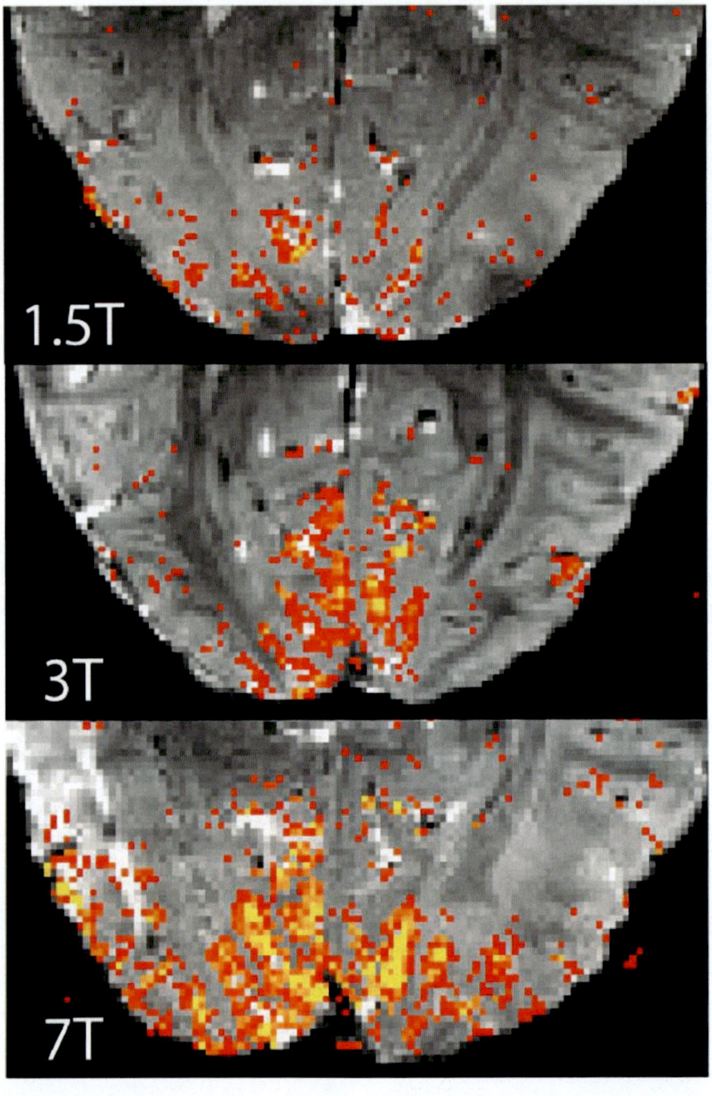


Figure 18. Transition-band SSFP fMRI at high-resolution (1 x 1 x 1mm$^3$) for three different field strengths in the same subject. Data was acquired using 3D stack-of-EPI (TR = 30 ms, $\alpha = 10^o$, 4.0-6.3 s/vol). Unlike the data shown in Fig. 6, the increase in field strength significantly improves the quality of activation maps, which may reflect the reduced dominance of physiological noise at high resolution (which has been previously documented for GRE [88]). The long TR used for this data may also cause a significant contribution from $T_2^*$ BOLD at high field.

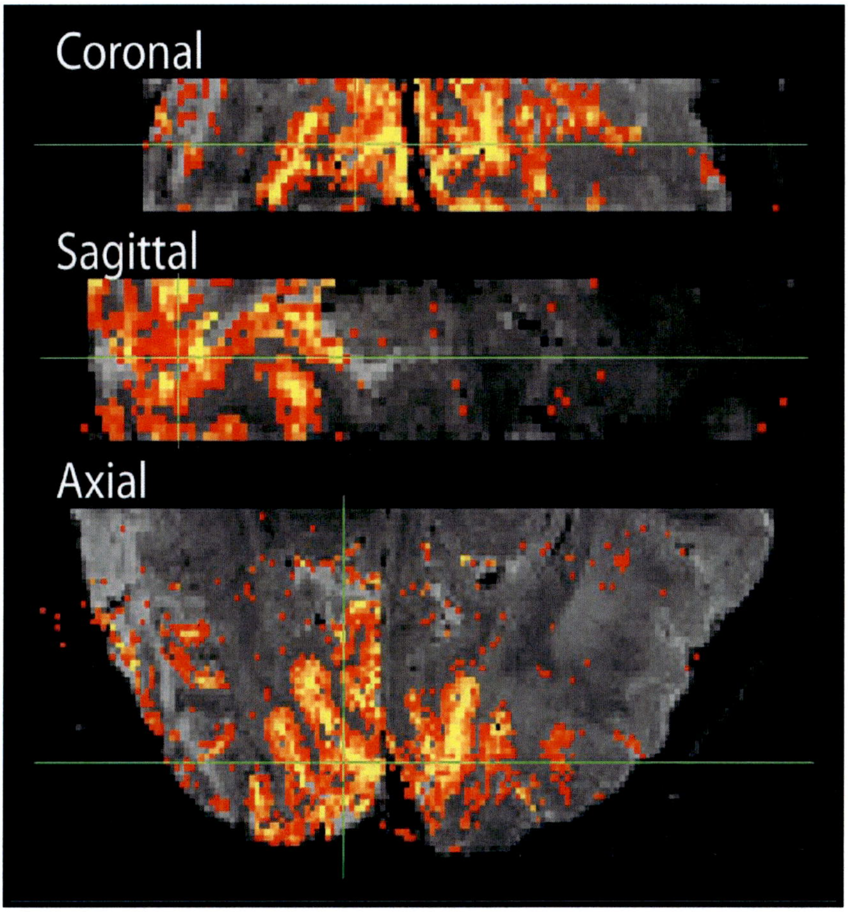


Figure 19. Transition-band SSFP fMRI at high-resolution (0.75 x 0.75 x 0.75mm$^3$) at 7 T. Data was acquired using 3D stack-of-EPI (TR = 30 ms, $\alpha$ = 10°, 7.2 s/volume). The importance of acquiring isotropic resolution is highlighted by the non-planar activation patterns in the sagittal and coronal planes: the undulations of the calcarine fissure would not be visible in conventional 2D data with thick slices (2-3 mm).

## Conclusion and Future Work

In this chapter, two new fMRI methods that are based on the balanced SSFP technique are introduced and their characteristics are explored. These SSFP fMRI methods provide an increased SNR with reduced image artifacts compared to conventional fMRI methods. With these advantages, one can use SSFP fMRI for high-resolution fMRI, reduction of distortion/blurring artifacts and acquisition of signal in areas that experience dropout in GRE BOLD.

There are still many improvements that can be made to satisfy various needs in this fast growing field. Some technical improvements that will broaden the applications of the methods include the parallel transmission and acquisition, an efficient activation band design, and new interleaving methods. Some future research directions that will deepen the understanding of the signal characteristics of SSFP fMRI include the temporal signal correlation, hemodynamic response function, intra- and extra-vascular contrast characteristics.

Judging from the benefits of SSFP and the recent results, we expect that the SSFP fMRI methods will have an important role in fMRI studies in the near future.

## References


[1] Ogawa S, Lee TM, Kay AR, Tank DW. Brain magnetic resonance imaging with contrast dependent on blood oxygenation. *PNAS.* 1990;87(24):9868-9872.

[2] Ogawa S, Tank DW, Menon R, Ellermann JM, Kim S, Merkle H, Ugurbil K. Intrinsic signal changes accompanying sensory stimulation: functional brain mapping with magnetic resonance imaging. *PNAS.* 1992;89(13):5951-5955.

[3] Kwong KK, Belliveau JW, Chesler DA, Goldberg IE, Weisskoff RM, Poncelet BP, Kennedy DN, Hoppel BE, Cohen MS, Turner R. Dynamic magnetic resonance imaging of human brain activity during primary sensory stimulation. *PNAS.* 1992;89(12):5675-5679.

[4] Glover GH, Lee AT. Motion artifacts in fMRI: comparison of 2DFT with PR and spiral scan methods. *Magn. Reson. Med.* 1995;33(5):624-635.

[5] Jezzard P, Clare S. Sources of distortion in functional MRI data. *Human Brain Mapping.* 1999;8(2-3):80-85.

[6] Cho ZH, Ro YM. Reduction of susceptibility artifact in gradient-echo imaging. *Magn. Reson. Med.* 1992;23(1):193-200.

[7] Yang QX, Williams GD, Demeure RJ, Mosher TJ, Smith MB. Removal of local field gradient artifacts in T2*-weighted images at high fields by gradient-echo slice excitation profile imaging. *Magn. Reson. Med.* 1998;39(3):402-409.

[8] Glover GH, Law CS. Spiral-in/out BOLD fMRI for increased SNR and reduced susceptibility artifacts. *Magn. Reson. Med.* 2001;46(3):515-522.

[9] Wilson JL, Jenkinson M, Jezzard P. A bit of a mouth full: susceptibility artifact reduction using diamagnetic passive shims. *Proceedings of the 10th Annual Meeting of ISMRM*; Honolulu, USA. 2002; p 205.

[10] Hsu JJ, Glover GH. Mitigation of susceptibility-induced signal loss in neuroimaging using localized shim coils. *Magn. Reson. Med.* 2005;53(2):243-248.

[11] Krueger G, Kastrup A, Glover GH. Neuroimaging at 1.5 T and 3.0 T: Comparison of oxygenation-sensitive magnetic resonance imaging. *Magn. Reson. Med.* 2001;45(4):595-604.

[12] Yacoub E, Shmuel A, Pfeuffer J, Van De Moortele PF, Adriany G, Andersen P, Vaughan JT, Merkle H, Ugurbil K, Hu X. Imaging brain function in humans at 7 Tesla. *Magn. Reson. Med.* 2001;45(4):588-594.

[13] Ogawa S, Menon RS, Tank DW, Kim SG, Merkle H, Ellermann JM, Ugurbil K. Functional brain mapping by blood oxygenation level-dependent contrast magnetic resonance imaging. A comparison of signal characteristics with a biophysical model. *Biophysical Journal.* 1993;64(3):803-812.

[14] Lee SP, Silva AC, Ugurbil K, Kim SG. Diffusion-weighted spin-echo fMRI at 9. 4 T: Microvascular/tissue contribution to BOLD signal changes. *Magn. Reson. Med.* 1999;42(5):919-928.

[15] Yacoub E, Van De Moortele PF, Shmuel A, Ugurbil K. Signal and noise characteristics of Hahn SE and GE BOLD fMRI at 7 T in humans. *Neuroimage.* 2005;24(3):738-750.

[16] Duong TQ, Yacoub E, Adriany G, Hu X, U urbil K, Kim SG. Microvascular BOLD contribution at 4 and 7 T in the human brain: Gradient-echo and spin-echo fMRI with suppression of blood effects. *Magn. Reson. Med.* 2003;49(6):1019-1027.

[17] Vaughan JT, Garwood M, Collins CM, Liu W, DelaBarre L, Adriany G, Andersen P, Merkle H, Goebel R, Smith MB. 7 T vs. 4 T: RF power, homogeneity, and signal-to-noise comparison in head images. *Magn. Reson. Med.* 2001;46(1):24-30.

[18] Van de Moortele PF, Akgun C, Adriany G, Moeller S, Ritter J, Collins CM, Smith MB, Vaughan JT, Ugurbil K. Destructive Interferences and Spatial Phase Patterns at 7 T with a Head Transceiver Array Coil. *Magn. Reson. Med.* 2005;54:1503-1518.

[19] Cho ZH, Ro YM, Chung SC, Chung JY. A direct susceptibility measurement in fMRI using SSFP interferometry (SSFPI) technique. *Proceedings of the Society of Magnetic Resonance*; Nice, France. 1995; p 806.

[20] Scheffler K, Seifritz E, Bilecen D, Venkatesan R, Hennig J, Deimling M, Haacke EM. Detection of BOLD changes by means of a frequency-sensitive trueFISP technique: preliminary results. *NMR in Biomedicine.* 2001;14(7-8):490-496.

[21] Miller KL, Hargreaves BA, Lee J, Ress D, Christopher deCharms R, Pauly JM. Functional brain imaging using a blood oxygenation sensitive steady state. *Magn. Reson. Med.* 2003;50(4):675-683.

[22] Bowen CV, Menon RS, Gati JS. High field balanced-SSFP fMRI: a BOLD technique with excellent tissue sensitivity and superior large vessel suppression. *Proceedings of the 13th Annual Meeting of ISMRM*; Miami Beach, USA. 2005; p 119.

[23] Carr HY. Steady-state free precession in nuclear magnetic resonance. *Physical Review.* 1958;112(5):1693-1701.

[24] Freeman R, Hill HDW. Phase and intensity anomalies in Fourier transform NMR. *J. Magn. Reson.* 1971;4:366-383.

[25] Oppelt A, Graumann R, Barfuss H, Fischer H, Hartl W, Shajor W. FISP- new fast MRI pulse sequence. *Electromedica.* 1986;54:15-18.

[26] Scheffler K, Lehnhardt S. Principles and applications of balanced SSFP techniques. *European Radiology.* 2003;13(11):2409-2418.

[27] Hargreaves BA, Gold GE, Beaulieu CF, Vasanawala SS, Nishimura DG, Pauly JM. Comparison of new sequences for high-resolution cartilage imaging. *Magn. Reson. Med.* 2003;49(4):700-709.

[28] Nayak KS, Hargreaves BA, Hu BS, Nishimura DG, Pauly JM, Meyer CH. Spiral balanced steady-state free precession cardiac imaging. *Magn. Reson. Med.* 2005;53:1468-1473.

[29] Scheffler K. A pictorial description of steady-states in rapid magnetic resonance imaging. *Concepts in Magnetic Resonance.* 1999;11(5):291-304.

[30] Fuchs F, Laub G, Othomo K. TrueFISP-technical considerations and cardiovascular applications. *European Journal of Radiology.* 2003;46(1):28-32.

[31] Gold GE, Hargreaves BA, Reeder SB, Block WF, Kijowski R, Vasanawala SS, Kornaat PR, Bammer R, Newbould R, Bangerter NK. Balanced SSFP imaging of the musculoskeletal system. *J. Magn. Reson. Imaging.* 2007;25(2):270-278.

[32] Chu SC, Xu Y, Balschi JA, Springer Jr CS. Bulk magnetic susceptibility shifts in NMR studies of compartmentalized samples: use of paramagnetic reagents. *Magn. Reson. Med.* 1990;13(2):239-262.

[33] Boxerman JL, Hamberg LM, Rosen BR, Weisskoff RM. MR contrast due to intravascular magnetic susceptibility perturbations. *Magn. Reson. Med.* 1995;34(4):555-566.

[34] Lee J, Shahram M, Schwartzman A, Pauly JM. Complex data analysis in high-resolution SSFP fMRI. *Magn. Reson. Med.* 2007;57(5):905-917.

[35] Miller KL, Smith SM, Jezzard P, Wiggins GC, Wiggins CJ. Signal and noise characterics of passband SSFP FMRI: A comparison with GRE at multiple field strengths *Neuroimage.* 2007(in press).

[36] Gati JS, Menon RS, Ugurbil K, Rutt BK. Experimental determination of the BOLD field strength dependence in vessels and tissue. *Magn. Reson. Med.* 1997;38(2):296-302.

[37] Miller KL, Smith SM, Jezzard P, Pauly JM. High-Resolution FMRI at 1.5 T Using Balanced SSFP. *Magn. Reson. Med.* 2006;55:161-170.

[38] Lee J, Lee JH, Hargreaves BA, Miller KL, Pauly JM. High resolution 3D spiral trajectory BOSS FMRI. *Proceedings of the 13th Annual Meeting of ISMRM*; Miami Beach, USA. 2005; p 120.

[39] Lee J, Santos JM, Conolly SM, Miller KL, Hargreaves BA, Pauly JM. Respiration-induced B0 field fluctuation compensation in balanced SSFP: Real-time approach for transition-band SSFP fMRI. *Magn. Reson. Med.* 2006;55(5):1197-1201.

[40] Lee J, Santos JM, Pauly JM. An interleaved center frequency acquisition method in transition-band SSFP fMRI: Increased spatial off-resonance coverage. *Proceedings of the 14th Annual Meeting of ISMRM*; Seattle, USA. 2006; p 3366.

[41] Zhong K, Leupold J, Hennig J, Speck O. Systematic investigation of balanced steady-state free precession for functional MRI in the human visual cortex at 3 Tesla. *Magn. Reson. Med.* 2007;57(1):67-73.

[42] Lee JH, Gurney PT, Dumoulin SO, Wandell BA, Shankaranarayanan A, Nishimura DG, Pauly JM. BOX fMRI using multiple-acquisition steady-sate free precession imaging for full-brain coverage *Proceedings of the 14th Annual Meeting of ISMRM*; Seattle, USA. 2006; p 3297.

[43] Bowen CV, Mason J, Menon RS, Gati JS. High field balanced-SSFP fMRI: Examining a diffusion contrast mechanism using varied flip-angles. *Proceedings of the 14th Annual Meeting of ISMRM*; Seattle, USA. 2006; p 665.

[44] Kim T, Lee J, Pauly JM. Analysis of the BOLD Signal Characteristics in balanced SSFP fMRI: a Monte-Carlo Simulation *Proceedings of the 15th Annual Meeting of ISMRM*; Berlin, Germany. 2007; p 696.

[45] Gasparovic C, Matwiyoff NA. The magnetic properties and water dynamics of the red blood cell: a study by proton-NMR lineshape analysis. *Magn. Reson. Med.* 1992;26(2):274-299.

[46] Weisskoff RM, Zuo CS, Boxerman JL, Rosen BR. Microscopic susceptibility variation and transverse relaxation: theory and experiment. *Magn. Reson. Med.* 1994;31(6):601-610.
[47] Bandettini PA, Wong EC, Jesmanowicz A, Hinks RS, Hyde JS. Spin-echo and gradient-echo EPI of human brain activation using BOLD contrast: a comparative study at 1.5 T. *NMR Biomed.* 1994;7(1-2):12-20.
[48] Dharmakumar R, Hong J, Brittain JH, Plewes DB, Wright GA. Oxygen-sensitive contrast in blood for steady-state free precession imaging. *Magn. Reson. Med.* 2005;53:574-583.
[49] van Zijl PCM, Eleff SM, Ulatowski JA, Oja JME, Ulu gcaron AM, Traystman RJ, Kauppinen RA. Quantitative assessment of blood flow, blood volume and blood oxygenation effects in functional magnetic resonance imaging. *Nature Medicine.* 1998;4(2):159-167.
[50] Boxerman JL, Bandettini PA, Kwong KK, Baker JR, Davis TL, Rosen BR, Weisskoff RM. The intravascular contribution to fMRI signal change: Monte Carlo modeling and diffusion-weighted studies in vivo. *Magn. Reson. Med.* 1995;34(1):4-10.
[51] Peters DC, Korosec FR, Grist TM, Block WF, Holden JE, Vigen KK, Mistretta CA. Undersampled projection reconstruction applied to MR angiography. *Magn. Reson. Med.* 2000;43(1):91-101.
[52] Gurney PT, Hargreaves BA, Nishimura DG. Design and analysis of a practical 3D cones trajectory. *Magn. Reson. Med.* 2006;55:575-582.
[53] Lee JH, Dumoulin SO, Glover GH, Wandell BA, Nishimura DG, Pauly JM. Full-brain coverage and high-resolution imaging capabilities of passband SSFP fMRI at 3 T. *Proceedings of the 15th Annual Meeting of ISMRM*; Berlin, Germany. 2007; p 694.
[54] Schneider E, Glover G. Rapid in vivo proton shimming. *Magn. Reson. Med.* 1991;18(2):335-347.
[55] Reese TG, Davis TL, Weisskoff RM. Automated shimming at 1.5 T using echo-planar image frequency maps. *J. Magn. Reson. Imaging.* 1995;5(6):739-745.
[56] Irarrazabal P, Meyer CH, Nishimura DG, Macovski A. Inhomogeneity correction using an estimated linear field map. *Magn. Reson. Med.* 1996;35(2):278-282.
[57] Kim DH, Adalsteinsson E, Glover GH, Spielman DM. Regularized higher-order in vivo shimming. *Magn. Reson. Med.* 2002;48(4):715-722.
[58] Foerster BU, Tomasi D, Caparelli EC. Magnetic field shift due to mechanical vibration in functional magnetic resonance imaging. *Magn. Reson. Med.* 2005;54(5):1261-1267.
[59] Sumanaweera TS, Glover GH, Binford TO, Adler JR. MR susceptibility misregistration correction. *IEEE Trans. Med. Imag.* 1993;12(2):251-259.
[60] Jehenson P, Syrota A. Correction of distortions due to the pulsed magnetic field gradient-induced shift in B0 field by postprocessing. *Magn. Reson. Med.* 1989;12(2):253-256.
[61] Noll DC, Schneider W. Respiration artifacts in functional brain imaging: sources of signal variation and compensation strategies. *Proceedings of the Society of Magnetic Resonance*; San Francisco, USA. 1994; p 647.

[62] Durand E, van de Moortele PF, Pachot-Clouard M, Le Bihan D. Artifact due to B0 fluctuations in fMRI: correction using the k-space central line. *Magn. Reson. Med.* 2001;46:198-201.

[63] Weisskoff RM, Baker J, Belliveau J, Davis TL, Kwong KK, Cohen MS, Rosen BR. Power spectrum analysis of functionally-weighted MR data: what's in the noise. *Proceedings of the Society of Magnetic Resonance*; New York, USA. 1993; p 7.

[64] Raj D, Paley DP, Anderson AW, Kennan RP, Gore JC. A model for susceptibility artefacts from respiration in functional echo-planar magnetic resonance imaging. *Phys. Med. Biol.* 2000;45(12):3809-3820.

[65] Van de Moortele PF, Pfeuffer J, Glover GH, Ugurbil K, Hu X. Respiration-induced B0 fluctuations in the human brain at 7 Tesla and its spatial distribution. *Magn. Reson. Med.* 2002;47(5):888-895

[66] Henry PG, van de Moortele PF, Giacomini E, Nauerth A, Bloch G. Field-frequency locked in vivo proton MRS on a whole-body spectrometer. *Magn. Reson. Med.* 1999;42(4):636-642.

[67] Benner T, van der Kouwe AJW, Kirsch JE, Sorensen AG. Real-time RF pulse adjustment for B0 drift compensation. *Magn. Reson. Med.* 2006;56:204-209.

[68] Woolrich MW, Ripley BD, Brady M, Smith SM. Temporal autocorrelation in univariate linear modeling of FMRI data. *Neuroimage.* 2001;14(6):1370-1386.

[69] Biswal B, DeYoe AE, Hyde JS. Reduction of physiological fluctuations in fMRI using digital filters. *Magn. Reson. Med.* 1996;35(1):107-113.

[70] Buonocore MH, Maddock RJ. Noise suppression digital filter for functional magnetic resonance imaging based on image reference data. *Magn. Reson. Med.* 1997;38(3):456-469.

[71] Hu X, Kim SG. Reduction of physiological noise in functional MRI using navigator echo. *Magn. Reson. Med.* 1994;31:495-503.

[72] Hu X, Le TH, Parrish T, Erhard P. Retrospective estimation and correction of physiological fluctuation in functional MRI. *Magn. Reson. Med.* 1995;34(2):201-212.

[73] Le TH, Hu X. Retrospective estimation and correction of physiological artifacts in fMRI by direct extraction of physiological activity from MR data. *Magn. Reson. Med.* 1996;35(3):290-298.

[74] Wowk B, McIntyre MC, Saunders JK. k-Space detection and correction of physiological artifacts in fMRI. *Magn. Reson. Med.* 1997;38(6):1029-1034.

[75] Noll DC, Genovese CR, Vazquez AL, O'Brien JL, Eddy WF. Evaluation of respiratory artifact correction techniques in multishot spiral functional MRI using receiver operator characteristic analyses. *Magn. Reson. Med.* 1998;40(4):633-639.

[76] Frank LR, Buxton RB, Wong EC. Estimation of respiration-induced noise fluctuations from undersampled multislice fMRI data. *Magn. Reson. Med.* 2001;45(4):635-644.

[77] Pfeuffer J, Van de Moortele PF, Ugurbil K, Hu X, Glover GH. Correction of physiologically induced global off-resonance effects in dynamic echo-planar and spiral functional imaging. *Magn. Reson. Med.* 2002;47(2):344-353.

[78] Glover GH, Li TQ, Ress D. Image-based method for retrospective correction of physiological motion effects in fMRI: RETROICOR. *Magn. Reson. Med.* 2000;44(1):162-167.

[79] Chuang KH, Chen JH. IMPACT: Image-based physiological artifacts estimation and correction technique for functional MRI. *Magn. Reson. Med.* 2001;46(2):344-353.

[80] Bandettini PA, Jesmanowicz A, Wong EC, Hyde JS. Processing strategies for time-course data sets in functional MRI of the human brain. *Magn. Reson. Med.* 1993;30(2):161-173.

[81] Worsley KJ, Liao CH, Aston J, Petre V, Duncan GH, Morales F, Evans AC. A general statistical analysis for fMRI data. *NeuroImage.* 2002;15(1):1-5.

[82] Wu ML, Wu PH, Huang TY, Shih YY, Chou MC, Liu HS, Chung HW, Chen CY. Frequency stabilization using infinite impulse response filtering for SSFP fMRI at 3T. *Magn. Reson. Med.* 2007;57(2):369-379.

[83] Santos JM, Wright GA, Pauly JM. Flexible real-time magnetic resonance imaging framework. *IEEE EMBS 26th Annual International Conference*; San Francisco, USA. 2004; p 1048.

[84] Lai S, Glover GH. Three-dimensional spiral fMRI technique: a comparison with 2D spiral acquisition. *Magn. Reson. Med.* 1998;39(1):68-78.

[85] Hu Y, Glover GH. Partial-k-space acquisition method for improved SNR efficiency and temporal resolution in 3 D fMRI. *Magn. Reson. Med.* 2006;55:1106-1113.

[86] Devlin JT, Russell RP, Davis MH, Price CJ, Wilson J, Moss HE, Matthews PM, Tyler LK. Susceptibility-induced loss of signal: comparing PET and fMRI on a semantic task. *Neuroimage.* 2000;11(6):589-600.

[87] Tracey I, Ploghaus A, Gati JS, Clare S, Smith S, Menon RS, Matthews PM. Imaging attentional modulation of pain in the periaqueductal gray in humans. *Journal of Neuroscience.* 2002;22(7):2748-2752.

[88] Triantafyllou C, Hoge RD, Wald LL. Effect of spatial smoothing on physiological noise in high-resolution fMRI. *Neuroimage.* 2006;32(2):551-557.

In: Research Topics on Brain Mapping
Editor: Yuanzhu Liáng, pp. 87-111
ISBN: 978-1-60456-001-5


*Chapter IV*

# Phase Synchronization at Different Frequency Bands Induced by the Emotional Film Stimuli of Happiness, Sadness and Fear

***Tommaso Costa, Elena Rognoni, Dario Galati and Manuella Crini***
Department of Psychology, University of Turin, Italy

## Abstract

The neural large-scale dynamics and the connectivity pathways among spatially separated neural groups are conceived as a fundamental brain mechanism to integrate and process information.

The new measures of nonlinear interdependencies applied to EEG recordings, such as phase synchronization, have been recently shown to be highly sensitive to detect the dynamical change underlying the brain functions.

In the present chapter, the patterns of interdependency among different brain regions were investigated extracting the Synchronization Index (SI) from EEG response to different emotional and non-emotional film stimuli. The three basic emotions of happiness, fear and sadness were induced with the goal to investigate the synchronization patterns at different frequencies bands specifically associated with the valence dimension (positive vs. negative) and with the distinct basic emotional systems.

The comparisons among the experimental conditions showed several significant SI changes. The results demonstrated an overall decrease of SI during emotional stimulation compared to neutral, indicating an increase of complexity in the cortical dynamics. Further differences were found among the specific emotions, involving a distinct couple of electrodes with topographical effects at the frequencies bands examined. During happiness, we found a large pattern of synchronization in the left frontal hemisphere, especially in delta and theta waves, while fear, compared to neutral stimuli, showed a higher right synchronization, especially in beta waves. Largely different SI patterns emerged in the comparisons between the two negative emotions of fear and sadness, suggesting that the basic emotions are mediated by specific synchronized activity. The observed emotion-related SI change supports the view that coupling-decoupling patterns among the neural networks may be a relevant neural mechanism for the emotional processing and that SI nonlinear analysis may contribute to describe how the brain generates the emotion.

# Introduction

## Neural Synchronization

The intricate connectivity among functionally specialized groups of neurons is an outstanding characteristic of mammalian brains, which are primarily characterized by the ability to integrate information (Tononi and Edelman, 1998). According to the functional integration approach (Frackowiak et al., 2004), the distributed networks of neurons transiently linked by reciprocal dynamic connections, defined neural assemblies (Hebb, 1949), are thought to be the basic functional mechanism mediating the wide sort of behaviors and mental processes. Integration is based on the positive and negative feedback among neural structures on different scale levels: on a small scale, the reentrant processes occurred at the level of cells and cell assemblies, while on a large scale, there were loops formed by reciprocal projections among brain structures distributed along the entire neuraxis, including limbic, cortical, and brain stem structures (Lewis, 2005).

Over the past years, a large body of empirical studies employing electro- and magneto-encephalography (EEG, MEG) or functional Magnetic Resonance Imaging (fMRI) have begun to explore the functional integration among the reentrant circuits and the neural networks on higher levels of brain functioning. In particular, the neurophysiological techniques such as EEG and MEG are highly suitable to capture these macroscopic spatial temporal dynamics, whose prevalent feature is the presence of metastable spatio-temporal pattern of neural activity distributed over many distinct brain regions.

Numerous mathematical methods have been devised to extract information on the various modes of reciprocal interaction from the EEG oscillations.

Since biological systems such as the neural networks are likely to be nonlinear, dissipative and stochastic systems (Rosenblum et al., 2004), nonlinear analysis may be particularly useful to describe the large-scale dynamics of the brain, as well as to define how much the system is deterministic or stochastic (Stam, 2005).

The phase synchronization among participating neuronal groups is one of the new nonlinear measures that has been proposed to play a key role in the integrative brain functions (Singer, 1999; Tononi and Sporns, 2003; Hebb, 1949). It specifically detects the interdependencies of instantaneous phases of two time series (Rosenblum et al., 1996). According to Boccaletti et al. (2002), a broad neurophysiological definition for neural synchronization refers to "the adjustment of time-varying properties between two or many subsystems (either equivalent or nonequivalent) to a common behavior through a coupling or an external forcing (periodical or noisy)" (see also Brown and Kocarev, 2000). Phase synchronization is characterized by a non uniform distribution of the phase difference between two signals, with the important advantage that it not only occurs between linear oscillators, but also between irregular and chaotic systems (Pecora and Carroll, 1990) and when the amplitudes of coupled chaotic oscillators remain uncorrelated (Rosenblum et al., 1996).

Much effort has recently been focused on detecting and quantifying synchronization within non-stationary noisy systems (Pikovsky et al., 2001). In such systems, the traditional cross-correlation technique may not assure appropriate detection in all cases of interdependency. Recent advances in synchronization analyses turn out to detect the direction of coupling between two systems, defining which signal becomes synchronized with another one and otherwise (Rosenblum and Pikovsky, 2001).

Direct evidence supporting phase synchrony as a basic mechanism for brain integration has recently been provided in relation to memory (Klimesh, 1999), learning (Singer, 1993), visual perception (Bressler et al. 1993; Rodriguez et al. 1999), binding processes (Tallon-Baudry and Bertrand, 1999), selective attention (Desmedt and Tomberg, 1994; Klimesch et al., 1998; Tallon-Baudry et al., 2001) and musical hearing (Bhattacharya, 2001). Although several cognitive processes have been linked to synchronization change, emotions have received relatively little attention in synchronization EEG studies. Nonetheless, synchronization may offer a highly informative tool to investigate the neural process underlying the emotion, that is overall recognized as a complex and multi-componential response produced by the different interconnecting neural systems. As the emotion involves cognitive, behavioral, expressive, sensory-motor and psychophysiological components, as it is mediated by largely distributed neural circuits extended along the cerebral neuraxis exerting effect on cortical dynamics detectable by synchronization analysis on EEG signals. In accordance with these considerations, investigations on synchronized activity performed by nonlinear analysis methods may extensively contribute to describe how emotions are generated and organized in the brain.

## The Models of Emotion

How can we define emotion? Since James posed the question in 1884, the definition of emotion has been long debated and, at the same time, holds one of the most relevant issues for psychological disciplines and neuroscience. Emotion holds a salient evolutionary function regulating the adaptation to the environment; furthermore, emotion deeply interacts and influences a lot of psychological processes such as perception, memory, attention and reasoning, representing an essential function of the whole system. On this basis, it seems unrealistic to achieve a full model of the mind, behavior and brain, excluding emotion.

Several theories have attempted to provide a comprehensive definition of emotion and describe the complex emotional domain. Three main models of emotion represent the theoretical backgrounds to investigate the distinct neuroanatomical underpinnings of emotion: the dimensional models, the discrete multi-systems models and the dual systems models of approach and withdrawal.

### *Dimensional Emotions*

In the past the cognitive approach to the studies of emotion in humans has developed the so-called dimensional theory that considers all emotions to be organized around a limited number of underlying dimensions: the valence or pleasantness dimension distinguishes positive (or pleasant) and negative (or unpleasant) emotions, and arousal dimension distinguishes emotion in terms of bodily activation (excitement) or deactivation (calm) (e.g. Russell, 1980). This account of emotion is based on results obtained by factor analysis on verbal assessments of emotional experiences. Several neuroimaging investigations supported a neural specialization associated with emotions with different subjective valence and arousal values (for a meta-analytic review, see Murphy et al., 2003). Lang and co-workers (1998a) have developed a neurobiological model of emotional dimensions, often referred to as the "bio-informational theory of emotion". Emotions are viewed as action dispositions, containing cognitive, motivational, physiological and behavioural components. These dispositions are organized as being either consummatory/appetitive tendencies or defensive/aversive tendencies. Consequently, this approach is associated with a two dimensional model of emotion: the valence dimension is related to variations on the level of the two motive systems, i.e. "appetitive" and "aversive"; the arousal dimension, adds to the two-dimensional affective space a component that modulates the emotional behaviour with respect to activation or intensity (Lang et al., 1998b). The two systems are thought to have different neural substrates, namely widespread networks involving a number of neocortical and subcortical structures. Variations in arousal are considered to reflect changes in the activation intensity of the aversive or appetitive subsystems.

### *Discrete Emotions*

In opposition with dimensional approach, some theorists hypothesized a limited number of emotions that differ one from another, called "basic" emotions, from which the wide range of more complex emotions are derived (e.g., Ekman, 1992). According to this theorization, basic emotions are innate, universal and biologically given, selected along the evolutionary history of species for their specific adaptive function in promoting the survival and adaptation goal. Each emotion is characterized by specific physiological, behavioural and expressive patterns, that predispose the adaptive response, as well as by universal signals, antecedent events, distinctive thoughts, memories and images, different subjective experiences. According to the evolutionary approach, basic emotions share automatic appraisal, presence in other primates, quick onset, brief duration and unbidden occurrence (Ekman, 1992).

The basic emotions are though to be generated by specific and at least in part dissociable central affective programs involving widely distributed neural circuits, that mediate the several components of response and integrate all the process that, from perception to appraisal, contribute to emotion (e.g. Ekman and Davidson, 1994; Panksepp, 1998).

The definition of the types and the number of basic emotional system is of crucial interest for affective neuroscience. Neuroimaging researches have recently supported a neural specialization for distinct basic emotions such as fear, sadness, happiness, anger and disgust (Murphy et al., 2003; Barrett and Wager, 2006).

### *The Approach - Withdrawal Emotional System*

Further models argue that the broad emotional domain may be organized around the basic and evolutionarily ancient systems of approach and withdrawal, associated to specific action tendencies (Davidson, 2003). The approach system facilitates appetitive or goal-directed behavior; it mainly generates the approach-related positive affect (like desire but not satisfaction), and also some negative affect that, like anger, predispose to approach the stimuli. The withdrawal system predisposes an organism to draw away from aversive stimuli, generating avoidance- related negative affect, such as fear and disgust (Davidson and Irwin, 1999).

## Emotions and EEG Cortical Dynamics

Emotion have been stimulating the neurophysiological research on EEG cortical dynamics investigated both in the domain of amplitudes and frequencies with linear measures, and with nonlinear measures that capture the dynamical complexity of the system and the mutual synchronization across cortical areas. The power spectral analysis measures the event-related de-synchronization (ERD) and synchronization (ERS) – in other words, the decrease and the increase in power distribution (Pfurtscheller and Lopes da Silva, 1999). It was consistently found that emotion induced significant alpha, theta and beta ERD as respect to neutral processing, indicating an higher level of the overall cortical activations (Krause et al., 2000), with topographical effects dependent on the valence in prefrontal and posterior regions (Aftanas et al., 2001; Aftanas et al., 1998b; Aftanas et al., 2004). Emotional states were found to exert a significant impact on EEG coherence (Tucker and Dawson, 1984; Hinrichs and Machleidt, 1992), a linear measure based on the cross- and auto-correlations of power spectral densities (Thatcher et al., 1986) and, hence, on the Fourier transform that disregards the non linear properties of EEG signal. The recent discoveries of the properties of the new nonlinear measures have producing a renewed interest in the EEG response during emotions, in order to complete the neurobiological models formulated on the basis of high spatial resolution neuroimaging techniques. Interesting findings were gathered by non-linear measures that detect the dynamical complexity of the system. Emotional stimulations were associated with a more posterior increase in dimension when compared with perceptual tasks (Aftanas et al., 1994). The dimensional complexity was proven to increase with emotional arousal, whereas no specific changes were clearly associated with emotional valence (Aftanas et al., 1997a). The estimates of nonlinear forecasting and chaoticness were shown to be associated with higher EEG predictability in posterior regions during negative emotion; in turn, the dynamical complexity increased over posterior areas during positive emotions and decreased over frontal areas (Aftanas et al., 1997b). It was claimed that dynamical complexity decreases as the brain processes become more bound to low degrees of freedom and that this effects could be due to the subcortical activation and vertical synchronization (Aftanas et al., 1998b). On this basis the findings obtained by EEG nonlinear analyses are surprisingly consistent with those obtained by neuroimaging studies referring both to localization and functional integration approach. In particular high arousing and negative emotions were found to induce an increased activity in the posterior perceptual cortical areas, such as the extrastriate cortex (Lang et al., 1998b; Surguladze et al., 2003). In a previous work (Costa et al, 2006) we investigated the patterns of EEG synchronization in response to positive and negative emotional film stimuli and we found differences in cortical activity related not only to the emotional arousal, but also to the emotional valence.

The findings collected so far consistently sustain that the enhancement of dynamical complexity could be an important functional mechanism to process emotion. The future investigations on how the neural networks become coupled and decoupled should represent a crucial issue to understand the functional organization of emotions in the brain. Nonetheless, several questions remain to be answered, in particular with reference to which effects could be attributed to different type of emotions. The most of the studies were concerned with dimensional models, disregarding more specific differences related to basic emotions with the same valence or arousal, as well as to emotions associated to approach and withdrawal systems.

## Objectives and Hypotheses

The present study addressed to investigate the neural synchronization on a large scale during emotional and non emotional processing and to evaluate the specific neural dynamics related to different basic emotions. The main goal was twofold: first, we intended to assess the nonlinear phase synchronization change generally associated with emotional processing; second, we intended to evaluate the synchronization patterns induced by specific basic emotions, in order to disambiguate whether the neural distinctions could be ascribed to the valence dimension or there were more subtle differences that could be better explained by the discrete models or by approach – whitdrawal system theory.

To accomplish these goals, phase synchronization was estimated by the synchronization index (SI) on EEG response to emotional film clips of fear, happiness and sadness. In addition, psychometrical ratings were collected after the experimental conditions, in order to acquire information about self-reported emotional experience and the subjective quality of emotion. The basic emotions investigated highly differ both for the specific biological function, as it was claimed by discrete models of emotion, for their valence and arousal values on the dimensional space, and for their association with approach and withdrawal systems. Hence they allow to compare the predictions drawn from the different models of emotion.

One of the main advantages of EEG measures is their ability to allow the estimation of the functional state different frequency bands with specific functional value: the reduction or desynchronization of alpha activity (8-12 Hz) is known to be a marker of the general brain activation occurring when subjects become engaged in mental tasks (Pfurtscheller and Lopes da Silva, 1999); theta rhythm (4-7 Hz) is particularly interesting for research on emotion, for its limbic origin and its association with the cortico-hippocampal-limbic interactions (Basar et al., 1999; Basar et al., 2001); delta rhythm (0,5-4 Hz) was generally associated to a decrease of the functional state of the brain, but recently it was reported that delta power increased as subjects processed emotional stimuli (Aftanas et al., 2004); a desynchronization of the beta rhythm(13-30 Hz) that is mainly generated in the motor cortex, was observed during the motor tasks (Basar et al., 2001), as well as during emotional processing (Aftanas et al., 1998b). For each of these frequency bands the fast Fourier-based power distribution was calculated in order to have a basic information on the cortical activation, and then the nonlinear synchronization analysis was performed in order to acquire information on the more subtle dynamics underlying the emotional response.

On the basis of the theoretical and empirical backgrounds, the main hypotheses to test were that: (a) significant changes of synchronized activity occurred during emotional processing as respect to non emotional processing; (b) the valenced emotions and the basic emotions differed in their synchronized activity within the functionally specific frequency bands and with topographical effects involving in particular frontal and occipital regions, that previous researches found to be relevant structures underlying emotion.

A neural correlate of valence dimension should be reflected in differences between happiness and the two negative emotions included in the study, sadness and fear. On the contrary, if there are more specific patterns of synchronized activity correlated with the arousal, we should find primarily differences between emotional and neutral stimuli processing, with a greater distinctions related to an highly arousing and activating emotion like fear. Otherwise, the distinctions among emotions, in particular between the two negative emotion of fear and sadness, may indicate that the discrete and dissociable systems, could reflect more subtle aspects of synchronization change, not fully reducible to more general dimensions. and of the functional basis of human emotion.

# Method

## Participants

Thirty-one healthy, right-handed (as measured by Edimburgh Handedness Inventory (Oldfield, 1971) volunteers participated in the experiment (16 males, 15 females), ranging in age from 20 to 30 years (mean $\pm$ S.D. age, 24.5 $\pm$ 2.4). All subjects underwent a physical evaluation to screen out chronic diseases, mental disorders, medication, head injury, drug or alcohol abuse. All had normal or corrected to normal vision.

The study was carried out in accordance with the Declaration of Helsinki principles, approved by the ethics committee of the University of Turin. All subjects gave written, informed consent and were informed of their right to discontinue participation at any time.

## Film Stimuli

Stimuli consisted of 48 sequences (10 sec long) representing different emotional scenarios of happiness, sadness, fear and neutral content (12 per condition). The stimuli were extracted from commercial films and then edited in order to exclude any element that differs from the target emotional content. In a pilot study the stimuli were validated by 30 judges that rated each clip on a 9-point Likert scale for the valence and arousal level and for the intensity of the basic emotions subjectively experienced. The happiness sequences depicted lovers' encounters, amusement scenes and successful moments. The sadness sequences depicted scenes of death, loss, sickness and sorrow. The fear sequences depicted people's or animals' aggressions and dangerous situations such as falling down and drowning. The neutral sequences depicted a series of routine actions. All the stimuli were in color and were presented without sound and balanced in relation to the presence of human beings and complexity.

## Self-Report of Emotional Experience

A self-report was used to assess the subjective emotional response to film stimuli. Subjects had to rate the pleasantness of their own emotional experience on a 9-point Likert scale ranging to 1 (very unpleasant) to 9 (very pleasant) and the arousal level from 1 (not at all, very calm) to 9 (fully experienced emotion, very excited). Finally, they indicated the intensity of the emotional state they experienced on a rating scale, including five primary emotions in random order: happiness, sadness, anger, fear, and disgust (from 1 indicating that the emotion was not at all present, to 9 indicating that it was felt very strongly).

## Procedures

The subjects were seated on comfortable chairs in the recording room and they were told to look at the TV screen placed in front of them both during the film clips and the black screen which separated each sequence.

Stimuli were presented in a block design with a regular baseline between each block. The experiment included 16 blocks including three stimuli of the same condition. Hence, there were 8 blocks for the 4 experimental conditions of neutral, happiness, sadness and fear, presented in two subsequent runs. Each run included two blocks of the same conditions. Stimuli were randomly assigned to blocks and run in random order both among and within subjects. An optimized random sequence was obtained with the restriction that no more than one block of the same condition was repeated in succession.

The experiment began with a 30-second baseline recording of resting EEG, followed by the emotional film clips in random order. Each trial consisted of: (1) a brief time (200 msec.) when a cross appeared on the screen; (2) one experimental block including three clips of the same emotional condition; (3) a 30 sec. post-film rest period.

At the end of the experimental session after a resting period, the subjects were asked to view again the stimuli and to rate the pleasantness level, the arousal or excitement level and the intensity level of the basic emotion experienced during a vision of each stimulus.

## Recordings and Data Pre-Processing

EEG was recorded from 19 sites (Fp1, Fp2, F7, F8, F3, F4, Fz, C3, C4, Cz, T3, T4, T5,T6, P3, P4, Pz, O1, O2), which refer to a ground electrode to the center of the forehead.

EEG and EOG signals were amplified by a multi-channel bio-signal amplifier (bandpass 0.3-70 Hz) and A/D converted at 256 Hz per channel with a 12-bit resolution. The impedance of recording electrodes was monitored for each subject prior to data collection and the threshold was always kept below 5 KOhms. EEG data was pre-processed using ICA (Independent Component Analysis) (Jung et al., 1998) removing artifacts from the traces. ICA is generally applicable for removal of a wide variety of EEG artifacts. It simultaneously separates the EEG and its artifacts into independent components based on the statistics of the data. ICA does this without relying on the availability of one or more reference channels for each type of artifact. This avoids the problem of the potential mutual contamination of regressing and regressed channels. We applied the ICA to remove ocular artifacts. We discarded all the distinct artifactual components through visual inspection. After the ICA-component removing process, a second stage of visual inspection of the EEG data was conducted. If any further artifact was present, the data was discarded. Then, data was band-pass filtered with a forward reverse filtering algorithm in the following five frequency-bands of interest: delta (0.5-3), theta (4-7 Hz), alpha (8-12 Hz) and beta (13-30 Hz).

## Extraction of Instantaneous Phase at Different Oscillations

Two signals are said to be synchronous if their rhythms coincide. In its classical sense, the term synchrony has been applied to the signal that had a dominant oscillatory mode around a chosen frequency $f$. Such a signal $x(t)$ can be written in the frequency domain as:

$$\widetilde{x}(f,t) = |\widetilde{x}(f,t)| \exp(i\phi(f,t))$$

in which the instantaneous amplitude $a(t)$ and phase $\phi(t)$ of $x(t)$ appear as separated entities. From this equation the amplitude of the signal is the absolute value of the spectro-temporal representation and the phase as the complex argument:

$$\varphi(f,t) = \arg(\widetilde{x}(f,t))$$

Phase synchronization is usually defined as the locking of the phase of two oscillators:

$$\varphi_{x,y} = n\phi_x(t) - m\phi_y(t) = const$$

where $n$ and $m$ are integers. Rosenblum et al.(1996) replaced this condition of phase locking by the weaker condition of phase entrainment:

$$|\varphi_{x,y}| = |n\phi_x(t) - m\phi_y(t)| < const$$

To investigate whether two systems show phase synchronization, it is first necessary to know their phase variables. This is non-trivial for many non-linear model systems and even more difficult when dealing with noisy time-series of unknown origin. In this work we have used the wavelet method to determine the phase of an arbitrary signal *x(t)*. Specifically, let *x(t)* be an EEG signal, then the wavelet transform is:

$$W(f,t) = \int_{-\infty}^{+\infty} x(t)\psi^{*}_{f,t}(u)du$$

where $\psi^{*}_{f,t}(u)$ is the complex conjugate of the Morlet wavelet defined by:

$$\psi_{f,t} = \sqrt{f}\exp(i2\pi f(u-t))\exp(-\frac{(u-t)^2}{2\sigma^2})$$

A good estimator of the degree of phase synchronization is the synchronization index (SI) (Rosemblum et al., 2001a; Rosemblum et al., 2001b) defined as:

$$\gamma^2_{n,m} = \langle\cos\phi_{n,m}(t)\rangle^2 + \langle\sin\phi_{n,m}(t)\rangle^2$$

where the brackets denote the average over time; it varies from 0 to 1. The advantage of this index, with respect to other ones (Rodriguez et al., 1999), is that its computation involves no parameters. In this study the changes of SI patterns were analyzed during responses to emotional-laden external stimulation, using non-emotional and emotional film stimuli differentiated for valence.

# Data Analysis and Results

## Behavioral Results

Figure 1 depicts the mean values and the standard deviation of the self reported valence and arousal attributed by subjects to the emotional and neutral stimuli. The ratings of pleasantness and arousal were submitted to repeated measures analyses of variance with condition as within-subject factor (4 levels: happiness, fear, sadness and neutral). The pleasantness resulted to be significantly different among conditions ($F(3, 54)= 47.76$; $p<0.05$), as well as the arousal ($F(2.3,54)= 38.97$; $p<0.05$). Mean comparisons performed as post-hoc analysis, using Bonferroni correction for multiple comparisons, showed that pleasantness was significantly higher for happiness as respect to all the other conditions ($p<.001$). The post-hoc analysis on arousal ratings showed that the significance of the overall model was due to differences between emotional conditions and neutral conditions ($p<.001$), whereas there were no significant differences among the specific emotions.

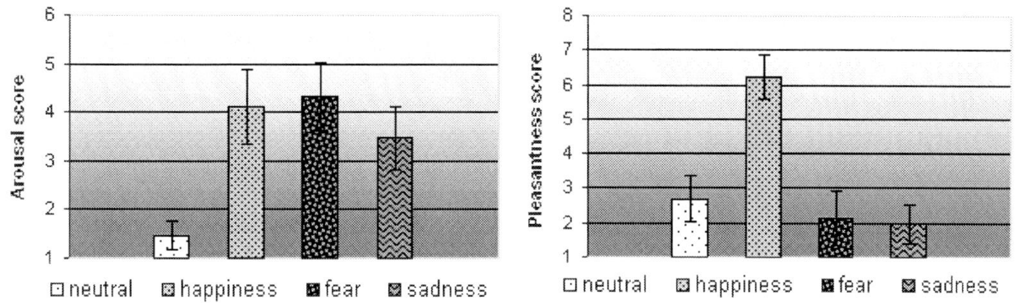


Figure 1. Mean and standard deviation of self-reported arousal (left panel) and pleasantness (right panel) of subjectively experienced emotion during the vision of the four categories of film clips.

In order to evaluate the validity of experimental conditions, a further ANOVA was performed on intensity scores given to basic emotions included in the scale, expecting that the target emotion was to be experienced more intensely than all the others. Two within-subjects factors were entered in the model: Condition (4 levels: neutral, happiness, fear, and sadness) and Emotion (5 levels: happiness, fear, anger, disgust and sadness). Results revealed a significant interaction effect of Condition X Emotion ($F(6.6; 79.4) = 65.54$, $p < .001$, $\eta^2 = .84$), confirming that the emotions more intensely experienced during the vision of the stimuli were the expected ones ($p < 0.001$, Bonferroni corrected).

## EEG Power Distribution Results

The spectral power ($\mu V^2$) was estimated on the artefact free EEG signals segmented in overlapped epoch (1 s. each), through the Fast Fourier Transform (FFT), using a Hamming window.

Power values within each epoch were averaged, converted to power density ($\mu V^2$/Hz) and grouped into the frequency ranges of interest: delta (0,5–4), theta (4–7 Hz), alpha (8–12 Hz) and beta (13–30 Hz). A log-transformation was performed on the row data in order to normalize the distribution, then the values were averaged across the different recording sites, obtaining five clusters corresponding to regional means of interest: frontal (F), central (C), temporal (T), parietal (P) and occipital (O). In addition, two clusters were obtained to perform the analysis of frontal lateralization: right frontal ($_{R}F$) and left frontal ($_{L}F$). The averaged power distribution across the respective electrode sites were calculated for these regional means for the three frequency bands of interest and each film category. These data were then entered in the subsequent statistical analyses.

In order to test the change between conditions across the different cortical areas, a 4 X 5 repeated measure ANOVA was performed including two factors within subjects: Condition (4 levels: neutral, happiness, sadness and fear) and Localization (5 levels: frontal, central, temporal, parietal and occipital). When the sphericity assumption was not met, the Huynh-Feldt correction on degree of freedom was adopted. As expected a mean effect of Frequency was significant $F(3;72)=93.69$; $p<.001$; $\eta^2=.8$). Further, highly significant results were found for the mean effect of Condition $F(1.6;38.49)=11.65$; $p<.001$; $\eta^2=.33$), Localization

$F(2.33;72)=4.22$; $p<.05$; $\eta^2=.15$) and, more interesting, the interaction effect of Condition X Frequency $F(6.3;152.7)=5.71$; $p<.001$; $\eta^2=.2$), indicating that the specific basic emotion induced a change in cortical activation, as it is depicted in figure 2.

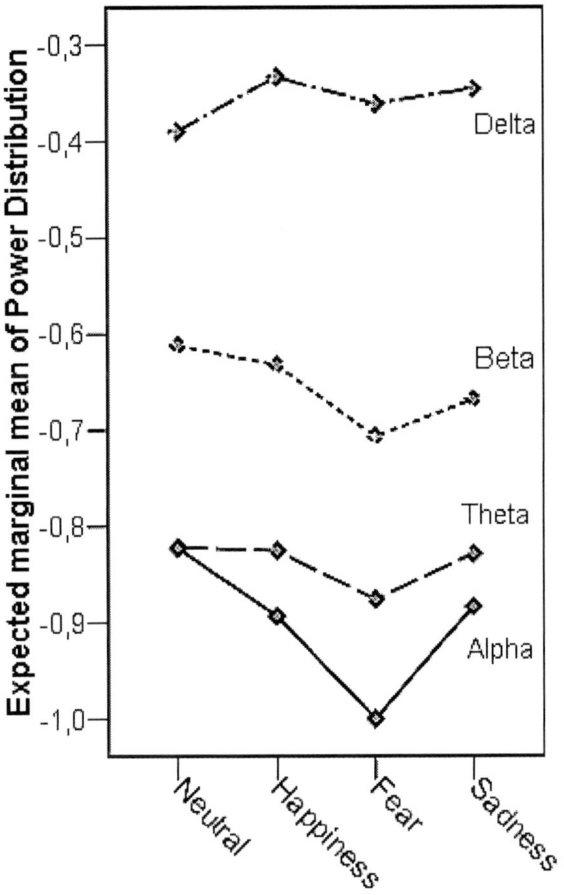


Figure 2. Expected marginal mean of the power distribution ($\mu V^2$) at the different frequency rhythms associated with processing neutral and emotional stimuli.

## EEG Phase Synchronization Results

The SI was calculated at each frequency band between each electrode paired to all other electrodes, obtaining a synchronization matrix for each subject and each condition. The statistical analysis was performed independently for the different frequency bands on the synchronization matrices for all the couples of channel locations, entering the SI values into repeated-measures ANOVAs with Condition as within-subject factor (4 levels: neutral, sadness, happiness and fear). The main effect of Condition was found to be statistically significant for a number of frontal and posterior couples of electrodes. The couples of electrodes that significantly differed among conditions are depicted in figure 3.

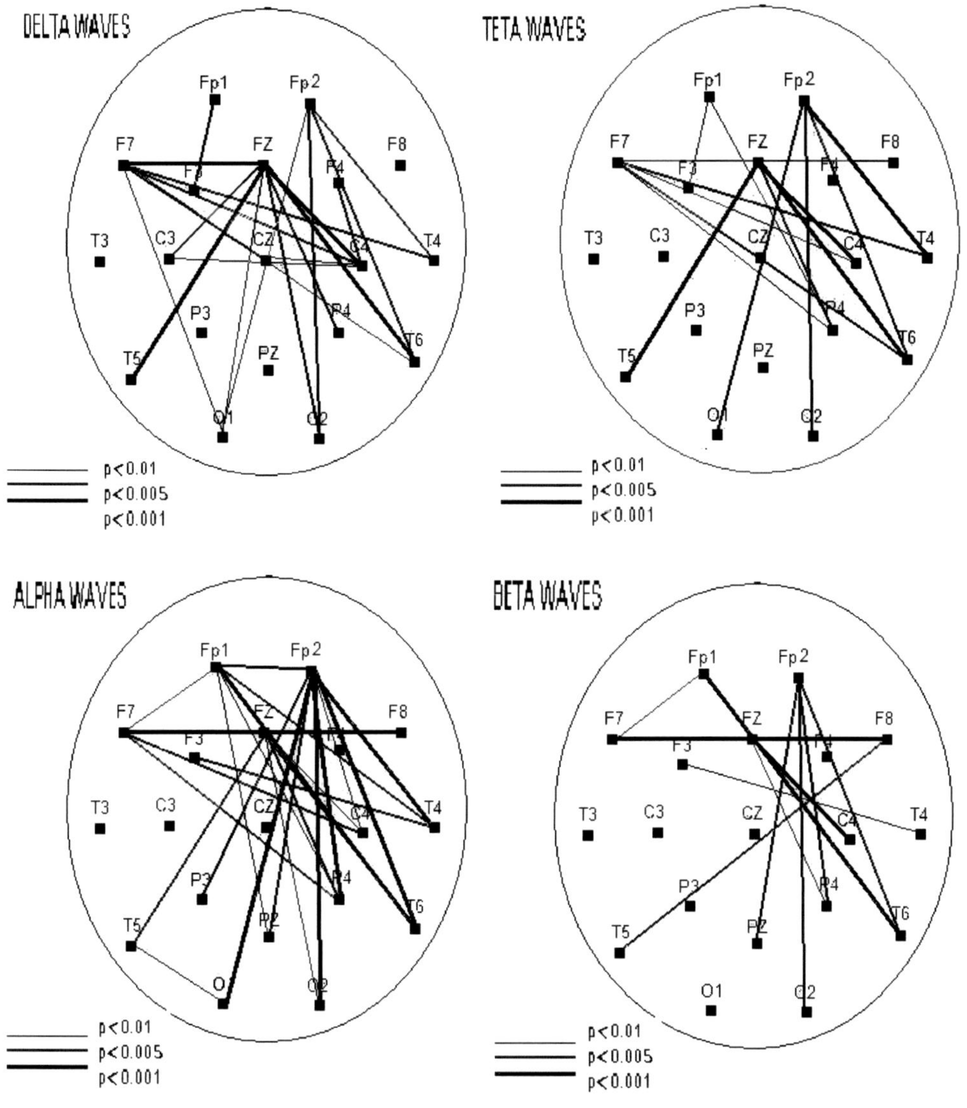


Figure 3. Images depicted the couples of electrodes whose synchronization index resulted to significantly differ among the four film clips categories at each frequency band in response. The different thickness of lines indicates the significance level of the F ratio.

Following, in order to assess the differences between conditions that contributed to the overall significance of the ANOVA models, post-hoc analyses were performed using the paired Tukey Test, that corrects for the multiple comparisons. Figure 4 depicts the synchronization patterns that resulted to be specifically associated with each emotion contrasted with neutral and figure 5 depicts the significant differences emerged from contrasts performed between the emotions.

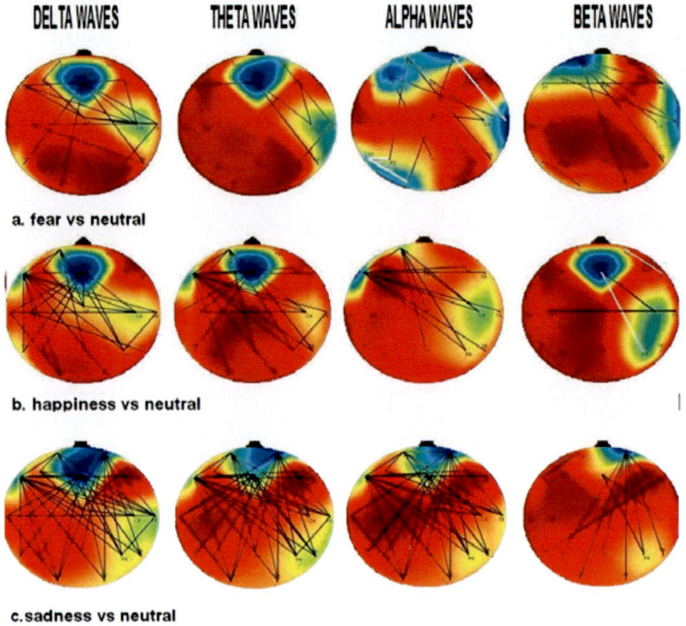


Figure 4. Map series representing significant (p<0.005) increases of SI between couples of electrodes associated with each emotion contrasted with neutral at different bands. Black lines represent a greater SI for neutral condition, while white SI represent a greater SI for emotional condition except for [a] at beta band in which SI is lower in the neutral condition respect to the fear stimuli.

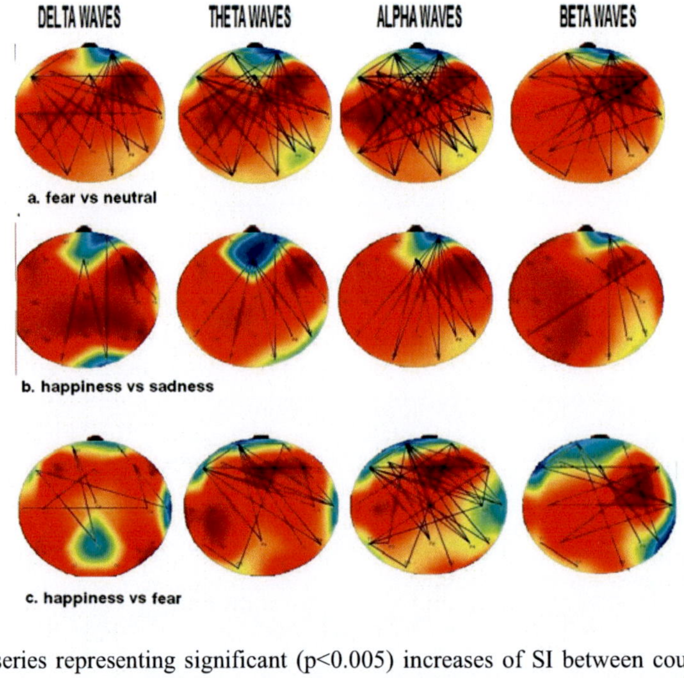


Figure 5. Map series representing significant (p<0.005) increases of SI between couples of electrodes associated with each emotion contrasted with others at different bands. The lines represent a greater SI

for [a] fear contrasted with sadness; [b] happiness contrasted with sadness and [c] fear contrasted with happiness.

## Discussion

The present work addressed to investigate the phase synchronization change across the local and distal EEG sites in response to film-induced basic emotions, differentiated for their valence and action tendency, in order to test which models of emotion best predicted the dynamical coupling and decoupling patterns.

The preliminary analysis on the self-reported emotional response and on the power distribution confirmed that our stimuli were able to induce the expected emotions, as well as to elicit change in the neural activity at the different frequency bands across all the cortical areas. In particular, the alpha rhythm, whose reduction is known to be a marker of the brain activation, significantly decreased during all the emotion as respect to neutral: fear resulted in the higher activation; happiness and sadness were associated with a mean level, whereas neutral response was associated to the lower level of brain activation. The observed alpha power change across conditions reflected the typical arousal level that the dimensional model ascribed to the three basic emotions here investigated (Russell, 1880). Beta and theta power also showed the expected patterns of reduction during emotion and in particular in fear. This effect was elsewhere reported (e.g., Aftanas et al., 1998b) and it was explained as a product of the cortical desynchronization induced by subcortical activity change induced by emotion (Davidson, 1990).

As respect to the power distribution analysis that informs on the quantitative brain activation change during mental engagement, the synchronization index (SI) informs on the qualitative change concerning the interconnecting patterns among different neural networks. The nonlinear analysis on synchronization deals with states in state space and not with amplitudes, power and frequencies and states may provide more information on the underlying system than amplitudes (Stam, 2005).

The present SI analysis turned out to detect at each frequency bands several significant synchronization changes during emotional and non emotional film-induction, involving local and distal couples of electrodes corresponding to different cortical regions.

In order to interpret the obtained results and compare them with previous findings, the notion of synchronization needs a clarification, as well as its relationship with the notion of dynamical complexity, that was the property more diffusely investigated in the literature on emotion. More than one meaning has been ascribed so far to complexity: nonetheless, all nonlinear analyses measures the complexity defined as degrees of freedom (or randomness) in a large system of interacting elements (Tononi et al., 1998). It refers to the lack of interactions between the elements of a dynamical system, exiting in an enhancement of the unpredictability and chaoticness of time series. As regard to a functional network, it is related to the lack of correlations between its functional sources. So, the higher the level of synchronization between functional sources in a functional network, the lower its dynamical complexity (Stam, 2005).

Like other non-linear measures of dynamical interaction, such as the Mutual Dimension (Dm), SI increases indicated an enhanced interaction between two dynamical systems or spatially separated cortical regions, corresponding to a lower dynamical complexity.

Conversely, SI decrease indicates that two dynamical system become functionally separated and process more independently the information (higher dynamical complexity). A further information could be extracted from the number of synchronization changes (both increase and decrease) centred around a specific electrode, named "center of gravity" or "main processing node", whose corresponding cortical region is thought to play a specific functional role in the mental task examined (see Aftanas et al. 1998a).

Accounting for these meanings of SI, results from the present study evidenced that each emotion, compared with neutral, was accompanied by a significant decrease of synchronization across several cortical regions, indicating that the emotional processing induced an higher dynamical complexity in the EEG signals. This effect was observed at alpha, theta and delta frequency bands and it could be ascribed to the general emotional arousal. Interestingly, the significant changes mainly occurred within the frontal sites and between the frontal and occipital sites, that recent neuroimaging studies demonstrated to be associated with emotional arousal (Murphy et al., 2003; Phan et al., 2002).

According with the hypothesis stated by the authors and with the expectations drawn from the theoretical background, the observed SI changes support the view that coupling-decoupling patterns between different neural networks could be a relevant neural mechanism underlying the emotional processing and that emotion induces an increase of complexity in the cortical dynamics. This result is quietly consistent with previous evidences on the dynamical complexity of EEG response to positive and negative film-induced emotions. Aftanas and co-workers found that the Dimensional Complexity (DCx), that measures the global complexity's degree of EEG dynamics reconstructed in state space (Elbert et al.,1994), increased during both positive and negative emotional stimuli processing, as respect to neutral; furthermore, authors found that DCx positively correlated with the self-reported emotional arousal (Aftanas et al., 1998b). Similar results were obtained with different classes of nonlinear measures, such as: i) the Lyapunov exponents, that inform on the dynamical properties of the system orbiting within the attractor (Elbert et al. 1994), providing an estimate of the mean exponential divergence or convergence of nearby trajectories in phase space and expressing the sensitive dependence of the system on initial conditions (Rosenstein et al. 1993); ii) the Kolmogorov entropy metric (K2), that evaluates the degree of "chaoticness" of the system, or the average rate at which information is generated by the system, or, equivalently, the rate at which current information about system is lost (Schouten et al. 1994); iii) nonlinear forecasting, that measures the deterministic structure of the time series, through an average analysis of the temporal variations of structures in the phase space, evaluating the loss of information during the system's evolution or, in other words, quantifying the memory loss of the past states during the evolution of the system.

The Kolmogorov entropy and the principal Lyapunov exponent (L1) were found to increase after viewing positive or negative movies compared to neutral movies, indicating an enhancement of cortical dynamics during emotion, independently on valence (Aftanas et al., 1997b). The same increase of dimensional complexity with emotional arousal was also observed with different emotional induction procedures, such as the memory for personal pain (Lutzenberger et al., 1997). An enhancement of complexity was also found during the emotional imagery when compared with a cognitive task, like mental arithmetic calculus

(Birbaumer et al., 1993), as a further suggestion that this effect could reflect, up to a certain level, an emotion-specific brain mechanism.

The results presented in this chapter and the previous findings converge to sustain that the neural information processing of non emotional stimuli was linked to an higher extend of degrees of freedom and, hence, to an higher predictability, while emotional processing is accompanied by an higher unpredictability and complexity of EEG signals, reflected in decreased cortical synchronization. Such a decoupling effect indicates that, at the cortical level, emotion was processed by more independent, parallel and active neural processes, involving more separated neural assemblies: it is arguable that an enlarging of the overall chaoticness, able to generate information at an higher rate, could be a functional mechanism necessary to process the salient value of emotional stimuli. Furthermore, it was underscored that decreased interconnections at the cortical level could indicate an enhancement of the functional connectivity between the given cortical area and subcortical regions (Aftanas et al. 1998b; Davidson, 1990), as well as of the vertical integration typical of emotion (Lewis, 2005). The subcortical information exchange is diffusely described during emotion by neuroimaging studies and increasing evidences have been recently collecting applying the dynamical causal model (e.g. Williams et al., 2006). In turn, processing a visual stimulus without an emotional salience could be more strongly constrained to the low degrees of freedom that characterize the information exchange among neural pathways involved at the cortical level in the perceptual object recognition.

Besides the emotional arousal effect, the present SI analysis succeeded also in detecting different synchronization patterns, at least in part specific for the basic emotions examined, as emerged from the synchronization maps associated with each single emotion contrasted with neutral, as well as from the significant contrasts between happiness, sadness and fear. The differences were both quantitative, referring to decrease or increase of SI, and qualitative, referring to the couples of electrodes involved in the SI patterns. The emotion-related effects mainly regarded (i) inter-hemispheric interactions, (ii) rostro-caudal interactions, and (iii) frontal lateralization effects.

Sadness was the emotion with the lower synchronized activity, happiness showed to be more synchronized than sadness, and fear showed the higher synchronized activity. At alpha frequency bands, and rather similarly, at delta and theta, the synchronization analyses showed that happiness and sadness, when compared with neutral, induced a wide number of significant decreases of the dynamical coupling within the left frontal region, between righ and left frontal regions and between the frontal and occipital regions. In turn, fear appeared not specifically associated with the left frontal and inter-hemispheric patterns, whereas it showed a specific change in right frontal sites.

Sadness specifically involved an overall ipsi-and controlateral decoupling across the frontal-parietal-occipital pathways, that was not observed, or there was at a lesser extend, in happiness and fear. This rostro-caudal effect was more pronounced at alpha band, with a main processing node in Fp2 and, at a lesser extend, in F7. Differently, happiness showed a specific rostro-caudal decoupling involving a more anterior left laterizated pathway (Fp1-Pz), with processing nodes in Fp1 and F7. Direct comparisons between happiness and sadness resulted in distinct patterns within the right frontal loci and between the frontal and posterior sites with right-sided processing nodes. As regard to the inter-hemispheric synchronization, sadness showed to produce a decoupling between the more anterior sites, such as the prefrontal loci Fp1-Fp2; conversely, happiness involved more posterior frontal sites and fear did not show to be associated with this network.

Fear appeared highly dissociable both from sadness and happiness, also presenting variation across the different frequency bands. At the delta and theta band, fear showed a restricted rostro-caudal desynchronization pattern and a specific right frontal pattern (F4-Cz). More interestingly, at the alpha band fear showed a specific effect of increased synchronization within the left posterior region (T5-P3 and T5-01), when compared to neutral, that did not occurred in happiness or in sadness (nor SI decrease or increase). This alpha synchronization pathway indicates lower degrees of freedom in posterior temporal and occipital areas during fear, that could be reconducted to a full visual elaboration of a stimulus with an high adaptive value.

At the beta band, fear response resulted highly different from happiness, sadness and neutral response, showing a specific increase of synchronization, involving short-distance interconnections within the right frontal regions, within posterior regions, as well as long-distance inter-hemispheric and rostro-caudal interconnections. The widely distributed EEG beta activity was found to be functionally related to increased alertness and cognitive processes (Steriade, 1999) and to emotional response, showing a desynchronization effect, in particular during highly aorusing negative emotions (Aftanas et al., 2006; Aftanas et al., 1998b). A circumscribed centrally distributed cortical beta rhythm was proven to be strongly related to motor functions and to originate from primary motor cortex (Pfurtscheller and Lopes da Silva, 1999), as well as from the supplementary motor area (Pfurtscheller et al., 2003). The emotional response of fear is strictly associated with the adaptive action tendency, that allows to face off a threath and achieve a safety condition. Considering this impelling/urgent adaptative value, the neural pathway of fear could necessarily reclutate the motor areas to prepare the movement, succeeding in cortical dynamics characterized by an higher predictability of information processing and a decreased complexity. A role of the motor component is sustained by the evidence that the significant contrasts involved the sites closed to the motor cortex (F8-F7, Fz-C4, Fp1 and F3 with T4). Furthermore, SI change during happiness, that is related to the behavioural activation as fear, showed a similar pattern of increased synchrony at beta band, although limited to the right prefrontal region (Fp2 -F8 and Fz-C4), whereas sadness, that is associated to behavioural inhibition, did not.

With regards topographical differences, previous studies reported that positive emotion induced a lower dynamical complexity over frontocortical regions, and an increase over posterior regions, whereas an opposite pattern was found for negative emotions, with a complexity increase over frontocortical regions, and a decrease over posterior regions (Aftanas et al., 1997b). Investigations on Dm reported that during positive emotion the central, parietal and posterior temporal areas became more coupled. In contrast, negative emotions produced a general dynamical decoupling over posterior regions, indicating that they were processed by more independent cortical networks (Aftanas et al., 1998a).

The present SI analysis on EEG response to happiness, sadness and fear just in part matched these findings: the increased complexity during positive emotions compared with negative was replicated considering the contrast between happiness and fear, while sadness clearly elicited a wider desynchronization. The wide posterior decoupling was instead observed during sadness, but not during fear. Hence, the present study succeeded in finding significant differences between emotions with the same valence: sadness and fear extensevely differed, but these specific patterns could not be detected in the perspective of dimensional models; rather they emerge when a more subtle distinction between basic emotions is done in the perspective of the discrete models.

The evidence that specific basic emotions with the same valence induce different EEG response could explain some of the divergences across the results collected so far. Most of the studies used video-clips with an highly arousing and aversive content (usually burn victims) inducing negative emotions linked to the withdrawal system and, in the basic emotion perspective, similar to fear and/or disgust. This type of stimuli are very different from ours, as well as the type of emotion induced. The negative emotion previously studied was similar enough, but not at all, to our film-induced fear. In fear, but not in sadness, we observed the similar synchronization increase (or dynamical complexity decrease) that previous studies found for negative emotion. Nonetheless, the present SI analysis did not find the topographical effect described elsewhere. The decreased dynamical complexity of negative emotion over frontocortical regions have been explained with the higher attentional constraints that negative emotion may put on the frontocortical activity: according to this hypothesis, the attentional resources should be allocated to process the attractive stimuli inducing pleasant emotion and retained from the aversive stimuli that subjects attempt to withdraw (Aftanas et al., 1997a; 1998a).

An alternative interpretative hypothesis refers to the different adaptive value of emotions and to their evolutionary hystory. For its basic role in the survival, fear is though to be one of the most ancient emotion: the neural substrates should be highly conserved along the evolutionary history and shared by several species as evolutionary homology (Panksepp, 1998). The adaptive value of a stimulus is evaluated by innate neural circuits underpinning the fear response, and this automatic appraisal process could be linked to more restrained processing patterns. Automatic processing pathways could imply a lesser extend of degrees of freedom of the information processing, explaining the higher synchronization and a lower dynamical complexity. Conversely, the neural substrates of happiness and sadness could be thought as more recent and more differentiated among the species, and in particular in the human beings: these two emotions could also linked to a more complex process for appraisal of the stimuli, more linked to a integration with memories and, in particular, with symbolic knowledge stored in the system (Leventhal and Scherer, 1987).

The lower frontal synchronization, and the higher complexity, of happiness and sadness, not observed in fear, suggest that these two emotions, especially sadness, could involve a larger evaluation component mediated by frontal cortex. Several findings from neuroimaging research reported that frontal regions are involved in the evaluation processes of an emotional response and in the emotional regulation through "top – down" connectivity circuits (Miller and Cohen, 2001).

Because of the urgent adaptive value of fear response, this emotion could not be necessarily linked to the evaluation process mediated by higher-level structures, such as frontal cortex, but it could be primarily elaborated by the subcortical structures such as the amygdala, as it was described by LeDoux (2000). In the present study, the film sequencies of fear depicted scenarios of danger and threath with a tipically evolutionary value, so that it could be expected that these stimuli induced an automatic elaboration in the subcortical structures with a diminished intervent of the more recent structures, like the frontal lobes. The scenarios of happiness and sadness sequences could have a more complex content that requested wider processing resources, exiting in more complex EEG dynamics.

Considering the present SI results as a whole, it has to be underscored the difference found between the two negative emotions included in the study and the higher similarity between sadness and happiness as respect to fear. In particular happiness and fear shared left-sided frontal synchronization pathways and frontal inter-hemispheric interconnections, whereas highly differed in the rostro-caudal pathways, with happiness more synchronized than sadness. The approach-withdrawal model of emotion could explain the observed dissociation between fear, on one side, and happiness and sadness, on the other side, instead of the dimensional model. Although the two models have been often overlapped reporting positive emotions to approach system and negative emotions to withdrawal system, there were some relevant differences. For example, the negative emotion of anger is associated with an approach tendency, as well as sadness is associated with a de-activation of the approach system (Davidson and Irwing, 1999; Davidson, 2003).

The present findings matched the predictions from this model of emotion: happiness and sadness were mediated by a frontal pattern that respectively showed an increase and decrease of synchronized activity. Interestingly, the lateralization pattern emerged in the present analysis is coherent with the hypothesis of a role of the left frontal region in the approach emotions, while the right frontal region would be involved in the withdrawal emotions: sadness and happiness showed several significant SI change with processing node in the left frontal hemisphere; on turn, fear showed processing nodes in the right hemisphere (mainly F4 and then Fp2).

Our results also showed that fear was associated with a larger involvement of the posterior regions in front of the larger involvement of anterior lobes in sadness and happiness, sustaining the hypothesis of a deeper involvement of the high order evaluation processes, while fear appears to be associated with a low-order sensory-motor evaluation.

Future research could advance these discoveries by including more differentiated emotions in the experimental designs, and comparing discrete emotions with the same valence. Further investigations could be concerned with disgust (negative emotion of withdrawal system) and anger (negative emotion of approach system) to disentangled the functional organization of emotion in the brain predicted by theoretical models.

## Conclusion

As far as we know, the present study is the first that investigated EEG cortical responses to emotional stimulation, using the Synchronization Index as a measure of the synchronized activity within the different frequency bands. The SI index here proposed contributes to the view of nonlinear interaction process occurring in cortical activity during emotional processing: SI had been shown to be sensitive to detecting the change in cortical dynamics related to emotional processing, differentiating the neural response induced by emotional arousal, by the emotional valence and in particular by specific basic emotions.

Results of this study support the view that synchronization provides an interesting and useful tool for studying and more deeply understanding the variation in brain activity that occurs during mental processes. Moreover, it was demonstrated that synchronization change could be considered as a relevant and necessary neural mechanism to generate emotion. The application of SI analysis to the EEG has been shown to offer information beyond that provided by linear EEG measures, as well as by nonlinear measures that estimate complexity from the individual signal. A meaningful information about cortical networks functioning in relation to emotion can be obtained, and it seems to be necessary for a deep understanding of neural activity underlying emotion.

If we consider the complex nature of emotion, which involves several biological systems as well as several neural circuits at different cerebral levels, we can conclude that synchronization seems to be a relevant topic for this field of research.

The results presented in this chapter also show the importance of investigating basic emotion, with respect to the more diffusely studied emotional valence dimension. It is arguable that the valence-specific effect expected on the basis of the dimensional model of emotion do not fully explain the data. The alternative model of approach-withdrawal better fits the present data as well as the model of discrete emotions. It is possible that there are brain mechanisms underlying the valence-process and that these mechanisms are further differentiated with respect to the specific kinds of emotion. Following our results, we can conclude that the model of basic emotions is more suitable than the dimensional model.

# References

Aftanas, L.I., Koshkarov, V.I., Mordvintsev, Y.N., and Pokrovskaja, V.L., (1994). Dimensional analysis of human EEG during experimental affective experience. *International Journal of Psychophysiology*, Volume: 18, pp. 67-70.

Aftanas, L.I., Lotova, N.V., Koshkarov, V.I., Pokrovskaja, V.L., Popov, S.A., and Makhnev, V.P., (1997a). Non-linear analysis of emotion EEG: calculation of Kolmogorov entropy and the principal Lyapunov exponent. *Neuroscience Letters*, Volume: 226, pp. 13-16.

Aftanas, L.I., Lotova, N.V., Koshkarov, V.I., Popov, S.A., and Makhnev, V.P., (1997b). Nonlinear forecasting measurements of the human EEG during evoked emotions. *Brain Topography*, Volume: 10, pp. 155-162.

Aftanas, L.I., Lotova, N.V., Koshkarov, V.I., and Popov, S.A., (1998a). Non-linear dynamical coupling between different brain areas during evoked emotions: an EEG investigation. *Biological Psychology*, Volume: 48, pp. 121-138.

Aftanas, L. I., Reva, N. V., Varlamov, A. A., Pavlov, S. V., and Makhnev, V. P., (2004). Analysis of Evoked EEG Synchronization and Desynchronization in Conditions of Emotional Activation in Humans: Temporal and Topographic Characteristics. *Neuroscience and Behavioural Physiology*, Vol. 34, No. 8.

Aftanas, L. I., Varlamov, A.A., Pavlov, S.V., Makhnev, V., and Reva, N., (2001). Event-related synchronization and desynchronization during affective processing: emergence of valence-related time-dependent hemispheric asymmetries in theta and upper alpha band. *International Journal of Neuroscience*, 110: 197–219.

Aftanas, L.I., Lotova, N.V., Koshkarov, V.I., Makhnev, V.P., Mordvintsev Yu. N., and Popov, S.A. (1998b) Non-linear dynamic complexity of the human EEG during evoked emotions. *International Journal of Psychophysiology*, 28(1):63-76.

Aftanas, L. I., Reva, N. V., Savotina, L. N., and Makhnev, V. P.(2006). Neurophysiological Correlates of Induced Discrete Emotions in Humans: An Individually Oriented Analysis. *Journal Neuroscience and Behavioral Physiology,* Volume 36, Number 2, pp.119-130

Barrett, L.F., and Wager, T.D., (2006). The Structure of Emotion: Evidence From Neuroimaging Studies. *Current Directions in Psychological Science*, Volume 15, Number 2, pp. 79-83(5).

Basar, E., Basar-Eroglu, C., Karakas, S., and Schurmann, M., (1999). Oscillatory brain theory: a new trend in neuroscience. *IEEE England. Med. Biol. Mag.*, 18:56–66.

Basar, E., Basar-Eroglu, C., Karakas, S. and Schurmann, M., (2001). Gamma, alpha, delta, and theta oscillations govern cognitive processes. *International Journal of Psychophysiology*, 39:241-8.

Bhattacharya, J., H., Petsche, H., and Pereda, E., (2001). Long-Range Synchrony in the γ Band: Role in Music Perception. *Journal of Neuroscience*, 21(16) :6329–6337.

Birbaumer, N., Lutzenberger, W., Elbert, T., Flor, H., and Rockstroh, B., (1993). Imagery and brain processes. In: N. Birbaumer and A. Ohman (Eds.). *The Structure of Emotion*, Hogrefe and Huber, Toronto,122-138.

Boccaletti, S., Kurths, J., Osipov, G., Valladares, D.L., Zhou, C.S., (2002). The synchronization of chaotic systems, *Physics Reports,* 366 (2002), 1–101.

Bressler, S.L., Coppola, R. and Nakamura, R., (1993). Episodic multiregional cortical coherence at multiple frequencies during visual task performance. *Nature*, 366:153-156.

Brown, R., and Kocarev, L., (2000). A unifying definition of synchronization for dynamical systems. *Chaos*, Volume: 10, pp. 344-349.

Costa, T., Rognoni, E., and Galati, D. (2006). EEG phase synchronization during emotional response to positive and negative film stimuli. *Neuroscience Letters*, 406:159-164.

Crawford, H.J., Clarke, S.W. and Kitner-Triolo, M. (1996). Self-generated happy and sad emotions in low an highly hypnotizable persons during waking and hypnosis: laterality and regional EEG activity differences. *International Journal of Psychophysiol*ogy, 24: 239-266.

Davidson, R.J, Chapman, J.P., Chapman, L.J., and Henriques, J.B., (1990) Asymmetrical brain electrical activity discriminates between psychometrically-matched verbal and saptial cognitive tasks. *Psychophysiology*, 27, 528-543.

Davidson, R. J., and Irwin, W., (1999). The functional neuroanatomy of emotion and affective style. *Trends in Cognitive Sciences*, 3, 11-21.

Davidson, R.J., (2003). Affective neuroscience and psychophysiology: Toward a synthesis. *Psychophysiology*, 40 (2003), 655–665.

Desmedt, J.E., and Tomberg, C., (1994). Transient phase-locking of 40 Hz electrical oscillations in prefrontal and parietal human cortex reflects the process of conscious somatic perception, *Neuroscience Letters*, 168: 126-129.

Ekman, P, and Davidson, R.J., (1994). *The nature of emotion: fundamental questions*. Oxford University Press.

Ekman, P., (1992). An argument for basic emotions, Cognition and emotion, 3:169-200.Ekman P., (1999) Basic Emotions In T. Dalgleish and M. Power (Eds.). *Handbook of Cognition and Emotion*. Sussex, U.K.: John Wiley and Sons, Ltd.

Elbert, T., Ray, W.J, Kowalik, Z.J., Skinner, J.E., Graf, K.E., and Birbaumer, N., (1994). Chaos and physiology: deterministic chaos in excitable cell assemblies. *Physiological Reviews*, Vol 74, 1-47.

Frackowiak, R.S.J., Friston, K.J., Frith, C., Dolan, R., Friston, K.J., Price, C.J., Zeki, S., Ashburner, J., and Penny, W.D., editors, (2004). *Human Brain Function*. Academic Press, 2nd edition.

Hebb, D.O., (1949). *The Organization of Behavior*. Wiley, New York.

Hinrichs, H. M., and Machleidt, W., (1992). Basic Emotions reflected in EEG-coherences, *International Journal of Psychophysiology*, 3:225-232.

Jung, T-P., Humphries, C., Lee T-W., Makeig, S., McKeown, M.J., Iragui, V., and Sejnowski, T.J., (1998). Extended ICA Removes Artifacts from Electroencephalographic Recordings, in D. Touretzky, M. Mozer and M. Hasselmo (Eds), *Advances in Neural Information Processing Systems*, 10:894-900.

Klimesch, W., (1999). EEG alpha and theta oscillations reflect cognitive and memory performance: a review and analysis. *Brain Research Review*, 291 :169-195.

Klimesch, W., Doppelmayr, M., Russagger, H., Pachinger, T. and Schwaiger, J., (1998). Induced alpha band power changes in the human EEG and attention. *Neuroscience Letters*, 244 :73-76.

Krause, C.M., Viemerö, V., Rosenqvist, A., Sillanmäki, L., Aström, T., (2000). Relative electroencephalographic desynchronization and synchronization in humans to emotional film content: an analysis of the 4±6, 6±8, 8±10 and 10±12 Hz frequency bands. *Neuroscience Letters*, 26;286(1):9-12.

Lang, P.J., Cuthbert, B.N., and Bradley, M.M., (1998a). Measuring emotion in therapy: Imagery, activation and feeling. *Behavior Therapy*, 29, 655–674.

Lang, P.J., Bradley, M.M., Fitzsimmons, J.R., Cuthbert, B.N., Scott, J.D., Moulder, B. and Nangia, V., (1998b). Emotional arousal and activation of the visual cortex: An fMRI analysis. *Psychophysiology*, 35:199–210.

LeDoux, J., (2000). Emotion Circuits in the Brain. *Annual Review of Neuroscience*, 23, 155-184.

Leventhal, H., and Scherer, K.R., (1987). The relationship of emotion to cognition: a functional approach to a semantic controversy, *Cognition and Emotion* 1, pp. 3–28.

Lewis, M.D., (2005). Bridging emotion theory and neurobiology through dynamic systems modeling, *Behavioral and Brain Sciences*, 28: 169-194.

Lutzenberger, W., Flor, H., and Birbaumer, N., (1997). Enhanced dimensional complexity of the EEG during memory for personal pain in chronic pain patients, *Neuroscience Letters*, Volume: 266, pp. 167-170.

Miller, E.K., and Cohen, J.D., (2001). An integrative theory of prefrontal cortex function. *Annual Review of Neuroscience*, 24:167-202.

Murphy, F.C., Nimmo-Smith, I., and Lawrence, A.D., (2003). Functional neuroanatomy of emotions: A meta-analysis. *Cognitive, Affective, and Behavioral Neuroscience*, 3 (3), 207-233.

Oldfield, R.C., (1971). The assessment and analysis of handedness: the Edinburgh Inventory. *Neuropsychologia*, 6, 97-113.

Panksepp, J., (1998). Affective neuroscience: The foundations of human and animal emotions. New York: Oxford University Press.

Pecora, L.M., and Carroll, T.L., (1990). Synchronization in chaotic systems, Phys Rev Lett, Volume: 64, pp. 821-824.

Pfurtscheller, G., and Lopes da Silva, F. H., (1999). Event-related EEG/EMG synchronization and desynchronization. Basic principles. *Clinical Neurophysiology*, 110: 1842–1857.

Pfurtscheller, G., Woertz, M., Supp, G., and Lopes da Silva, F.H., (2003). Early onset of post-movement beta electroencephalogram synchronization in the supplementary motor area during self-paced finger movement in man. *Neuroscience Letters*, 20;339(2).

Phan, L.K., Wager, T., Taylor, S.F. and Liberzon, I., (2002). Functional Neuroanatomy of Emotion: A Meta-Analysis of Emotion Activation Studies in PET and fMRI. *NeuroImage*, 16:331–348.

Pikovsky, A.S., Rosemblum, M.G. and Kurths, J., (2001). *Synchronization – A universal Concept in Nonlinear Science.* Cambridge.

Rodriguez, E., George, N., Lachaux, J.P., and Martinerie, J., (1999). Perception's shadow: long-distance synchronization of human brain activity. *Nature* 397: 430-433.

Rosenblum, M., Pikovsky, A., and Kurths, J., (1996). Phase synchronization of chaotic oscillators. *Physical Review Letters*, 76:1804-1807.

Rosenblum, M., Pikovsky, A., Kurths, J., Schafer, C., and Tass, P.A., (2001a). Phase synchronization: from theory to data analysis, in F. Moss and S. Gielen (eds.), *Handbook of Biological Physics*, Elsevier Science.

Rosenblum, M.G., Pikovsky, A.S., (2001b). Detecting direction of coupling in interacting oscillators, *Physical Review*, Volume: 64, 045202.

Rosenblum, M.G., Pikovsky, A.S., Kurhts J., (2004). Synchronization approach to analysis of biological systems. *Fluctuation Noise Lett*ers, Volume: 4, pp. L53-L62.

Rosenstein, M.T., Collins, J.J. and De Luca, C.J., (1993). A practical method for calculating largest Lyapunov exponents from small data sets, *Physica D,* Volume: 65, pp. 117-134.

Russell, J.A., (1980). A Circumplex Model of Affect. *International Journal of Psychophysiology*, 39: 1161-1178.

Schouten, J., Takens, F., van den Bleek, and C.van.den, (1994). Maximum-likelihood estimation of the entropy of an attractor, *Physical Review E,* Volume: 49, pp. 126-129.

Singer, W., (1993). Synchronization of cortical activity and its putative role in information processing and learning. *Annual Review of Physiology*, 55:349-374.

Singer, W., (1999). Neurobiology: Striving for coherence. *Nature*, 397:391– 393.

Stam, C.J. (2005). Nonlinear dynamical analysis of EEG and MEG: Review of an emerging field. *Clinical Neurophysiology*, Vol: 116 Issue: 10, pp: 2266-2301

Steriade, M., (1999). Cellular substrates of brain rhythms. In: Niedermeyer E, Lopes da Silva F (eds) *Electroencephalography. Basic principles, clinical applications and related* Welds, 4th edn. Williams and Wilkins, Baltimore, pp 28–75.

Surguladz, S.A., Brammer, M.J., Young, A.W., Andrew, C., Travis, M.J., Williams, S.C.R., and Phillips, M.L., (2003). A preferential increase in the extrastriate response to signals of danger *NeuroImage*, 19 1317–1328.

Tallon-Baudry, C., Bertrand, O., and Fischer, C., (2001). Oscillatory Synchrony between Human Extrastriate Areas during Visual Short-Term Memory Maintenance. *Journal of Neuroscience*, 21:1-5.

Tallon-Baudry, C., and Bertrand, O., (1999). Oscillatory gamma activity in humans and its role in object representation, *Trends in Cognitive Science*, 3,4:152-163.

Tononi, G. and Edelman, G.M., (1998). Consciousness and complexity. *Science*, 282:1846-51.

Tononi, G. and Sporns, O., (2003). Measuring information integration. *BMC Neuroscience*, 4-31.

Tononi, G., Edelman,G.M., Sporns, O., (1998). Complexity and coherency: integrating information in the brain, *TICS*, Volume: 2, pp. 474-484

Tucker, D.M., and Dawson, S.L., (1984). Asymmetric EEG changes as method actors generated emotions. *Biological Psychology*, 19, 63–75.

Thatcher, R.W., Krause, P.J., and Hrybyk, M., (1986). Cortico-cortical associations and EEG coherence: a two-compartmental model. *Electroencephalogr. Clin. Neurophysiol.* 64, 123–143.

Williams, L.M., Das, P., Liddell B.J., , Kemp, A.H., Rennie, C.J., and Gordon, E., (2006). Mode of Functional Connectivity in Amygdala Pathways Dissociates Level of Awareness for Signals of Fear *The Journal of Neuroscience*, 6, 26(36):9264-9271.

In: Research Topics on Brain Mapping
Editor: Yuanzhu Liáng, pp. 113-134
ISBN: 978-1-60456-001-5


*Chapter V*

# Sensori-Motor Integration in the Somatosensory Areas During the Preparatory Period of Self-Initiated Voluntary Movement

***Toshiaki Wasaka and Ryusuke Kakigi***
Department of Integrative Physiology,
National Institute for Physiological Sciences, Okazaki, JAPAN

## Abstract

The somatosensory information processing during its course from the peripheral to the somatosensory areas is influenced by top-down modulation (centrifugal mechanism) mediated by a network comprising brain structures, motor and higher-order brain systems. However, little is known about the property of sensori-motor integration in the somatosensory cortices during the preparatory period of voluntary movement in humans. To elucidate the mechanisms underlying sensori-motor integration in the primary (SI) and secondary somatosensory cortex (SII), we investigated the temporal change in somatosensory evoked magnetic fields (SEFs) using a self-initiated voluntary movement task. Electrical stimulation of the right median nerve was applied continuously, while the subjects performed a self-initiated finger extension every 5 to 7 sec. They were instructed not to pay attention to the electrical stimulation. The preparatory period of self-initiated finger extension was divided into subperiods from the onset of the electromyogram, and the magnetoencephalogram signals following stimulation in each subperiod were averaged. In SI, three equivalent current dipole (ECD) components (N20m, P30m and P60m) were recognized. Although the ECD moment for N20m and P60m was not significantly changed in the preparatory period, that for P30m was significantly smaller in the 0- to -500-ms subperiod. As for bilateral SII, the ECD moment for the SII ipsilateral to movement (SIIi) showed no significant change, while that for the contralateral SII (SIIc) was significantly larger in the same subperiod. Voluntary movement is associated with both the actual motor command and a copy of the motor command (efference copy and corollary discharge) providing information about the expected sensory consequences of the movement. The opposite effects of voluntary movement on SI and SII indicated that these cortical areas are affected differently by the centrifugal mechanism and play a different role in the function of the sensori-motor integration.

## Introduction

Recognizing one's own movement is essential to the control of voluntary movement. For precise movement, a motor program requires sensory signals from the target body area to be moved, and the appropriate integration of sensory and motor signals is essential. The movement of one's body parts is perceived not only by visual information but also by somatosensory feedback from muscles, skins and tendons which provide us information on the status of each part being moved in a moment. The motor and higher-order brain systems regulate sensory information at several processing stages. The existence of interactions between motor commands and somatosensory information processing in the sensory and motor cortices has been investigated. The recent studies have demonstrated this sensori-motor interaction and suggest that cortical mechanisms such as corollary discharge [88] and efference copy [100] related to movement generation and execution modify the somatosensory information processing (for a review, [72]).

Somatosensory information is modulated by the effect of voluntary movement during its course from the peripheral to the somatosensory cortical areas. This phenomenon has been reported as modulation in the short- and long-latency components of somatosensory evoked potentials (SEPs) and somatosensory evoked magnetic fields (SEFs). With regard to the modulation in somatosensory cortices produced by voluntary movement, change of the SEP/SEF amplitude was found not only during movement [5][15][46][68][81] but also just prior to it (preparatory period) [4][9][26][91][103][104][105]. It is assumed that these electrophysiological changes are associated with a decrease in tactile sensitivity commonly observed before the onset of movement of the limb that received the sensory stimulation [10][75][83]. However, the property of activation in the somatosensory cortices during the preparatory period remained unknown.

In previous studies, premovement modulation of the somatosensory information processing has been investigated using reaction time tasks [4][9][26][52][54][65][86][91]. However, a reaction time task evokes various cognitive brain activities, such as attention, expectancy and motivation, and may change the sensori-motor activities. In fact, the neuronal effect of attention on the somatosensory information processing has been addressed with various methods, including single unit recording in monkeys [31][37], SEPs/SEFs [13][18][62][63] and functional magnetic resonance imaging (fMRI) [40][70][90]. Using the self-initiated voluntary movement task without external cues, one can observe temporal modulation of somatosensory cortices activities with respect to movement onset and elucidate the neural interaction between somatosensory and motor areas in detail without affecting any neuronal activities, i.e., attention and expectancy, relating to external cues for the movement. The objective of this study was to discover the mechanism of sensori-motor integration in the primary (SI) and secondary somatosensory cortex (SII) during the preparatory period of self-initiated voluntary movement.

# Sensori-Motor Integration in Somatosensory Cortices

## The Modulation of Short-Latency SEP/SEF Components with Voluntary Movement

Since the first observation of SEP modulation with voluntary movement by Giblin in 1964 [20], it has been reported that active movements [5][6][59][93], passive movements [1][28][81] and continuous tactile stimulation [43][45][47] gave rise to reduction of the amplitude in the short-latency SEP/SEF components (for a review, see [7]). This effect is termed 'gating' and has been largely demonstrated in both upper [5][6][9][43][80][93][97] and lower limb SEP studies [8][14][64][67][82][84][89][94][98][103][104][105].

The gating effect of short-latency SEP/SEF component may occur via two major mechanisms: first, suppression of somatosensory response can be carried out by inhibitory interaction between the given sensory signals and the efferent signals induced by the motor command from the motor related areas (centrifugal mechanism), and second, modulation can be exerted by interaction between the given sensory afferents for producing SEPs/SEFs and the afferent signals evoked by the movement, i.e., afferent signals from the muscles, joint and skin (centripetal mechanism) [44][57].

## Effects of Pure Centrifugal Mechanism on SEPs/SEFs

A few studies have attempted to clarify the centrifugal mechanism of task-relevant somatosensory information processing, utilizing a forewarned reaction time paradigm where the somatosensory stimulation used to elicit the SEPs was also used as an imperative signal [52][54][65][86]. They reported that short-latency SEPs were attenuated when the somatosensory stimulation triggered voluntary movement. Moreover, timing of SEP modulation (gating) in concern to voluntary movement has been well explored by Starr and Cohen using reaction time task paradigm [9][91]. SEPs following stimulation of the median nerve were recorded at different time points during and after a response signal (auditory signal) to move the ipsilateral thumb. There is a clear attenuation of the P27 about 100 ms before the occurrence of the EMG. Since the centripetal mechanism can be excluded because of no occurrence of EMG activity in this premovement period, the pure centrifugal mechanism caused the attenuation of the short-latency SEP component.

## Modulation in Long-Latency SEP/SEF Components with Voluntary Movement

Although much attention has been given to sensori-motor integration between somatosensory information processing and voluntary movement in the short-latency component of SEPs, the consistent result was not reported in concern of the modulation of the long-latency SEP components in humans. It has been reported that long-latency SEPs were attenuated [43][81] or enhanced [4][25][52][54][59][68] before and during voluntary movement. In addition to these SEP studies, magnetoencephalography (MEG) studies have shown that the short-latency SI activities were attenuated with voluntary movement [15][46][53], whereas the long-latency SII activities were enhanced [15][29][53][60]. However, some researchers showed an attenuation of the SII activation [3][33].

## The Modulation of SI Activation During the Preparatory Period of Self-Initiated Voluntary Movement (Experiment 1)

Evidence of 'gating' between the somatosensory afferent signals and voluntary movement has been reported [1][5][20][28][48][81][93][99]. Two major mechanisms for gating effects, centrifugal and centripetal effect, have been discussed in previous studies [44][57]. During voluntary movement, both mechanisms involving centrifugal and centripetal effect might occur. To separate centrifugal from centripetal mechanism, we designed the present study, in which the SEFs were recorded in the preparatory period. Since no afferent signals were evoked by voluntary movement, the modulation of activation in somatosensory areas that occurred during the preparatory period was considered due to the interaction between the sensory activities for motor preparation. However, most previous studies investigating the premovement modulation of somatosensory areas used a reaction time task with an external cue signal for voluntary movement, but it was difficult to exclude the effect of the cognitive activity after the cue signal or the direct effect of the sensory activity following the signal itself. To resolve this problem, we used a self-initiated voluntary movement task. The stimulation for SEFs was delivered randomly during the movement execution, and the voluntary movement was self-paced. We collected the premovement epochs and analyzed them to elucidate when the SEF modulation occurred during the preparatory period of the voluntary movement. Furthermore, since Berietschaftspotential (BP) is recorded in the preparatory period of self-initiated voluntary movement [56][85], we can investigate the relationship between the activation of SI and motor-related areas [101].

## Experimental Condition

### *Subjects*

Nine healthy volunteers participated in the present study (mean age 33.0, range 24-49, S.D. 8.5 years). All subjects were right-handed males. Written informed consent was obtained from each participant prior to the study. No medication was given to the subjects before the experiment.

### *Median Nerve Stimulation*

The right median nerve was stimulated on the palm side at the wrist with a saddle type electrode. The electrode was fixed to the wrist using a belt to prevent it moving during the finger movement. The cathode was placed proximal to the anode. Constant current square wave pulses (duration, 0.2 ms) were provided, and the intensity was adjusted to produce a slight twitch of the muscle (abductor pollicis brevis). The interstimulus interval (ISI) of the stimulation was changed randomly from 600 to 800 ms (mean ISI, 700 ms).

### *Experimental Paradigm*

The subjects sat on a recording chair in the MEG device in a magnetically shielded room. The SEFs were recorded using two conditions. One condition (rest condition) was under the stationary condition as the control, in which the subjects kept their arms relaxed on a table in front of them. In the other condition (movement condition), the subjects performed a voluntary finger extension during the continuous electrical stimulation of the median nerve. In the movement condition, the subjects were instructed to extend the right index finger as quickly as possible for a short time and then to relax. They were instructed to repeat the movement every 5 to 7 s, but were allowed to perform the movement at their own pace. The subjects were asked to concentrate on the movement and not to pay attention to the continuous electrical stimulation

### *MEG Equipment*

The SEFs were recorded with a helmet-shaped 306 channels detector array (Vectorview, Elekta Neuromag Oy, Helsinki, Finland), which comprised 102 identical triple sensor elements. Each sensor element consists of two orthogonal planar gradiometers and one magnetometer coupled to a multi-SQUID (Superconducting Quantum Interference Device). In the present study, we analyzed MEG signals recorded from 204 channels planar-type gradiometers. The signals were filtered with a bandpass filter of 0.03-300 Hz, and digitized at 995Hz. We also recorded an electromyogram (EMG) to determine the preparatory period of voluntary movement. The EMG was obtained from the right extensor indicis muscle in the forearm using a pair of disk electrodes.

Prior to the MEG recording, four head position indicator (HPI) coils were attached to the subject's head to measure with respect to the three anatomical landmarks using a 3 D digitizer to allow alignment of the MEG and magnetic resonance image (MRI) coordinate systems (3.0 T Siemens Allegra). Current was then fed to the HPI coils and the resulting magnetic fields were measured with the magnetometer, which allowed for aligning the individual head coordinate system with the magnetometer coordinate system.

### *Data Acquisition and Analysis*

The preparatory period of voluntary movement was temporally divided into six subperiods; 0 (EMG onset) to –500 ms, –500 to –1000 ms, –1000 to –1500 ms, –1500 to –2000 ms, –2000 to –3000 ms and –3000 to –4000 ms (figure 1). Since the electrical stimulation for the SEFs was delivered continuously, we collected the SEF epochs in each subperiod. The analysis time for SEF was 250 ms which included a prestimulus period of 50 ms.

Single equivalent current dipoles (ECDs) of N20m, P30m and P60m were estimated during six subperiods and Rest condition [21]. The head was modeled with a sphere best fitting the inner curvature of the skull in the SI region in the individual MR images. The ECDs best explaining the magnetic field distribution over SI were found by least-squares searches taking account of the signals from at least 20 channels around the signal maxima, so that these covered both field extremes of the local field distribution over SI. The goodness-of-fit (GOF) value of an ECD was calculated to indicate in percentage terms how much the dipole accounts for the measured field variance. Only ECDs explaining more than 90% of the GOF value at selected point of time over a subset of channels were used for further analysis. Peak amplitude of ECD moment for recognizable consistent components within 100 ms after stimulation of the median nerve, were compared using one-way repeated measured analysis of variance (ANOVA), with the subperiod and the Rest condition as the factor. The F values were obtained after Greenhouse-Geisser correction when appropriate and a correction coefficient epsilon was used. Post-hoc analysis followed by Fisher's PLSD was used for multiple comparisons. The level of statistical significance was set at 5% ($p<0.05$).

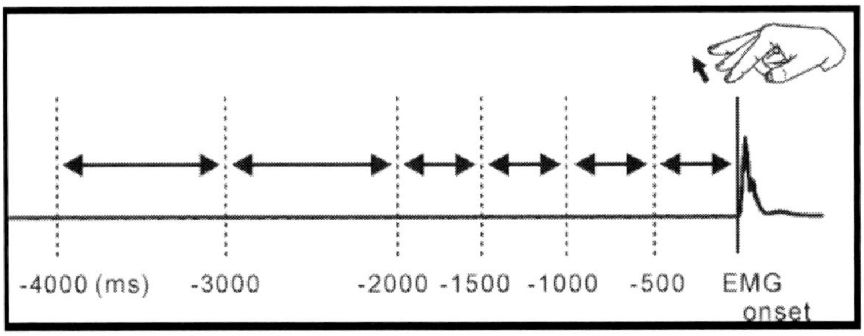


Figure 1. A schema of the premovement subperiods in this study. The premovement subperiods and the onset of the rectified EMG. The preparatory period was divided into five subperiods from the onset of EMG to 4000 ms before movement. The time scale is expressed in minus values before the onset of movement. Stimulation of the median nerve was applied at random and the MEG signals following stimulation were averaged separately depending on each subperiod to obtain the premovement somatosensory evoked magnetic fields (SEFs). Adapted from Wasaka et al. (2003) [101].

## Results

Figure 2 shows the SEF waveforms elicited by stimulation of the right median nerve in one subject. Clear deflections were obtained from the gradiometers on SI in the hemisphere contralateral to the stimulated side. The initial upward deflection, N20m, peaking at around 20 ms after the stimulation (mean, 20.7 ms), was followed by a downward deflection, P30m, around 30 ms (mean, 29.6 ms) and a downward deflection, P60m, around 60 ms after the stimulation (mean, 65.3 ms). One small upward deflection, N45m, was also identified between P30m and P60m, but it did not exceed the baseline in some subjects. Responses at a latency longer than 80 ms were recognized in the hemisphere contralateral and ipsilateral to the stimulated side, but the responses were not consistent among the subjects because of a short ISI [23][66][106].

We estimated the ECD of each component. Figure 3 shows the locations of the estimated dipoles on the MR images in one subject. N20m, P30m and P60m were generated in the postcentral wall in the hemisphere contralateral to the stimulated side in all subjects including this one. Peak ECD moment of P30m was significantly attenuated in the preparatory subperiod, whereas N20m and P60m were unchanged. The P30m evoked in the 0 to –500 ms subperiod was significantly attenuated in amplitude compared to that in the Rest sequence ($p<0.01$), and the P30m amplitude during 0 to –500 ms ($p<0.01$), –500 to –1000 ms ($p<0.01$) and –1000 to –1500 ms ($p<0.05$) subperiods were smaller than that during –3000 to –4000 ms subperiod (figure 3).

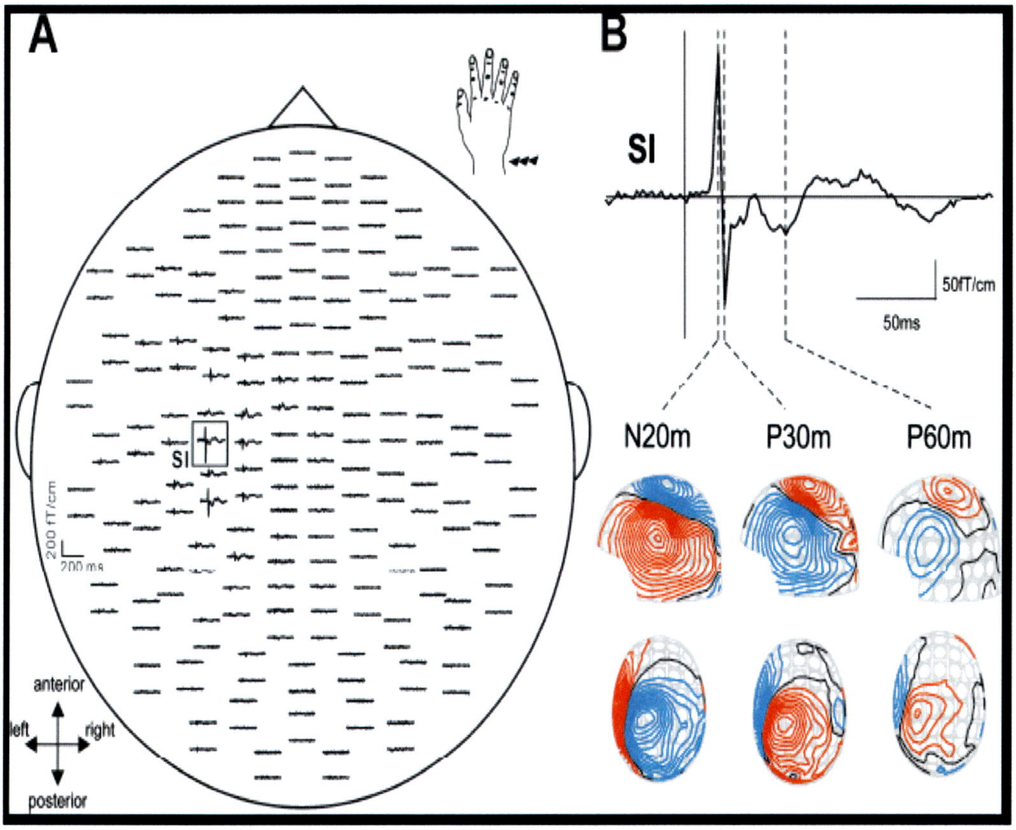


Figure 2. SEFs following stimulation of the median nerve at right wrist in a subject. A: 204 channel SEF waveforms viewed from the top of the head. B: An enlarged waveform obtained from one MEG channel in the primary somatosensory cortex (SI) (framed channel in A) and 3 dimensional (3D) isocontour maps of magnetic fields of each component recorded from the gradiometers. A vertical line indicates the stimulus. Three main components, N20m, P30m and P60m, were identified. The sensor array viewed from the left and top, with a field pattern of each component. Areas surrounded with red and blue contour lines show the outflux and influx of magnetic fields, respectively. Redrawn from Wasaka et al. (2003) [101].

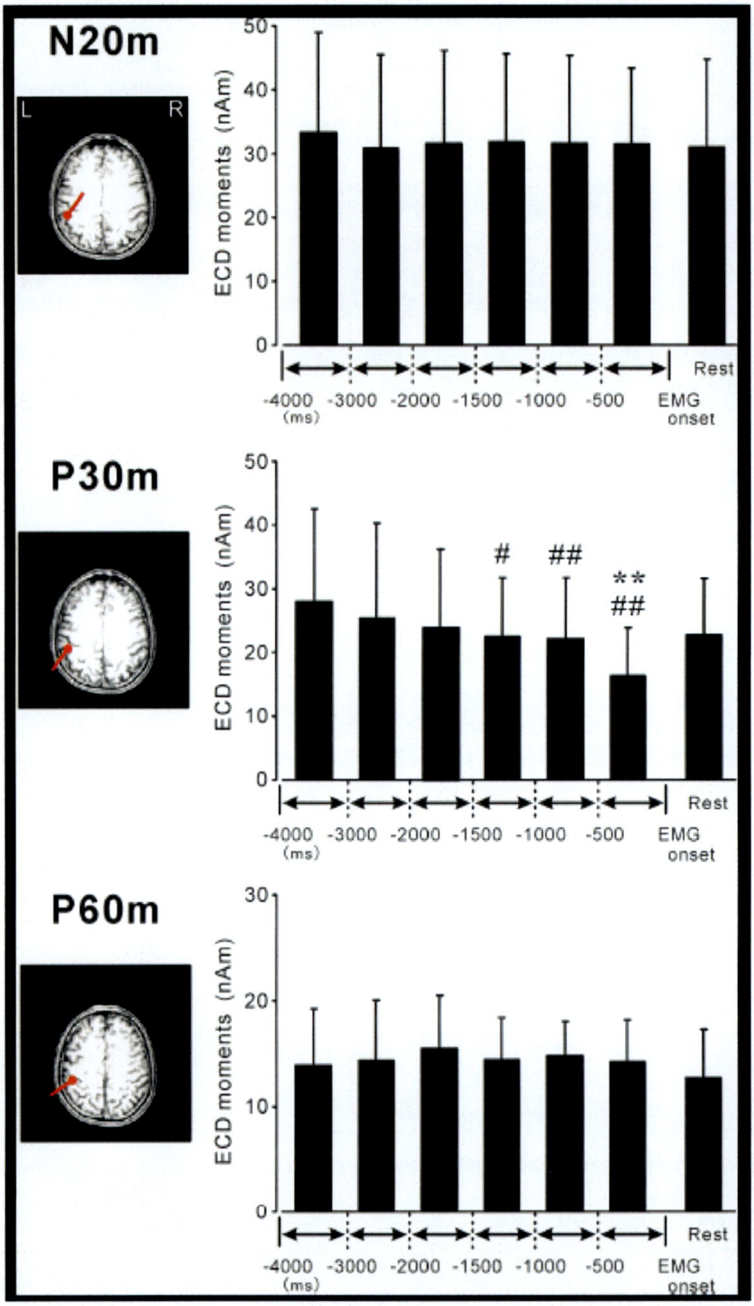


Figure 3. The localization and direction of ECD for each SEF component on MR images. All ECDs were located in the posterior bank of the central sulcus in the hemisphere contralateral to the stimulated side. The right graphs show the mean and standard deviation of the ECD moments of N20m, P30m and P60m components in the rest condition and premovement subperiods of the movement condition. * $p<0.05$, ** $p<0.01$; Statistical significance compared with the values in the rest condition, # $p<0.05$, ## $p<0.01$; Statistical significance compared with the values for the 4000 to 3000 ms subperiod before EMG onset. Two periods for P30m showed a significant reduction as compared with the rest condition and/or the 4000 to 3000 ms subperiod before EMG onset. N20m and P60m showed no significant change. Adapted from Wasaka et al. (2003) [101].

### *Discussion of Experiment 1*

Not all cortical responses reduce their amplitude before and during movement, the effect of which involves only selected components. The change in the N20 component of the SEP during the preparatory period was controversial in previous studies. Some authors reported that the amplitude did not change before movement [9][65][86][91], while others reported attenuation of the component just before the movement [26][74]. In the present study, the N20m ECD moment was unchanged in each subperiod. In contrast, ECD moment for P30m showed a clear and significant attenuation during the preparatory period. These results have been confirmed by human [52][54] and monkey studies [71][87]. In our self-initiated voluntary movement task, we considered that we could exclude the brain activity following the cue and the anticipatory effect evoked by a cue on the motor preparatory brain activity [38][58]. Therefore, it was possible that the attenuation of P30m was of selective gating between the self-initiated preparatory brain activity and applied sensory signal for SEFs.

Interestingly, the time course of the P30m modulation, starting from 1000 to 1500 ms before the movement and the remarkable attenuation just prior to the movement (0 to –500 ms subperiod), was similar to that of the activities of movement-related cortical potentials. In the preparatory period just before movement, the neural activity in the sensori-motor cortex seemed to change dramatically [11][19]. The supplementary motor area (SMA) and the primary motor cortex (MI) activities in this period were reported in humans recorded from the cortex [32][73][95]. Intracortical microstimulation of the neurons in MI in monkeys showed a profound decrease in the magnitude of the short-latency component of SEPs [39]. Moreover, in our previous study, the extent of the centrifugal gating effect on SEPs was dependent on the amplitude of the negative slope [103]. In addition, motor-related cortices, such as SMA and MI, have extensive cortico-cortical connections to other cortices such as SI [42] and possibly other sensory associated cortices. From these results, the activities in SMA and MI before voluntary movement could modulate the response in SI, especially the generator for the P30m component.

With regard to the ECD location for N20m, P30m and N60m, the present results were consistent with those of previous studies [24][30][49]. The ECDs of these components were identified around SI in the hemisphere contralateral to the stimulated side. In general, the primary component, N20/N20m, is generated in area 3b of SI [2][12][30]. However, the generator for P30m is still controversy. Inui et al. (2004) reported a temporal relation of activities among multiple cortical areas, Brodmann's areas 3b, 4 and 1, around 20 to 30 ms following stimulation of the dorsum of the hand [36]. Kawamura et al. (1996) suggested that area 4 of MI is involved in generating P30m [51]. Lin et al. (2005) reported that N20m and P35m (corresponding to P30m in our study) have different generators, with distinctive neurophysiological behaviors in response to varying stimulus intensity levels [61]. Furthermore, Wikström et al. (1996) who investigated the modulation of SEF components caused by the effect of ISI, proposed that the mechanism responsible for P35m was inhibitory postsynaptic potentials in the deeper layers in area 3b [106]. In the present study, although the ECD was estimated around SI in the hemisphere contralateral to the stimulated side, we could not separate the many sources in this time frame. However, the functional difference between N20/N20m and P30/P30m is evident from the results of previous studies [61][106] and a recovery function [27]. The activation of SI for P30m might be essential to control the motor performance in a feedforward manner, and the interaction taking place in the generator for P30m between such an intrinsic activity and the given afferent signals following stimulation of the median nerve might occur at an early stage of the preparatory period for voluntary movement.

# The Modulation of SII Activation During the Preparatory Period of Voluntary Movement (Experiment 2)

Compared with SI, SII was speculated to serve a higher level of cognitive function in somatosensory information processing, such as attention, decision-making, objective recognition and integration of nociceptive and non-nociceptive inputs [34][35][63][69][78][79][92][96]. However, in concern of sensori-motor integration, the role of SII has not been elucidated in humans. Previous studies investigating the modulation of SII with voluntary movement showed an enhancement of SII activation during the movement execution [15][30][60], but some researchers showed an attenuation of the activation [3][33]. We assumed that the reason for the discrepancy was that most previous studies utilized a paradigm where the modulation in SII activation was not investigated time-locked to the onset of movement. Therefore, it was impossible to analyze the timing of modulation in the somatosensory areas with respect to the onset of voluntary movement. Using a self-initiated voluntary movement task without external cues, one can observe temporal somatosensory modulation with respect to movement onset and elucidate neural interaction between SII and motor related areas. In this study, we investigated the SII modulation during the preparatory period of self-initiated voluntary movement [102].

## Experimental Condition

### *Subjects*

Eleven normal male volunteers participated in this study (mean age 31.1, range 25-42, S.D. 5.8 years). All subjects were right-handed. Written informed consent was obtained from each participant prior to the study.

### *Median Nerve Stimulation*

It was shown that neural activities in SII were affected by the ISI. The SEFs from SI can be obtained with short ISIs, while responses from SII require an ISI of at least 1000 ms [23][66][106]. To record the activation in SII clearly, we adopted longer ISI (mean ISI, 2000 ms). The ISI was changed randomly from 1800 to 2200 ms.

### *Experimental Paradigms*

We used the same task with previous experiment. The SEFs were recorded under the movement condition, in which the subject performed a voluntary index finger extension of right hand.

### *Data Acquisition and Analysis*

The preparatory period of voluntary movement was temporally divided into five subperiods; 0 (EMG onset) to –500 ms, –500 to –1000 ms, –1000 to –1500 ms, –1500 to –2000 ms and –2000 to –3000 ms (figure 4). Since the electrical stimulation for the SEFs was delivered continuously, we collected the SEF in each subperiod. We checked the EMG for every trial off-line after the experiment.

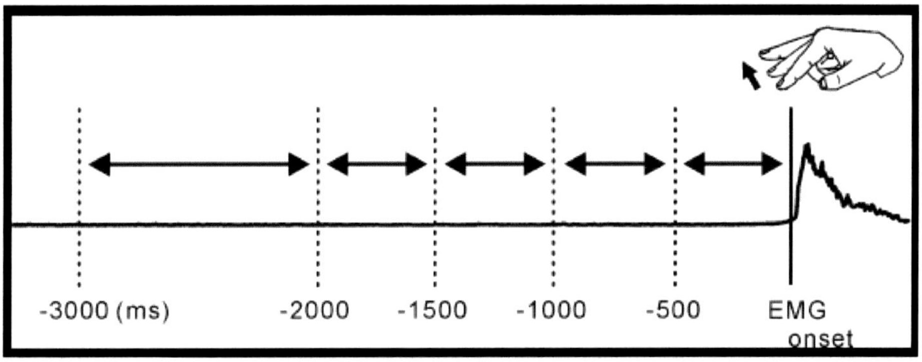


Figure 4. A schema of the premovement subperiods in this study. The premovement subperiods and the onset of the rectified EMG. The preparatory period was divided into five subperiods from the onset of EMG to 3000 ms before movement. The time scale is expressed in minus values before the onset of movement. Adapted from Wasaka et al. (2005) [102].

To identify the characteristics of the sources (SI and bilateral SII) of the measured responses to the electrical stimuli, time-varying ECDs were used [21]. The signals were evaluated over successive time periods, best describing the most dominant source of the response, by a least-squares search in a spherical volume conductor model for the head by using a subset of 14 to 18 channels including the local maximum response area, which was based on each subject's MRI scan. When necessary, the contribution of previously identified sources was subtracted from the measured response pattern using signal-subspace projection. Only ECDs which account for more than 80% of the field variance in the channel subset were accepted for further analysis. Finally, all channels were used to compute the time-varying multi-dipole model allowing the strengths of the previously found ECDs to change over the entire period of analysis while the source locations and orientations were kept fixed.

For the peak amplitude of the ECD moment, a two-way repeated measure ANOVA was performed with Subperiod and Component as the factors. To analyze the assumption of sphericity prior to the repeated measures ANOVA, we used Mauchly's test of sphericity. If the result of the test was significant and the assumption of sphericity was violated, the Greenhouse-Geisser adjustment was used to correct for the sphericity altering the degrees of freedom using a correction coefficient epsilon. A post-hoc analysis followed by the Tukey test was used for multiple comparisons. The level of statistical significance was set at 5% ($P < 0.05$).

## Results

Figure 5 shows the SEF waveforms elicited by stimulation of the right median nerve in one subject. Clear deflections were obtained from the gradiometers in the hemisphere contralateral to the stimulated side at a latency of less than 50 ms and in both hemispheres at around 80 to 100 ms. The earliest deflection N20m after the stimulation and the subsequent deflection P30m were identified in the anterior parietal cortex contralateral to the simulated side. The long-latency responses were identified in the bilateral temporal regions, corresponding to SII. The bilateral long-latency responses were estimated to occur in the upper bank of the Sylvian fissure, corresponding to SII (figure 6).

To compare the ECD moment for SII in the premovement subperiods, we used a two-way ANOVA concerning Subperiod and Component. A significant main effect was found for the SII contralateral to the side of the stimulation (SIIc) ($F(4, 40)=4.241$, $p<0.01$). In contrast, although the activation in the SII ipsilateral to the side of stimulation (SIIi) tended to increase in the 0 to –500 ms subperiod, there was no significant effect for SIIi ($F(4, 40)=2.337$, $p=0.072$). The ECD moment for SIIc was significantly larger in the 0 to –500 ms subperiod than –1500 to –2000 ms ($p<0.01$) or –2000 to –3000 ms subperiod ($p<0.05$, figure 6).

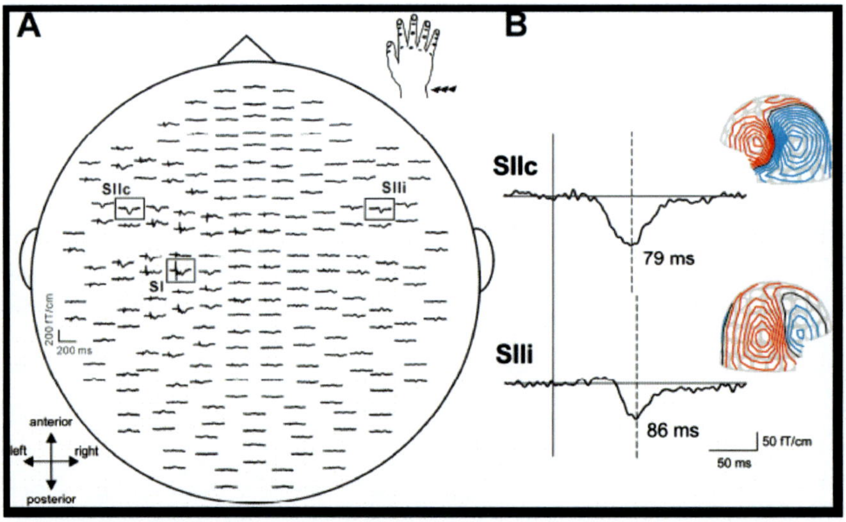


Figure 5. SEFs following stimulation of the right median nerve in one subject. A: 204 channel SEF waveforms viewed from the top of the head. Clear deflections were obtained from the gradiometers in the central region contralateral to the stimulated side and in the temporal regions in both hemispheres. B: Enlarged waveforms obtained from the MEG channels in the secondary somatosensory cortex contralateral (SIIc) and ipsilateral to the stimulation (SIIi). A vertical line indicates the stimulus. The sensor array viewed from the right (SIIi) and left (SIIc), with a field pattern of each component. Areas surrounded with red and blue contour lines show the outflux and influx of magnetic fields, respectively. Redrawn from Wasaka et al. (2005) [102].

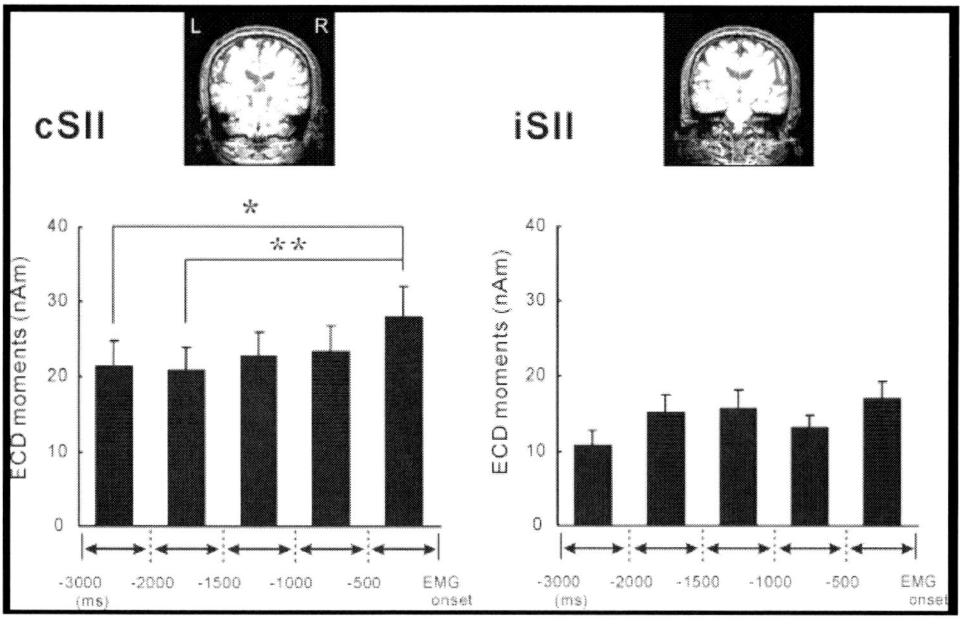


Figure 6. The localizations and directions of the ECD superimposed on the subject's MR image. The ECD for around 100 ms responses were identified in the bilateral temporal regions, corresponding to the SII cortices. The graph shows mean and standard error of the ECD moment of SIIc and SIIi in the premovement subperiods. * $p<0.05$, ** $p<0.01$; Statistical significance compared within two pairs. The ECD moment for SIIc was significantly larger in the 0 to 500 ms subperiod than the 1500 to 2000 ms or 2000 to 3000 ms subperiod before EMG onset, while that for SIIi was not significantly changed within the subperiods. Adapted from Wasaka et al. (2005) [102].

## Discussion of Experiment 2

This study showed that the modulation of SII ipsilateral and contralateral to finger extension differed during the preparatory period: ECD moment for SIIc showed a significant enhancement, while that for SIIi was unchanged. As far as we know, little attention has been given to the centrifugal mechanism on the activation of SII. In previous studies, there was no consistent agreement as to the function of SII concerning sensori-motor integration during voluntary movement. The long-latency components of SEPs were enhanced before and during voluntary movement [4][52][68]. Similarly, enhancement of SII activation was observed by MEG studies [15][48][53][60] and it was assumed that this phenomenon reflects tuning of the SII neurons to relevant somatosensory information from the regions of contracting muscle [29]. On the other hand, some researchers reported an attenuation of SII activation [3][33]. Using a self-initiated voluntary movement task, whereby the centripetal effect on the SEF response can be eliminated, one can mainly examine the centrifugal effect. We indicated an enhancement of SIIc activation in the 0 to –500 ms subperiod. Although the functional role of the human bilateral SII in sensori-motor integration has remained obscure, the activation of motor related areas prior to voluntary movement enhances the cortical effects of somatosensory information processing either by increasing synchronicity or by adding to the number of neurons activated in SIIc by the centrifugal mechanism.

It is generally agreed that attention to somatosensory information enhances activation of SII [17][22][55][62][63]. In the present study, we instructed the subjects to concentrate on the finger extension and not to pay attention to stimulation of the median nerve. In addition, subjects reported that they concentrated on the finger extension and did not turn their mind to the electrical stimulation throughout the recording session. However, a major effect of attention on the SII enhancement cannot be excluded. In fact, the amplitude of the long-latency SEP/SEF components may be modified not only when the subject's attention is focused on the electrical stimulation, but also when attention is directed toward the stimulated body part (spatial attention). Therefore, the spatial attention effect cannot be excluded from an enhancement of SII activation, since the subject was instructed to pay attention to press the button, thus to the stimulated body part.

Although the modulation in SIIi did not reach a level of significance, we observed that the activation in SIIi tended to increase. The reason why it did not reach a significant level is unknown, but we assumed that centrifugal mechanism acted differently on SIIc and SIIi. The interpretation for different centrifugal effect on SII is somewhat complicated. Since the peak latency of the ECD moment was longer for SIIi than for SIIc, activation of SIIi appeared to occur from the contralateral hemisphere via the corpus callosum [41][76]. However, if SIIi was driven by SIIc via the corpus callosum, we could not explain why SIIc activation was enhanced during the preparatory period while SIIi activation was not. To explain the mechanism, we considered that activation of SIIi would not necessarily depend on SIIc. Forss et al. (1999) showed in an MEG study that SIIi was activated in stroke patients even if the contralateral SI and SII areas were both damaged, and speculated that SIIi received direct inputs from the periphery in humans [16]. It was assumed that the activation of SIIi was induced by the projection from the ipsilateral thalamus and/or the contralateral hemisphere via the corpus callosum pathway. Although the sensori-motor function of SII was not fully clarified, we assumed that the function of SII in sensori-motor integration differed between the hemispheres contralateral and ipsilateral to the movement. To clarify the function of the bilateral activation of SII concerning sensori-motor integration, further research will be required.

## Conclusion

We observed a remarkable difference of modulation between SI and SII with voluntary movement, that is, an inhibition in SI and a facilitation in SII. A similar difference in modulation with voluntary movement has been reported in short- and long-latency SEP/SEF components [52][53][54][68]. In monkeys, the ablation of SI supported the notion of hierarchical processing of the somatosensory input. Removal of the SI area seriously impaired the processing of tactile information in the SII area in macaques [77]. However, deactivation of SI did not have clear effects on the responsiveness of SII [107] and a recent study in marmosets showed that the responsiveness of SII was largely independent of SI and tactile information could be directly conveyed to both the cortices from overlapping regions within the ventral posterior nucleus of the thalamus [108]. In humans, MEG responses from SII increased with active attention, while little effect of attention was observed in SI

[17][24][62][63]. Moreover, the finding of an MEG study was also in favor of parallel processing in SI and SII showing simultaneous activations in these areas [50]. From these results, we assumed that the somatosensory information processing concerning sensori-motor integration in SII would be independent of that in SI. Although the somatosensory information processing in SI and SII cortices was functionally different, the differential modulation in SI and SIIc, which started simultaneously in the 0 to –500 ms subperiod, was remarkable. In the 0 to –500 ms subperiod, although we did not record movement related cortical potential, it was speculated that the negative slope appeared [85]. In this period, since activities in SMA and MI were recorded from the cortex in humans [32], we speculated that the activities of SMA and MI might be important for the change in SI and SIIc during the preparatory period. Previously, efferent neural signals created by central motor networks in parallel with the motor commands were used to predict the sensory consequences of one's own motor acts, efference copy and corollary discharge. The different modulation in SI and SII is likely attributable to the effect of the neural mechanism such as efference copy and corollary diccharge on their areas.

# References

[1] Abbruzzese G., Ratto S., Favale E. and Abbruzzese M. (1981) Proprioceptive modulation of somatosensory evoked potentials during active or passive finger movements in man. *J. Neurol. Neurosurg. Psychiatry*, 44, 942-949.

[2] Allison T., McCarthy G., Wood C.C. and Jones S.J. (1991) Potentials evoked in human and monkey cerebral cortex by stimulation of the median nerve. A review of scalp and intracranial recordings. *Brain*, 114, 2465-2503.

[3] Avikainen S., Forss N. and Hari R. (2002) Modulated activation of the human SI and SII cortices during observation of hand actions. *NeuroImage*, 15, 640-646.

[4] Böcker K.B., Forget R. and Brunia C.H. (1993) The modulation of somatosensory evoked potentials during the foreperiod of a forewarned reaction time task. *Electroencephalogr. Clin. Neurophysiol.*, 88, 105-117.

[5] Cheron G. and Borenstein S. (1987) Specific gating of the early somatosensory evoked potentials during active movement. *Electroencephalogr. Clin. Neurophysiol.*, 67, 537-548.

[6] Cheron G. and Borenstein S. (1991) Gating of the early components of the frontal and parietal somatosensory evoked potentials in different sensory-motor interference modalities. *Electroencephalogr. Clin. Neurophysiol.*, 80, 522-530.

[7] Cheron G., Dan B. and Borenstein S. (2000) Sensory and motor interfering influences on somatosensory evoked potentials. *J. Clin. Neurophysiol.*, 17, 280-294.

[8] Cohen L.G. and Starr A. (1985) Vibration and muscle contraction affect somatosensory evoked potentials. *Neurology*, 35, 691-698.

[9] Cohen L.G. and Starr A. (1987) Localization, timing and specificity of gating of somatosensory evoked potentials during active movement in man. *Brain*, 110, 451-467.

[10] Coquery J.M. (1978) Role of active movement in control of afferent input from skin in cat and man, In Gordon G. (Eds.), *Active touch*, (pp. 161-169) New York: Pergamon Press.

[11] Deecke L., Scheid P. and Kornhuber H.H. (1969) Distribution of readiness potential, pre-motion positivity, and motor potential of the human cerebral cortex preceding voluntary finger movements. *Exp. Brain Res.*, 7, 158-168.

[12] Desmedt J.E., Nguyen T.H. and Bourguet M. (1987) Bit-mapped color imaging of human evoked potentials with reference to the N20, P22, P27 and N30 somatosensory responses. *Electroencephalogr. Clin. Neurophysiol.*, 68, 1-19.

[13] Desmedt J.E. and Tomberg C. (1989) Mapping early somatosensory evoked potentials in selective attention: critical evaluation of control conditions used for titrating by difference the cognitive P30, P40, P100 and N140. *Electroencephalogr. Clin. Neurophysiol.*, 74, 321-346.

[14] Dimitrov B., Gavrilenko T. and Gantchev G.N. (1996) Modulation of somatosensory evoked potentials during coordination between posture and movement. *Int. J. Psychophysiol.*, 22, 111-116.

[15] Forss N. and Jousmäki V. (1998) Sensorimotor integration in human primary and secondary somatosensory cortices. *Brain Res.*, 781, 259-267.

[16] Forss N., Hietanen M., Salonen O. and Hari R. (1999) Modified activation of somatosensory cortical network in patients with right-hemisphere stroke. *Brain*, 122, 1889-1899.

[17] Fujiwara N., Imai M., Nagamine T., Mima T., Oga T., Takeshita K., Toma K. and Shibasaki H. (2002) Second somatosensory area (SII) plays a significant role in selective somatosensory attention. *Brain Res. Cogn. Brain Res.*, 14, 389-397.

[18] García-Larrea L., Bastuji H and Mauguière F. (1991) Mapping study of somatosensory evoked potentials during selective spatial attention. *Electroencephalogr. Clin. Neurophysiol.*, 80, 201-214.

[19] Gerloff C., Uenishi N., Nagamine T., Kunieda T., Hallett M. and Shibasaki H. (1998) Cortical activation during fast repetitive finger movements in humans: steady-state movement-related magnetic fields and their cortical generators. *Electroencephalogr. Clin. Neurophysiol.*, 109, 444-453.

[20] Giblin D.R. (1964) Somatosensory evoked potentials in healthy subjects and patients with lesions of the nervous system. *Ann. N. Y. Acad. Sci.*, 112, 93-142.

[21] Hämäläinen M. Hari R. Ilmoniemi R. Kunuutila J. and Lounasmaa O.V. (1993) Magnetoencephalography-Theory, instrumentation, and application to noninvasive studies of the working human brain. *Rev. Mod. Phys.*, 65, 413-497.

[22] Hari R., Hämäläinen H., Hämäläinen M., Kekoni J., Sams M. and Tiihonen J. (1990) Separate finger representations at the human second somatosensory cortex. *Neuroscience*, 37, 245-249.

[23] Hari R., Karhu J., Hämäläinen M., Knuutila J., Salonen O., Sams M. and Vilkman V. (1993) Functional organization of the human first and second somatosensory cortices: a neuromagnetic study. *Eur. J. Neurosci.*, 5, 724-734.

[24] Hari R. and Forss N. (1999) Magnetoencephalography in the study of human somatosensory cortical processing. *Philos. Trans. R. Soc. Lond. B. Biol. Sci.*, 354, 1145-1154.

[25] Hazemann P., Audin G. and Lille F. (1975) Effect of voluntary self-paced movements upon auditory and somatosensory evoked potentials in man. *Electroencephalogr. Clin. Neurophysiol.*, 39, 247-254.

[26] Hoshiyama M. and Sheean G. (1998) Changes of somatosensory evoked potentials preceding rapid voluntary movement in Go/No-go choice reaction time task. *Brain Res. Cogn. Brain Res.*, 7, 137-42.

[27] Hoshiyama M. and Kakigi R. (2001) Two evoked responses with different recovery functions in the primary somatosensory cortex in humans. *Clin. Neurophysiol.*, 112, 1334-1342.

[28] Huttunen J. and Hömberg V. (1991) Modification of cortical somatosensory evoked potentials during tactile exploration and simple active and passive movements. *Electroencephalogr. Clin. Neurophysiol.*, 81, 216-223.

[29] Huttunen J., Wikström H., Korvenoja A., Seppalainen A.M., Aronen H. and Ilmoniemi R.J. (1996) Significance of the second somatosensory cortex in sensorimotor integration: enhancement of sensory responses during finger movements. *Neuroreport*, 7, 1009-1012.

[30] Huttunen J., Wikström H., Salonen O. and Ilmoniemi R.J. (1999) Human somatosensory cortical activation strengths: comparison between males and females and age-related changes. *Brain Res.*, 818, 196-203.

[31] Hyvärinen J., Poranen A. and Jokinen Y. (1980) Influence of attentive behavior on neuronal responses to vibration in primary somatosensory cortex of the monkey. *J. Neurophysiol.*, 43, 870-882.

[32] Ikeda A., Lüders H.O., Burgess R.C. and Shibasaki H. (1992) Movement-related potentials recorded from supplementary motor area and primary motor area. Role of supplementary motor area in voluntary movements. *Brain*, 115, 1017-1043.

[33] Inoue K., Yamashita T., Harada T. and Nakamura S. (2002) Role of human SII cortices in sensorimotor integration. *Clin. Neurophysiol.*, 113, 1573-1578.

[34] Inui K., Tran T.D., Qiu Y., Wang X., Hoshiyama M. and Kakigi R. (2003) A comparative magnetoencephalographic study of cortical activations evoked by noxious and innocuous somatosensory stimulations. *Neuroscience*, 120, 235-248.

[35] Inui K., Wang X., Qiu Y., Nguyen B.T., Ojima S., Tamura Y., Nakata H., Wasaka T., Tran T.D. and Kakigi R. (2003) Pain processing within the primary somatosensory cortex in humans. *Eur. J. Neurosci.*, 18, 2859-2866.

[36] Inui K., Wang X., Tamura Y., Kaneoke Y. and Kakigi R. (2004) Serial processing in the human somatosensory system. *Cereb. Cortex*, 14, 851-857.

[37] Iriki A., Tanaka M. and Iwamura Y. (1996) Attention-induced neuronal activity in the monkey somatosensory cortex revealed by pupillometrics. *Neurosci. Res.*, 25, 173-181.

[38] Jahanshahi M., Jenkins I.H., Brown R.G., Marsden C.D., Passingham R.E. and Brooks D.J. (1995) Self-initiated versus externally triggered movements. I. An investigation using measurement of regional cerebral blood flow with PET and movement-related potentials in normal and Parkinson's disease subjects. *Brain*, 118, 913-933.

[39] Jiang W., Chapman C.E. and Lamarre Y. (1990) Modulation of somatosensory evoked responses in the primary somatosensory cortex produced by intracortical microstimulation of the motor cortex in the monkey. *Exp. Brain Res.*, 80, 333-344.

[40] Johansen-Berg H. and Lloyd D.M. (2000) The physiology and psychology of selective attention to touch. *Front. Biosci.*, 5, 894-904.

[41] Jones E.G. and Powell T.P. (1969) Connexions of the somatic sensory cortex of the rhesus monkey. II. Contralateral cortical connexions. *Brain*, 92, 717-730.

[42] Jones E.G., Coulter J.D. and Hendry S.H. (1978) Intracortical connectivity of architectonic fields in the somatic sensory, motor and parietal cortex of monkeys. *J. Comp. Neurol.*, 181, 291-347.

[43] Jones S.J. (1981) An 'interference" approach to the study of somatosensory evoked potentials in man. *Electroencephalogr. Clin. Neurophysiol.*, 52, 517-530.

[44] Jones S.J., Halonen J.P. and Shawkat F. (1989) Centrifugal and centripetal mechanisms involved in the 'gating' of cortical SEPs during movement. *Electroencephalogr. Clin. Neurophysiol.*, 74, 36-45.

[45] Kakigi R. and Jones S.J. (1985) Effects on median nerve SEPs of tactile stimulation applied to adjacent and remote areas of the body surface. *Electroencephalogr. Clin. Neurophysiol.*, 62, 252-265.

[46] Kakigi R., Koyama S., Hoshiyama M., Watanabe S., Shimojo M. and Kitamura Y. (1995) Gating of somatosensory evoked responses during active finger movements magnetoencephalographic studies. *J. Neurol. Sci.*, 128, 195-204.

[47] Kakigi R., Koyama S., Hoshiyama M., Kitamura Y., Shimojo M., Watanabe S. and Nakamura A. (1996) Effects of tactile interference stimulation on somatosensory evoked magnetic fields. *Neuroreport*, 7, 405-408.

[48] Kakigi R., Shimojo M., Hoshiyama M., Koyama S., Watanabe S., Naka D., Suzuki H. and Nakamura A. (1997) Effects of movement and movement imagery on somatosensory evoked magnetic fields following posterior tibial nerve stimulation. *Brain Res. Cogn. Brain Res.*, 5, 241-253.

[49] Kakigi R., Hoshiyama M., Shimojo M., Naka D., Yamasaki H., Watanabe S., Xiang J., Maeda K., Lam K., Itomi K and Nakamura A. (2000) The somatosensory evoked magnetic fields. *Prog. Neurobiol.*, 61, 495-523.

[50] Karhu J. and Tesche C.D. (1999) Simultaneous early processing of sensory input in human primary (SI) and secondary (SII) somatosensory cortices. *J. Neurophysiol.*, 81, 2017-2025.

[51] Kawamura T., Nakasato N., Seki K., Kanno A., Fujita S., Fujiwara S. and Yoshimoto T. (1996) Neuromagnetic evidence of pre- and post-central cortical sources of somatosensory evoked responses. *Electroencephalogr. Clin. Neurophysiol.*, 100, 44-50.

[52] Kida T., Nishihira Y., Wasaka T., Sakajiri Y. and Tazoe T. (2004) Differential modulation of the short- and long-latency somatosensory evoked potentials in a forewarned reaction time task. *Clin. Neurophysiol.*, 115, 2223-2230.

[53] Kida T., Wasaka T., Inui K., Akatsuka K., Nakata H. and Kakigi R. (2006) Centrifugal regulation of human cortical responses to a task-relevant somatosensory signal triggering voluntary movement. *NeuroImage*, 32, 1355-1364.

[54] Kida T., Wasaka T., Nakata H. and Kakigi R. (2006) Centrifugal regulation of task-relevant somatosensory signals to trigger a voluntary movement. *Exp. Brain Res.*, 169, 289-301.

[55] Kida T., Inui K., Wasaka T., Akatsuka K., Tanaka E. and Kakigi R. (2007) Time-varying cortical activations related to visual-tactile cross-modal links in spatial selective attention. *J. Neurophysiol.*, 97, 3585-3596.

[56] Kornhuber H.H. and Deecke L. (1965) Hirnpotentialaenderungen bei willkuerbewegungen und passiven bewegungen des menschen: bereitschaftspotential und reafferente potentiale. *Pflügers Arch. Gesamte Physiol. Menschen Tiere*, 284, 1-17.

[57] Kristeva-Feige R., Rossi S., Pizzella V., Lopez L., Erné S.N., Edrich J. and Rossini P.M. (1996) A neuromagnetic study of movement-related somatosensory gating in the human brain. *Exp. Brain Res.*, 107, 504-514.

[58] Kutas M. and Donchin E. (1980) Preparation to respond as manifested by movement-related brain potentials. *Brain Res.*, 202, 95-115.

[59] Lee R.G. and White D.G. (1974) Modification of the human somatosensory evoked potentials during voluntary movement. *Electroencephalogr. Clin. Neurophysiol.*, 36, 53-62.

[60] Lin Y.Y., Simões C., Forss N. and Hari R. (2000) Differential effects of muscle contraction from various body parts on neuromagnetic somatosensory responses. *NeuroImage*, 11, 334-340.

[61] Lin Y.Y., Chen W.T., Liao K.K., Yeh T.C., Wu Z.A., Ho L.T. and Lee L.S. (2005) Differential generators for N20m and P35m responses to median nerve stimulation. *NeuroImage*, 25, 1090-1099.

[62] Mauguière F., Merlet I., Forss N., Vanni S., Jousmäki V., Adeleine P. and Hari R. (1997) Activation of a distributed somatosensory cortical network in the human brain: a dipole modelling study of magnetic fields evoked by median nerve stimulation. Part II: Effects of stimulus rate, attention and stimulus detection. *Electroencephalogr. Clin. Neurophysiol.*, 104, 290-295.

[63] Mima T., Nagamine T., Nakamura K. and Shibasaki H. (1998) Attention modulates both primary and second somatosensory cortical activities in humans: a magnetoencephalographic study. *J. Neurophysiol.*, 80, 2215-2221.

[64] Morita H., Petersen N. and Nielsen J. (1998) Gating of somatosensory evoked potentials during voluntary movement of the lower limb in man. *Exp. Brain Res.*, 120, 143-152.

[65] Murase N., Kaji R., Shimazu H., Katayama-Hirota M., Ikeda A., Kohara N., Kimura J., Shibasaki H. and Rothwell J.C. (2000) Abnormal premovement gating of somatosensory input in writer's cramp. *Brain*, 123, 1813-1829.

[66] Nagamine T., Makela J., Mima T., Mikuni N., Nishitani N., Satoh T., Ikeda A. and Shibasaki H. (1998) Serial processing of the somesthetic information revealed by different effects of stimulus rate on the somatosensory-evoked potentials and magnetic fields. *Brain Res.*, 791, 200-208.

[67] Nakajima T., Wasaka T., Kida T., Nishimura Y., Fumoto M., Sakamoto M. and Takashi E. (2006) Changes in somatosensory evoked potentials and Hoffmann reflexes

during fast isometric contraction of foot plantarflexor in humans. *Percept. Mot. Skills*, 103, 847-860.

[68] Nakata H., Inui K., Wasaka T., Nishihira Y. and Kakigi R. (2003) Mechanisms of differences in gating effects on short-and long-latency somatosensory evoked potentials relating to movement. *Brain Topogr.*, 15, 211-222.

[69] Nakata H., Inui K., Wasaka T., Tamura Y., Tran T.D., Qiu Y., Wang X., Nguyen T.B. and Kakigi R. (2004) Movements modulate cortical activities evoked by noxious stimulation. *Pain*, 107, 91-98.

[70] Nelson A.J., Staines W.R., Graham S.J. and McIlroy W.E. (2004) Activation in SI and SII: the influence of vibrotactile amplitude during passive and task-relevant stimulation. *Brain Res. Cogn. Brain Res.*, 19, 174-184.

[71] Nelson R.J. (1987) Activity of monkey primary somatosensory cortical neurons changes prior to active movement. *Brain Res.*, 406, 402-407.

[72] Nelson R.J. (1996) Interactions between motor commands and somatic perception in sensorimotor cortex. *Curr. Opin. Neurobiol.*, 6, 801-810.

[73] Neshige R., Lüders H. and Shibasaki H. (1988) Recording of movement-related potentials from scalp and cortex in man. *Brain*, 111, 719-736.

[74] Nishihira Y., Araki H. and Ishihara A. (1991) Attenuation of somatosensory evoked potentials immediately following rapid reaction movement. *Electromyogr. Clin. Neurophysiol.*, 31, 15-20.

[75] Ochoa J. and Torebjörk E. (1983) Sensations evoked by intraneural microstimulation of single mechanoreceptor units innervating the human hand. *J. Physiol. (Lond)*, 342, 633-654.

[76] Pandya D.N. and Vignolo L.A. (1969) Interhemispheric projections of the parietal lobe in the rhesus monkey. *Brain Res.*, 15, 49-65.

[77] Pons T.P., Garraghty P.E., Friedman D.P. and Mishkin M. (1987) Physiological evidence for serial processing in somatosensory cortex. *Science*, 237, 417-420.

[78] Qiu Y., Inui K., Wang X., Nguyen B.T., Tran T.D. and Kakigi R. (2004) Effects of distraction on magnetoencephalographic responses ascending through C-fibers in humans. *Clin. Neurophysiol.*, 115, 636-646.

[79] Romo R., Hernandez A., Zainos A., Lemus L. and Brody C.D. (2002) Neuronal correlates of decision-making in secondary somatosensory cortex. *Nat. Neurosci.*, 5, 1217-1225.

[80] Rossini P.M., Paradiso C., Zarola F., Mariorenzi R., Traversa R., Martino G. and Caramia M.D. (1990) Bit-mapped somatosensory evoked potentials and muscular reflex responses in man: comparative analysis in different experimental protocols. *Electroencephalogr. Clin. Neurophysiol.*, 77, 266-275.

[81] Rushton D.N., Rothwell J.C. and Craggs M.D. (1981) Gating of somatosensory evoked potentials during different kinds of movement in man. *Brain*, 104, 465-491.

[82] Sakamoto M., Nakajima T., Wasaka T., Kida T., Nakata H., Endoh T., Nishihira Y. and Komiyama T. (2004) Load- and cadence-dependent modulation of somatosensory evoked potentials and Soleus H-reflexes during active leg pedaling in humans. *Brain Res.*, 1029, 272-285.

[83] Schmidt R.F., Schady W.J. and Torebjörk H.E. (1990) Gating of tactile input from the hand. I. Effects of finger movement. *Exp. Brain Res.*, 79, 97-102.

[84] Seyal M., Ortstadt J.L., Kraft L.W. and Gabor A.J. (1987) Effect of movement on human spinal and subcortical somatosensory evoked potentials. *Neurology*, 37, 650-655.

[85] Shibasaki H., Barrett G., Halliday E. and Halliday A.M. (1980) Components of the movement-related cortical potential and their scalp topography. *Electroencephalogr. Clin. Neurophysiol.*, 49, 213-226.

[86] Shimazu H., Kaji R., Murase N., Kohara N., Ikeda A., Shibasaki H., Kimura J. and Rothwell J.C. (1999) Pre-movement gating of short-latency somatosensory evoked potentials. *Neuroreport*, 10, 2457-2460.

[87] Soso M.J. and Fetz E.E. (1980) Responses of identified cells in postcentral cortex of awake monkeys during comparable active and passive joint movements. *J. Neurophysiol.*, 43, 1090-1110.

[88] Sperry R.W. (1950) Neural basis of the spontaneous optokinetic response produced by visual inversion. *J. Comp. Physiol. Psychol.*, 43, 482-489.

[89] Staines W.R., Brooke J.D., Cheng J., Misiaszek J.E. and MacKay W.A. (1997) Movement-induced gain modulation of somatosensory potentials and soleus H-reflexes evoked from the leg. I. Kinaesthetic task demands. *Exp. Brain Res.*, 115, 147-155.

[90] Staines W.R., Graham S.J., Black S.E. and McIlroy W.E. (2002) Task-relevant modulation of contralateral and ipsilateral primary somatosensory cortex and the role of a prefrontal-cortical sensory gating system. *NeuroImage*, 15, 190-199.

[91] Starr A. and Cohen L.G. (1985) 'Gating' of somatosensory evoked potentials begins before the onset of voluntary movement in man. *Brain Res.*, 348, 183-186.

[92] Steinmetz P.N., Roy A., Fitzgerald P.J., Hsiao S.S., Johnson K.O. and Niebur E. (2000) Attention modulates synchronized neuronal firing in primate somatosensory cortex. *Nature*, 404, 187-190.

[93] Tapia M.C., Cohen L.G. and Starr A. (1987) Selectivity of attenuation (i.e., gating) of somatosensory potentials during voluntary movement in humans. *Electroencephalogr. Clin. Neurophysiol.*, 68, 226-230.

[94] Tinazzi M., Zanette G., La Porta F., Polo A., Volpato D., Fiaschi A. and Mauguière F. (1997) Selective gating of lower limb cortical somatosensory evoked potentials (SEPs) during passive and active foot movements. *Electroencephalogr. Clin. Neurophysiol.*, 104, 312-321.

[95] Toma K., Matsuoka T., Immisch I., Mima T., Waldvogel D., Koshy B., Hanakawa T., Shill H. and Hallett M. (2002) Generators of movement-related cortical potentials: fMRI-constrained EEG dipole source analysis. *NeuroImage*, 17, 161-173.

[96] Torquati K., Pizzella V., Della Penna S., Franciotti R., Babiloni C., Romani G.L. and Rossini P.M. (2003) "Gating" effects of simultaneous peripheral electrical stimulations on human secondary somatosensory cortex: a whole-head MEG study. *NeuroImage*, 20, 1704-1713.

[97] Touge T., Takeuchi H., Sasaki I., Deguchi K. and Ichihara N. (1997) Enhanced amplitude reduction of somatosensory evoked potentials by voluntary movement in the elderly. *Electroencephalogr. Clin. Neurophysiol.*, 104, 108-114.

[98] Valeriani M., Restuccia D., Di Lazzaro V., Barba C., Le Pera D. and Tonali P. (1998) Dissociation induced by voluntary movement between two different components of the centro-parietal P40 SEP to tibial nerve stimulation. *Electroencephalogr. Clin. Neurophysiol.*, 108, 190-198.

[99] Valeriani M., Restuccia D., Di Lazzaro V., Le Pera D. and Tonali P. (1999) Effect of movement on dipolar source activities of somatosensory evoked potentials. *Muscle Nerve*, 22, 1510-1519.

[100] von Holst E. and Mittelstaedt H. (1950) Das Reafferenzprinzip: Wechselwirkungen Zwischen Zentralnervensystem und Peripherie. *Natursissenschaften*, 37, 464-476.

[101] Wasaka T., Hoshiyama M., Nakata H., Nishihira Y. and Kakigi R. (2003) Gating of somatosensory evoked magnetic fields during the preparatory period of self-initiated finger movement. *NeuroImage*, 20, 1830-1838.

[102] Wasaka T., Nakata H., Akatsuka K., Kida T., Inui K. and Kakigi R. (2005) Differential modulation in human primary and secondary somatosensory cortices during the preparatory period of self-initiated finger movement. *Eur. J. Neurosci.*, 22, 1239-1247.

[103] Wasaka T., Nakata H., Kida T. and Kakigi R. (2005) Changes in the centrifugal gating effect on somatosensory evoked potentials depending on the level of contractile force. *Exp. Brain Res.*, 166, 118-125.

[104] Wasaka T., Nakata H., Kida T. and Kakigi R. (2005) Gating of SEPs by contraction of the contralateral homologous muscle during the preparatory period of self-initiated plantar flexion. *Brain Res. Cogn. Brain Res.*, 23, 354-360.

[105] Wasaka T., Kida T., Nakata H. and Kakigi R. (2006) Pre-movement modulation of tibial nerve SEPs caused by a self-initiated dorsiflexion. *Clin. Neurophysiol.*, 117, 2023-2029.

[106] Wikström H., Huttunen J., Korvenoja A., Virtanen J., Salonen O., Aronen H. and Ilmoniemi R.J. (1996) Effects of interstimulus interval on somatosensory evoked magnetic fields (SEFs): a hypothesis concerning SEF generation at the primary sensorimotor cortex. *Electroencephalogr. Clin. Neurophysiol.*, 100, 479-487.

[107] Zhang H.Q., Murray G.M., Turman A.B., Mackie P.D., Coleman G.T. and Rowe M.J. (1996) Parallel processing in cerebral cortex of the marmoset monkey: effect of reversible SI inactivation on tactile responses in SII. *J. Neurophysiol.*, 76, 3633-3655.

[108] Zhang H.Q., Murray G.M., Coleman G.T., Turman A.B., Zhang S.P. and Rowe M.J. (2001) Functional characteristics of the parallel SI- and SII-projecting neurons of the thalamic ventral posterior nucleus in the marmoset. *J. Neurophysiol.*, 85, 1805-1822.

In: Research Topics on Brain Mapping
Editor: Yuanzhu Liáng, pp. 135-152

ISBN: 978-1-60456-001-5


*Chapter VI*

# Quantitative Aspects of BOLD Functional MRI

***Norihiko Fujita*[*1], *Hisashi Tanaka*[1] *and Kenya Murase*[2]**
[1] Department of Radiology, Osaka University Graduate School of Medicine
[2] Department of Medical Physics and Engineering, Faculty of Health Science, Osaka University Graduate School of Medicine

## Abstract

BOLD (blood oxygenation level dependent) contrast based functional MRI (fMRI) has been established as a noninvasive tool for brain mapping research. For most applications of BOLD fMRI, the primary objective is simply to identify activated areas in response to a specific stimulation. The fractional BOLD signal change depends on the imaging parameters such as echo time and field strength, and only its relative magnitude to the time-course signal variation (noise) is used for a statistical inference to reveal focal area(s) of interest. While a quantitative and absolute evaluation of BOLD signal change in terms of physiological parameters usually does not need to be considered, recent theoretical and experimental studies for the quantitative use of BOLD fMRI have provided us with new opportunities: 1) mapping of hemodynamic parameters of the human brain in the baseline state, such as deoxyhemoglobin concentration, venous CBV (cerebral blood volume), OEF (oxygen extraction fraction) and oxidative energetics in terms of cerebral metabolic rate of oxygen ($CMRO_2$) 2) optimization of imaging parameters, e.g., the voxel volume and echo time for given hardware settings such as the field strength and coil sensitivity.

---

[*] Corresponding Author: Norihiko Fujita, M.D. Department of Radiology; Osaka University Graduate School of Medicine; 2-2 Yamadaoka, Suita, Osaka 565-0871, Japan; Phone: 81-6-6879-3434; Fax: 81-6-6879-3439; e-mail: nofujita@radiol.med.osaka-u.ac.jp; nofjt@nifty.com

# Introduction

We describe quantitative aspects of blood oxygenation level-dependent (BOLD) [1,2] contrast based functional MRI. We first explain the meaning of "quantitative" in comparison with "qualitative "functional MRI for identifying activated areas in response to stimulation. As shown in figure 1, BOLD contrast to noise ratio (CNR) is defined as the signal difference ($\Delta S$) between active and resting states in units of the standard deviation ($\sigma$) of time-course fMRI signal within each voxel [3, 4]. When these quantities, $\Delta S$ and $\sigma$ are normalized to the baseline signal ($S$), BOLD CNR is expressed by:

$$\text{BOLD CNR} = \Delta S/\sigma = \text{BOLD signal change}/\ ^{(n)}\sigma, \tag{1}$$

where 'BOLD signal change' represents the stimulation-induced fractional signal change, $\Delta S/S$ , and $^{(n)}\sigma$ is the signal variation relative to the baseline signal, $\sigma/S$, which corresponds to the reciprocal of the time-course signal to noise ratio (SNR).

BOLD CNR, i.e., the magnitude of BOLD signal change relative to $^{(n)}\sigma$ is generally used for a statistical inference in order to reveal focal area(s) of interest in response to stimulation. In the context of qualitative functional MRI, BOLD CNR is therefore viewed as merely a statistical measure for extracting activated areas. In this article, we evaluate separately the two terms of BOLD CNR, i.e., BOLD signal change and fMRI time-course signal variation (noise) in a quantitative manner, which provides us with new opportunities: 1) mapping of hemodynamic parameters of the human brain in the baseline state, such as deoxyhemoglobin concentration, oxygen extraction fraction (OEF) and oxidative energetics in terms of cerebral metabolic rate of oxygen ($CMRO_2$) if combined with a cerebral blood flow (CBF) measurement [5-9] and 2) optimization of imaging parameters, e.g., the voxel volume and echo time for given hardware settings such as the field strength and coil sensitivity [10, 11].

The latter issue relates to the quantitative characteristics of BOLD fMRI noise [12-14] rather than BOLD contrast, which will be described later. We first provide a brief review on BOLD contrast mechanisms with a particular emphasis on the importance of gradient-echo extravascular BOLD signal, which is the basis for the quantitative evaluation of BOLD contrast.

# BOLD Contrast

BOLD contrast depends on the amount of deoxyhemoglobin within an imaging voxel [1,2]. The presence of paramagnetic deoxyhemoglobin leads to perturbations of the magnetic field both in and around the vessels, and therefore it affects the signal in both extravascular and intravascular compartments. The relative contribution of these origins to the total BOLD signal change is significantly affected by the specifics of a fMRI measurement [15-20]. The intravascular contribution, which is substantially identical to venous blood signal, can be significantly reduced or removed with the use of very high magnetic fields, diffusion weighting/velocity sensitization [17] and/or an inversion recovery technique such as vascular space occupancy (VASO) [20]. Recent studies with the use of a conventional gradient-echo

echo-planar image acquisition [20, 21] indicated that the extravasular contribution to the total BOLD signal was relatively dominant in the range of 50% to 70 % even at as low as 1.5T, and the extravasular contribution would predominate much more with the increase of magnetic field strength [15, 19]. A BOLD signal model with both contributions is possible [9,17-19], but the model depends on many parameters, and therefore, it might complicate the fitting of the data acquired in order to extract relevant physiological parameters. We therefore consider only the extravascular BOLD contribution in the following.

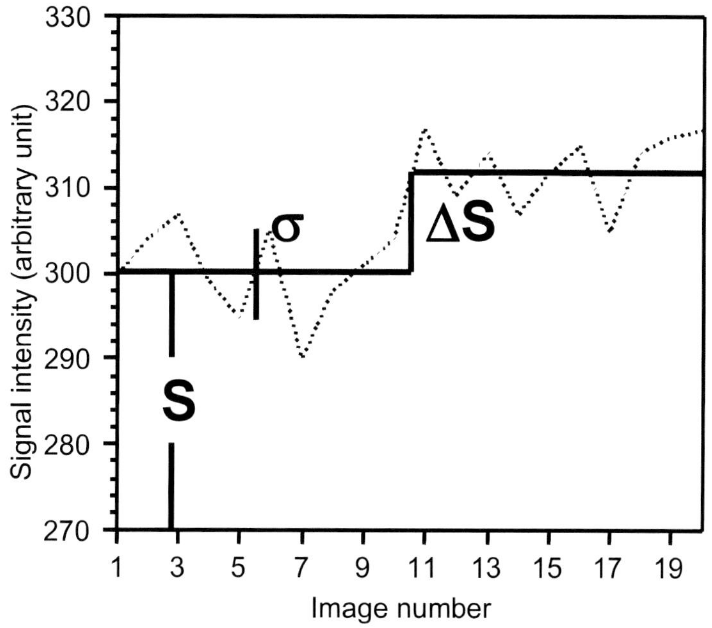


Figure 1. BOLD CNR and functional SNR. A hypothetical fMRI signal time course from a single voxel is shown (broken line). The first 10 images and the last 10 images correspond to the resting and active states, respectively. BOLD contrast to noise ratio (CNR) is defined as the signal difference ($\Delta S$) between active and resting states in units of the standard deviation ($\sigma$) of time course fMRI signal, i.e., $\Delta S/\sigma$. When these quantities, $\Delta S$ and $\sigma$ are normalized to the baseline signal ($S$), BOLD CNR is expressed by 'BOLD signal change'/ $^{(n)}\sigma$. 'BOLD signal change' represents, the stimulation induced fractional signal change, $\Delta S/S$ , and $^{(n)}\sigma$ is the signal variation relative to the baseline signal, $\sigma/S$, which corresponds to the inverse of the time-course (functional) signal to noise ratio (SNR).

Since the fundamental discovery of BOLD contrast [1, 2], the extravascular BOLD contrast mechanism has been studied extensively [5, 15-19]. The theoretical and numerical simulation results consistently showed that there exists a significant difference between gradient-echo and spin-echo signal acquisitions, as shown in figure 2. The spatial specificity may be significantly improved with the use of a spin-echo pulse sequence because of its selective sensitivity to microvessels [22], but it is explicit that the sensitivity for overall vessels is significantly reduced compared with the use of a gradient-echo. Spin-echo BOLD signal highly depends on vessel size, which substantially prevents its quantitative evaluation. In contrast, gradient-echo extravascular BOLD signal has an almost constant sensitivity for all sized vessels, except for very small capillary-sized vessels [5, 15, 19], as shown in figure

2. In view of its quantification, it can be approximately characterized by only a single parameter as determined by the constant BOLD sensitivity for relatively large sized vessels. This approximation may be justified by the large weight of the venous part in tissue vasculature and the greater BOLD signal change by veins as compared with capillaries [8, 15-19, 23]. In the next section, we describe details on the gradient-echo exravascular BOLD signal change, which is the basis for quantification of BOLD contrast.

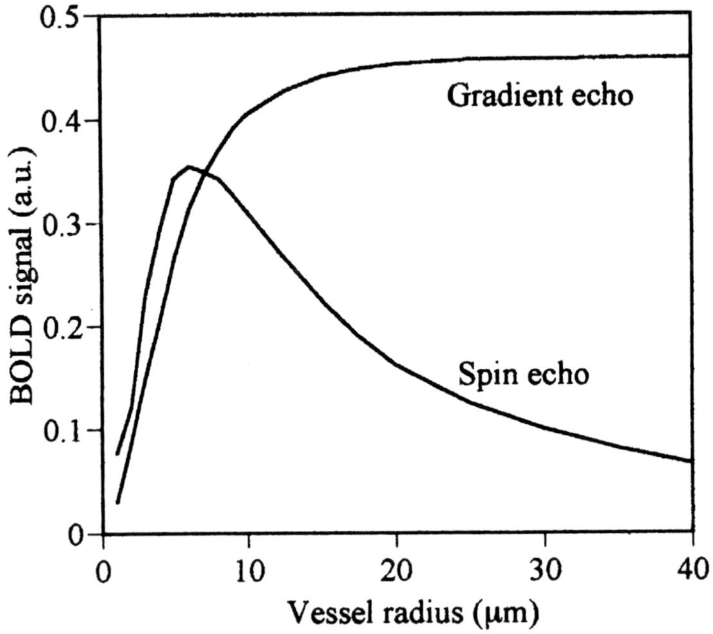


Figure 2. Gradient echo and spin echo extravascular BOLD signal as a function of vessel radius; A numerical simulation was performed assuming a vascular network model of randomly oriented paramagnetic vessels within an imaging voxel. In case of the gradient echo signal acquisition (*TE*=50 ms, at 1.5T), the BOLD signal change is almost constant for the radius greater than 10 μm, although it is significantly reduced for capillary sized microvessels. In case of the spin echo signal acquisition (*TE*=100 ms, at 1.5 T), the peak BOLD signal change occurred at the vessel radius of 7 μm. While this indicates its selective sensitivity to microvessels, it is explicit that the sensitivity for overall vessels is significantly reduced compared with the gradient echo case.

## Gradient-Echo Extravascular BOLD Signal Change

In BOLD contast-based fMRI, the typical pulse sequences used are gradient echoes with long echo times. In this case, the transverse signal decay is characterized by the effective relaxation rate, $R_2*$ . Then, the measured signal $S(t)$ can be approximately described in terms of a simple linear exponential function, exp $(-R_2*t)$, where $t$ is time from spin excitation, and $t$ is specifically designated as echo time (*TE*) when it defines the time between excitation and signal acquisition.

In general, $R_2*$ consists of two contributions, $R_2* = R_2 + R_2'$, on the assumption that the effect of macroscopic magnetic field inhomogeneities is negligible (figure 3). The $R_2$

relaxation rate constant describes the irreversible part with respect to a phase reversal π pulse and the $R_2'$ relaxation rate represents the reversible part of the MR signal decay that originates from relatively large scale field inhomogeneities. For simplicity, we consider that such large scale field inhomogeneities originate only from intravascular deoxyhemoglobin, and then, the $R_2'$ term is specifically denoted by $R_{2dHb}'$:

$$R_2^* = R_2 + R_2'_{dHb} . \tag{2}$$

Assuming a vascular model with randomly oriented paramagnetic vessels within an imaging voxel, Yablonskiy and Haccke [5] theoretically investigated purely extravascular BOLD signal change for gradient-echo signal acquisition. They showed that on the condition that the gradient-echo signal is measured at relatively long $TE$s, $R_2'_{dHb}$ is proportional to the total amount of deoxyhemoglobin within an imaging voxel. When we define venous part of CBV as $v$ and oxygen extraction fraction as OEF, the total amount of deoxyhemoglobin is proportional to the product of $v$ and OEF [7]. Therefore, $R_2'_{dHb}$ is expressed by

$$R_2'_{dHb} = k\, v\, \mathrm{OEF}, \tag{3}$$

where $k$ is the proportional constant that increases linearly with the static magnetic field strength [5, 7].

The BOLD fractional signal change ($\Delta S/S$) as shown in figure 1 is usually only a few percent. Therefore, it is approximately converted to the change in $R_2^*$, $\Delta R_2^* = -\Delta S/S/TE$, where $TE$ is the echo time. From equation (2), it is explicit that $\Delta R_2^*$ should consists of the stimulation-induced change of $R_2$, $\Delta R_2$ and that of $R_2'_{\mathrm{dHb}}$, $\Delta R_2'_{\mathrm{dHb}}$ (figure 3). However, it has been shown that $\Delta R_2$ is more than one order smaller than $\Delta R_2'_{\mathrm{dHb}}$ [16, 24] , which is compatible with the fact that the overall sensitivity for gradient-echo is much greater than that for spin-echo as noted previously (figure 2). Therefore, the change in the effective relaxation rate, $\Delta R_2^*$ primarily results from $\Delta R_2'_{\mathrm{dHb}}$, i.e.,

$$\Delta R_2'_{\mathrm{dHb}} = -\Delta S/S/TE. \tag{4}$$

Quantitatively, the stimulation-induced change, $\Delta R_2'_{\mathrm{dHb}}$ should be calibrated based on its baseline value, $R_2'_{\mathrm{dHb}}$ that corresponds to equation (3) [7, 8]. The calibrated BOLD signal change, $\Delta R_2'_{\mathrm{dHb}}/R_2'_{\mathrm{dHb}}$, has the quantitative relationship with CBF, CBV, and $CMRO_2$ [8, 15, 25-27]: From the representation of $R_2'_{\mathrm{dHb}}$ shown in equation (3) and a flow-volume relationship, $\Delta v/v = (1 + \Delta\mathrm{CBF/CBF})^{\alpha} - 1$, the conservation law for oxygen supply and consumption provides the following expression:

$$\Delta R_2'_{\mathrm{dHb}}/R_2'_{\mathrm{dHb}} = (1 + \Delta\mathrm{CBF/CBF})^{\alpha - 1}(1 + \Delta\, \mathrm{CMRO_2/CMRO_2}) - 1. \tag{5}$$

As for the parameter, α, characterizing the volume-flow relationship , $\alpha$=0.38 has been taken from a PET experiment on global CBF change with a respiratory $CO_2$ challenge [28]. This value of α may be appropriate for a total CBV change as measured by PET activation experiments [29], while recent studies with PET [30] and $^{19}$F NMR [31] have shown that it may result in overestimation for a change of BOLD-sensitive venous fraction of CBV. Therefore, $\alpha = 0.19$ may be appropriate for BOLD contrast [8].

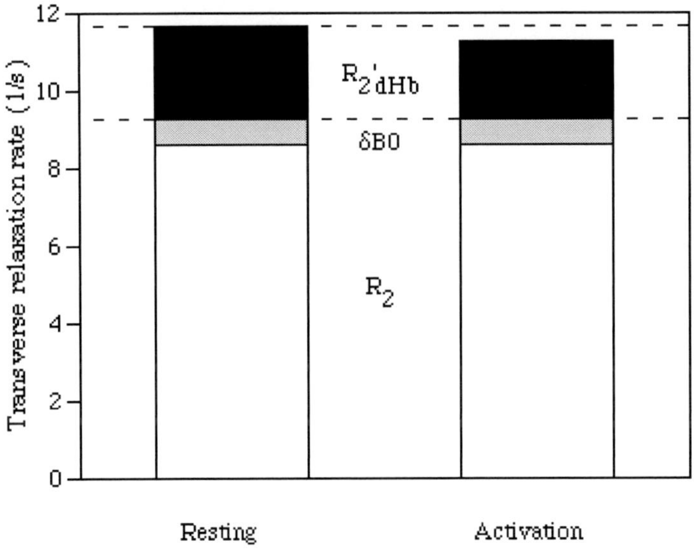


Figure 3. Transverse relaxation rate changes during resting and active states. The effective transverse relaxation rate, $R_2^*$, as measured by gradient echo sequences is generally represented by the sum of $R_2$, $R_2'$, and $\delta B_0$, each being the irreversible relaxation rate of tissues as measured by spin echo sequences, the reversible relaxation rate caused by tiny magnetic susceptibility sources within an imaging voxel, and macroscopic magnetic field inhomogeneities, respectively. If deoxyhemoglobin (dHb) is assumed to be the only susceptibility source, $R_2'$ specifically corresponds to $R_2'{}_{dHb}$, and $R_2^*$ is represented by the sum of $R_2$ (white), $\delta B_0$ (gray), and $R_2'{}_{dHb}$ (black). The basis of BOLD contrast is a decrease in dHb content during the active state compared with that during the resting state, which leads to a decrease in $R_2^*$. Since the contribution of $R_2$ to BOLD contrast is usually small and $\delta B_0$ does not change, the decrease in $R_2^*$ specifically corresponds to a decrease in $R_2'{}_{dHb}$, $\Delta R_2'{}_{dHb}$.

## Calibration of BOLD Signal and Quantitative Evaluation of Hemodynamic Parameters

From equation [4], the measured BOLD signal change is converted to the relaxation rate change, $\Delta R_2'{}_{dHb}$. This quantity should be normalized by its baseline value, $R_2'{}_{dHb}$, in order to evaluate the change of the cerebral metabolic rate of oxygen ($CMRO_2$), as shown in equation (5). In such a view of quantitative fMRI, the calibration of BOLD signal has been performed with the use of $CO_2$ breathing [25-27] or breath holding [32] as a physiological means of manipulating CBF independent of $CMRO_2$. The method consists of rather complex procedures, such as the requirement of a source of $CO_2$, the use of a facemask, and/or the low signal to noise ratio associated with additional BOLD and CBF measurement. Furthermore, the procedure of $CO_2$ challenge may modulate the normal state of oxygen metabolism and perfusion, which may significantly affect subsequent activation experiments [33, 34].

On the other hand, direct approaches for calibrating BOLD signal have been recently proposed [6-9]. The methodology is commonly based on a time-efficient measurement of the reversible contribution of the transverse relaxation rate, $R_2'$ with a modified spin-echo pulse sequence [35, 36]. The $R_2$ term in equation (2) is the major contribution to the total relaxation rate, $R_2*$, and the contribution due to deoxyhemoglobin, $R_2'_{dHb}$ is relatively small. Therefore, careful treatments should be done for an accurate measurement of this quantity. One such treatment is related to the fact that brain tissues display multi-compartment transverse signal decay, rather than a one-component structure similar to water in a phantom [7-9]. A method for correcting this effect has been devised by acquiring additional data on the multi-component $R_2$ decay [7]. Based on an MR signal model that incorporates the multi-compartment signal decay and other tissue factors, He and Yablonskiy [9] has recently proposed a method for a separate estimation of venous CBV and OEF, rather than $R_2'_{dHb}$ as their product.

Figure 4 shows an example of the quantitative fMRI study based on the direct measurement method of $R_2'_{dHb.}$ This subject showed a BOLD fractional signal increase of 1.52 ± 0.99% within the activated areas in the bilateral occipital lobe, while the calibrated BOLD signal map relative to the baseline $R_2'_{dHb}$ showed a one order of magnitude larger change, a 15.7 ± 12.8% decrease in the same area (figure 4a). The relative decrease in $R_2'_{dHb}$ corresponds to the same amount of decrease in deoxyhemoglobin, as shown in equation (3). The fractional CBF change map (figure 4b) showed a 79.7 ± 30.3% increase within the activated area. From the calibrated BOLD signal change as well as the CBF change, a fractional change of $CMRO_2$ (figure 4c) was calculated on a voxel-by-voxel basis using equation (5), assuming $\alpha = 0.19$. The fractional $CMRO_2$ change map represented in the scale of 0% to 50% showed a similar spatial pattern with the fractional CBF map in the scale of 0% to 100% (figure 4b). This means that the magnitude of the fractional $CMRO_2$ increase in the activated area, i.e., 38.3 ± 20.2% is approximately half that of the fractional CBF increase. Previous quantitative fMRI studies in humans [25-27] also have consistently shown that the ratio of CBF change to $CMRO_2$ change is 2 to 3:1 for a similar visual activation.

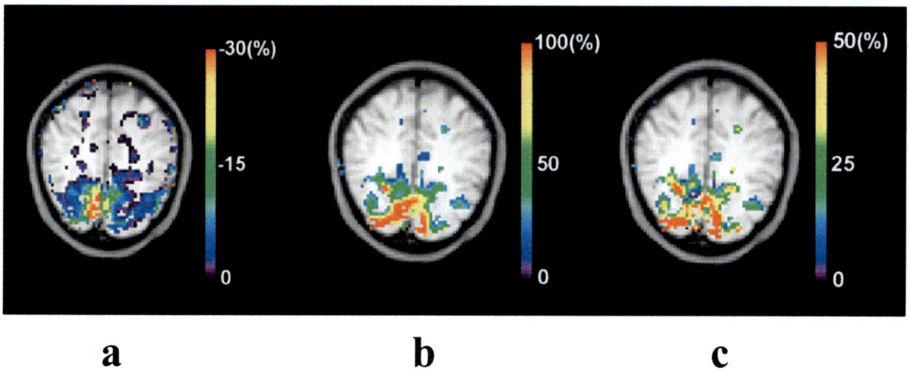


Figure 4. A representative case of quantitative functional MRI during visual stimulation. (a) calibrated BOLD signal change (b) fractional CBF change; (c) fractional $CMRO_2$ change calculated from equation (5) assuming $\alpha = 0.19$.

This sort of quantitative functional MRI has been achieved by the evaluation of physiological parameters such as $R_2'_{dHb}$ in the baseline state, either in an indirect manner [25-27] or a direct manner [8]. Recently, there has been a noticeable trend towards such quantitative measurements of the baseline states of the brain using MRI [37, 38]. This is ascribed to the fact that there have been arising some important questions to be answered on physiology of the brain in the baseline state. For example, during states of pharmacological perturbations such as anesthesia, $CO_2$/acetazolamide, hypoxia, or caffeine administration, or pathologic states such as hemodynamic impairment, BOLD signal in response to a given stimulation may be modulated compared with that during a normal physiologic state [39]. This indicates that alterations of the baseline states of the brain lead to a significant modulation of BOLD effect. In relation to negative BOLD signals, a recent study [40] has revealed that an understanding of its energetic basis can be obtained using the quantitative use of BOLD fMRI. Such an effort is also crucial for deciphering the consequences of baseline-state impairment by diseases of the brain such as stroke. For example, a MRI study [41] on patients with acute infarction of middle cerebral artery (MCA) distribution showed that a prominent low intensity on the $T_2$* weighted image was seen in the affected MCA territory. The low intensity was rationally explained due to an increased BOLD effect caused by the increase of the amount of deoxyhemoglobin. The increase of the amount of deoxyhemoglobin results from the increase of OEF and/or venous fraction of CBV, which is known to occur at the hyperacute stage of infarction using PET imaging techniques [42]. Such studies for patients will be more available for research and clinical applications, if they can be performed based on MRI methods rather than PET methods, in particular using the quantitative fMRI methods as described here.

## BOLD CNR and Noise in fMRI

So far, we have described quantitative aspects of BOLD signal change and the relevant physiological issues such as the quantitative evaluation of $CMRO_2$. In the following, we provide a quantitative description of BOLD CNR. BOLD CNR reflects how easily we can see differences between the resting and active states (figure 1), and therefore we exclusively discuss sensitivity issues of functional MRI. For a given BOLD signal change, BOLD CNR is determined by the noise magnitude which corresponds to the standard deviation of a series of time-course signal, as shown in equation [1]. We first describe some important characteristics of the noise in BOLD fMRI as related to its quantitative evaluation. Then, we show that a quantitative understanding of BOLD CNR is useful for optimization of imaging parameters such as voxel size, which is one of the most important imaging variables affecting activation detection in fMRI.

Noise in BOLD fMRI can generally be classified as thermal noise ($\sigma_T$), noise related to scanner instabilities ($\sigma_I$), and physiological noise ($\sigma_P$) [12]. Previous studies [12, 13] have reported that $\sigma_I$ is usually small compared with the other noise contributions when using a well-adjusted MR scanner, in particular under a careful quality assurance protocol for its stable performance [43]. Therefore, we consider only the two noise contributions, $\sigma_T$ and $\sigma_P$. Previous fMRI studies showed some distinctive differences exist between the characteristics of thermal noise and physiological noise. Weisskoff et al. [44] noted the specific frequency distributions to the physiological noise as related to cardiac pulsation and respiration, while because of its random nature, thermal noise has no specific frequency distributions. Krueger and Glover [12] showed that the difference in signal strength dependence could be used to estimate each noise contribution separately, which was the basis for a further quantitative evaluation. Recently, it has been experimentally demonstrated that the magnitudes of thermal and physiological noise depended differently on voxel size [14]. A quantitative analysis of the thermal and physiological noise contributions is provided, with a particular emphasis on the difference in voxel size dependence.

## Thermal Noise and Physiological Noise as a Function of Voxel Volume

A recent experimental study [14] showed that the magnitude of ${}^{(n)}\sigma_P$ was almost independent of the voxel volume, where ${}^{(n)}\sigma_P$ is the physiological noise relative to the baseline signal, i.e., $\sigma_P/S$,. This is because physiological noise has some correlation distance significantly greater than a single voxel, which may extend to the whole brain in case of changes in systemic physiological activities. As for the thermal noise contribution relative to the baseline signal, ${}^{(n)}\sigma_T$, its dependence on the voxel volume ($V$) has been well known from the early days of MRI: ${}^{(n)}\sigma_T(V)$ is inversely proportional to voxel volume, $V$, for initial settings of MR imaging parameters and ${}^{(n)}\sigma_T(V)$ is inversely proportional to the square root of voxel volume, $V^{1/2}$, for post-processing acquired MR images [45]. Taking into account such differences in voxel volume dependence between ${}^{(n)}\sigma_T$ and ${}^{(n)}\sigma_P$, the time-course signal variation , ${}^{(n)}\sigma(V)$, is given by:

$$ {}^{(n)}\sigma(V) = ({}^{(n)}\sigma_T(V)^2 + {}^{(n)}\sigma_P{}^2)^{1/2}. \quad (6) $$

Figure 5 shows an example of ${}^{(n)}\sigma(V)$ as calculated from equation (6). The relative physiological noise, ${}^{(n)}\sigma_P$ was assumed to be 1% , and ${}^{(n)}\sigma_T(V)$ was assumed to decrease as 1/ $V$ and take the same value with ${}^{(n)}\sigma_P$ of 1% at $V$=4. We define $V_E$ as the voxel size at which the magnitudes of physiological and thermal noise are equal, and $V_E$ is 4 for this case.

For the region of small voxel volumes of $V< V_E = 4$ in figure 5, the thermal noise contribution dominates over the total noise. We consider an initial choice of voxel volume in this thermal noise dominant regimen, $V< V_E = 4$. The use of a bigger voxel volume in comparison with the initial choice of voxel volume reduces the total noise efficiently, which will lead to an improved detection of activated areas. Figure 6 shows functional activation maps during visual stimulation as a function of voxel volume. At the relatively high spatial resolution (upper, 4x 2 mm; on the left, 128), the thermal noise contribution dominated over the total noise, and therefore, the choice of the voxel volume corresponds to $V< V_E = 4$ in figure 5. An increase in effective voxel volume with the use of spatial smoothing (upper, 4x 2 mm; Z-64 and Z-32) led to a significantly improved detection of activated voxels, as expected from the effective decrease of the total noise .

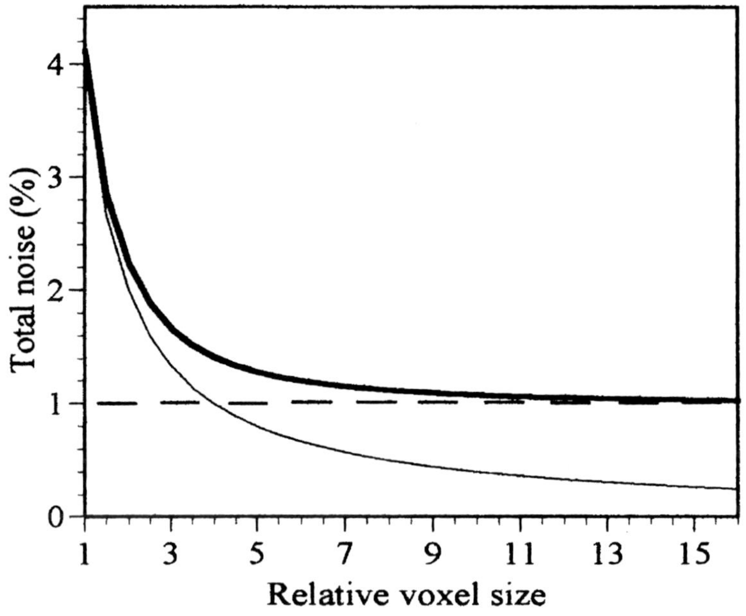


Figure 5. functional MRI noise calculated as a function of voxel volume ($V$). The bold line represents the total noise (${}^{(n)}\sigma$ ($V$) ) calculated from the two component noise model, ${}^{(n)}\sigma(V) = ({}^{(n)}\sigma_T(V)^2 + {}^{(n)}\sigma_P^{\,2})^{1/2}$ (See, equation(6)). The physiological noise relative to the baseline signal, ${}^{(n)}\sigma_P$ was assumed to be 1%, independent of the voxel size (broken line), while the relative thermal noise contribution (thin line), ${}^{(n)}\sigma_T(V)$ is assumed to decrease proportionally to $1/V$ and match the relative physiological noise of 1% when the relative voxel volume is 4.

For the region of large voxel volumes of $V \cong V_E = 4$ or $V > V_E = 4$ in figure 5, the physiological noise is comparable with the thermal noise or the physiological noise dominates over the total noise. We consider an initial choice of voxel volume of $V \cong V_E$. The use of a bigger voxel volume in comparison with the initial choice of voxel volume reduces the total noise, but the effect is significantly small and therefore it will not lead to an improved detection of activated voxels so much. Figure 6 clearly shows this. At the relatively low spatial resolution (lower, 8 mm; on the left, 128), the magnitudes of thermal noise and physiological noise were comparable, and therefore, the choice of the voxel volume corresponds to the voxel volume of $V \cong V_E = 4$ in figure 5. The increases of the number of activated voxels associated with an effective increase in voxel volume (lower, 8 mm; Z-64 and Z-32) were not so prominent in comparison with the above-mentioned thermal noise dominant case (upper, 4x 2 mm).

As shown in figure 6, the choice of voxel volume in BOLD fMRI is important, because it significantly affects the final outcome of detecting functional activations. The two-component noise model shown in figure 5 suggests that the voxel volume in which thermal noise matches physiological noise, i.e., $V_E$ can be viewed as an upper limit to voxel volume in fMRI. In other words, $V_E$ is the point at which one can get a relatively high SNR for the least loss in resolution [11]. However, $V_E$ may not be optimal for maximizing detection of functional activations. As for the optimization of voxel size in fMRI, a further discussion is possible with a quantitative BOLD CNR consideration.

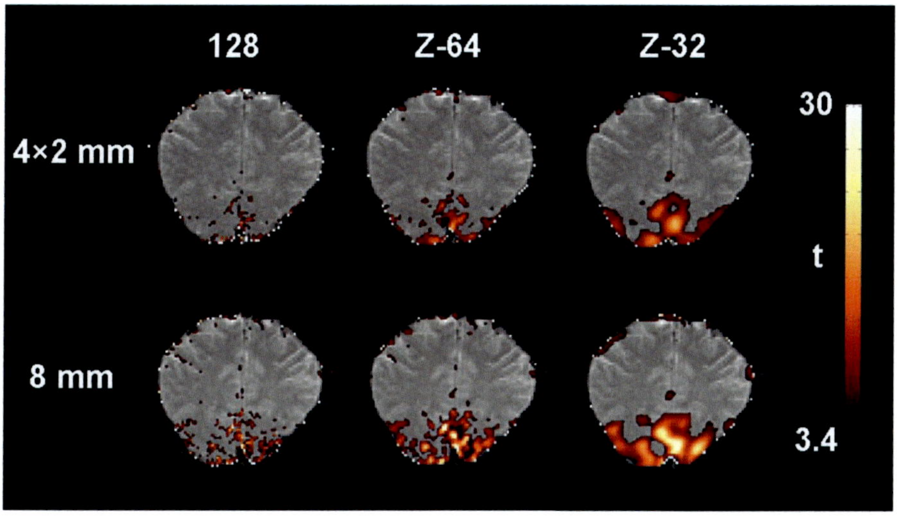


Figure 6. Functional MRI activation maps during visual stimulation. as a function of effective voxel volume. The lower activation maps were obtained from a time series of EPI image data of 8 mm slice thickness, while the upper from EPI image data of four contiguous slices of 2 mm slice thickness. The four slices were subslice averaged (4 x 2 mm) to obtain a slice of 8 mm thickness. The magnitude of the relative thermal noise for the 4x 2 mm image was twice greater that for the 8 mm image, as theoretically expected. The maps on the left were calculated from the original 8 mm and 4 x 2 mm image datasets with a 128 x 128 matrix (nominal in plane resolution = 2 mm x 2 mm). The original images were Fourier transformed into 128 x 128 k space data and spatially smoothed with the zero padding filter using 64 x 64 (Z 64) and 32 x 32 (Z 32) lines of central k space data, respectively. The effective in plane spatial resolution of the Z 64 and Z 32 image was 4 mm x 4 mm and 8 mm x 8 mm, respectively. Each activation map represents color coded $t$ values ($t$>3.4; p<0.001) superimposed on the corresponding original 128 x 128 or spatially smothed EPI image.

# BOLD CNR as a Function of Voxel Volume

In any imaging modality, an optimum voxel volume for maximizing CNR is determined as a compromise between two opposing effect: One is a modulation in noise as a function of voxel volume and the other is a modulation in contrast due to partial volume effects (PVE) [4]. We theoretically evaluated BOLD CNR, taking into account a BOLD contrast modulation due to PVE as well as the noise as a function of voxel volume shown in equation (6). For this purpose, we assumed a three-dimensional Gaussian distribution of BOLD signal [4]. The volume of hypothetical activation as determined by full width at half maximum was varied, and the contrast modulation with respect to the voxel volume was calculated, as shown in figure 7a. Based on its definition, we evaluated BOLD CNR as the ratio of the calculated BOLD contrast modulation due to PVE to the noise function shown in equation (6).

When only the thermal noise contribution is considered, the calculated BOLD CNR behavior significantly varied, depending on each size of activation (figure 7b). The calculated results indicate that the optimal voxel volume matches the volume of activation, because it represents the minimum voxel volume with nearly the maximum of the available BOLD CNR.

Thus the volume of activation, which is generally not known a priori, determines the optimum voxel volume. In contrast to this, the presence of physiological noise significantly reduced the dependence of BOLD CNR on the volume of activation (figures 7c). Thus, for a wide range of activation volumes, the relative BOLD CNR was maximized at a limited range of voxel volumes between each volume of activation and $V_E$. In other words, $V_E$ is essentially the optimal point at which one can get a sufficiently high BOLD CNR for a wide range of BOLD activation volumes, i.e., either the volume of activation smaller or greater than $V_E$ .

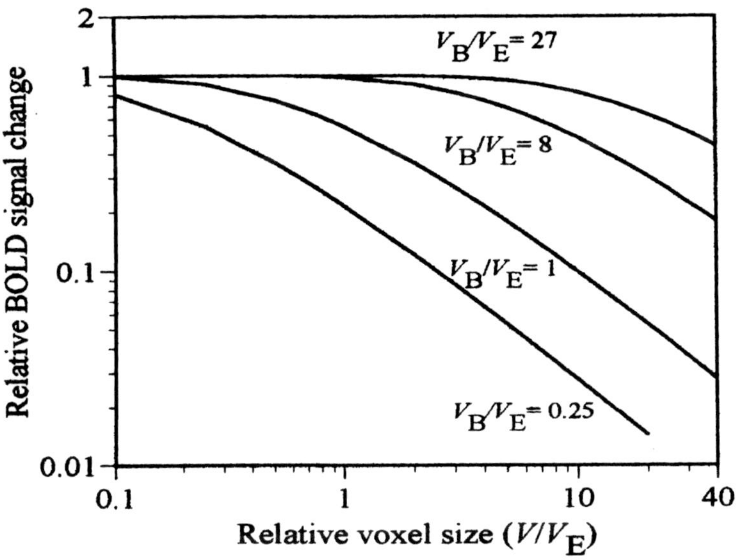


a.

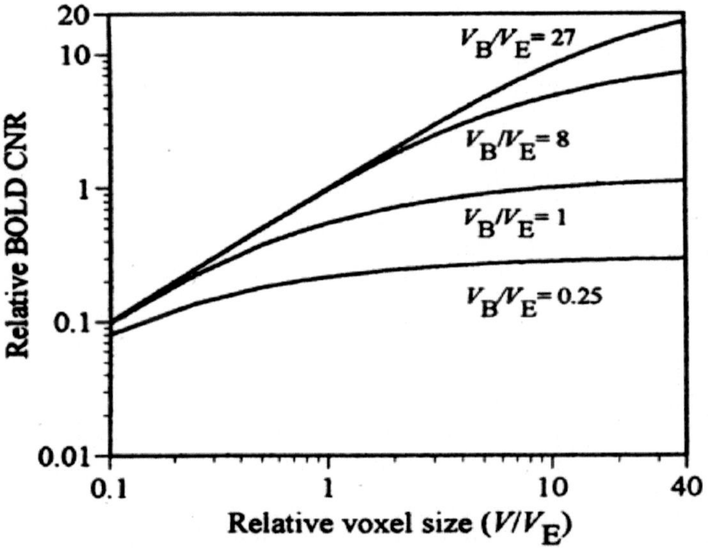


b.

Figure 7. Continued on next page.

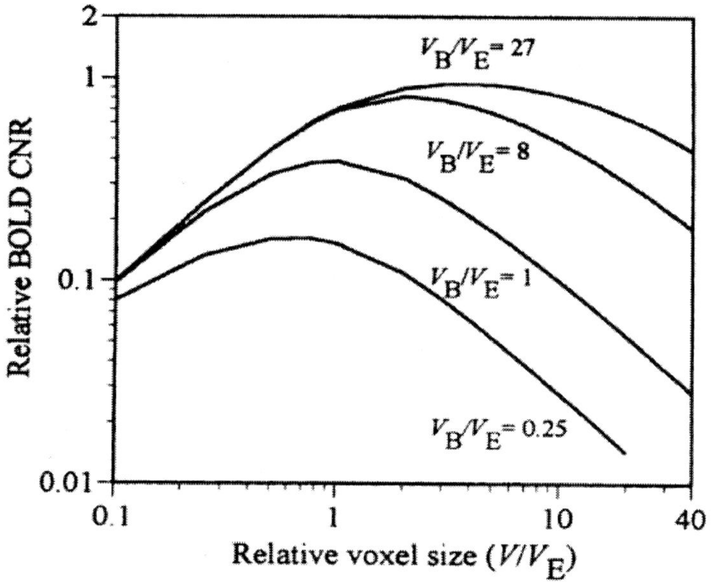


c.

Figure 7. Calculated BOLD CNR as a function of voxel volume 7a: BOLD contrast modulation due to partial volume effects (PVE). A three dimensional Gaussian distribution of BOLD signal was assumed. $V_B$ represents a characteristic volume for the hypothetical activation, and $V_E$ a reference voxel volume. Since $V_E$ can be set arbitrarily, it is assumed that $V_E$ represents the voxel size at which the magnitudes of physiological and thermal noise are equal, in the same way as Figures 7b and 7c. The abscissa represents a voxel volume relative to $V_E$, $V/V_E$, and each value of $V_B/V_E$ represents the volume of activation relative to $V_E$. For each relative volume of activation, BOLD contrast modulation due to PVE is represented. 7b: BOLD CNR in the absence of physiological noise. The abscissa represents a voxel volume relative to $V_E$, $V/V_E$, in the same way as figure 7a. The relative BOLD CNR values were calculated as the ratio of the BOLD contrast modulation shown in figure 7a to the noise function corresponding to equation (6). When thermal noise alone is considered, the noise function is simply given by $V_E/V$ for the case of initial imaging parameter settings for acquiring MR images. The calculated BOLD CNR results indicate that the optimal voxel volume matches the volume of activation, because it represents the minimum voxel volume with nearly the maximum of the available BOLD CNR. Thus the volume of activation, which is generally not known a priori, determines the optimum voxel volume. 7c: BOLD CNR in the presence of physiological noise. Taking into account the presence of physiological noise, the noise function is given by $((V_E/V)^2+1)^{1/2}$ for the case of initial imaging parameter settings for acquiring MR images. Note that the calculated BOLD CNR values do not exceed unity, and the scale of the ordinate is therefore set differently from those in figure 7b. For relative activation volumes of $V_B/V_E$ =0.25, 1, 8, and 27, maximal BOLD CNR values were obtained at a limited range of $V/V_E$, i.e., approximately 0.7, 1, 2, and 3, respectively.

From experimental data using a conventional volume head coil by Triantafyllou *et al* [14], $V_E$ was calculated to be about 50 (3.7 × 3.7 × 3.7) mm$^3$ at 1.5 T. We performed a similar measurement at 1.5 T and found that $V_E$ was 45 to 50 mm$^3$ for gray matter regions. On the assumption that the optimum voxel volume is given by $V_E$, this volume of $V_E$ at 1.5 T agrees well with the optimum voxel volume of 80 mm$^3$ experimentally determined for the detection of motor cortex activation under similar experimental conditions [46]. With the use of higher field strengths and /or highly sensitive multi-channel coils, $V_E$ can be reduced to as small as 6 mm$^3$ for gray matter regions [11, 14]. On the other hand, cognitive neuroscience applications of fMRI in the context of multiple-subject analysis tend to apply a Gaussian filter of 5–10 mm in width during postprocessing to project the data to a scale, where homologies in functional anatomy are expressed across subjects, and hence the effective voxel volume usually exceeds 100 $mm^3$. The optimum voxel volume as determined by $V_E$ may therefore be small enough for such cognitive neuroscience applications, even at 1.5 T.

Theoretical studies [10, 47] have shown that an optimal *TE* for maximizing BOLD CNR corresponds to the $T_2$* of gray matter when thermal noise dominates other noise. In contrast, BOLD CNR is independent of *TE* when physiological noise of BOLD origin is the dominant noise source [48]. This indicates that the use of a shorter *TE* would be beneficial because it minimizes susceptibility-related artifacts. As such, an optimal TE for maximizing BOLD CNR is determined by the relative contribution of these noise sources, and therefore, the choice of an optimal TE would vary, depending on the voxel volume.

In fMRI, the use of higher field strengths and/or highly sensitive multi-channel coils has improved the detection of subtle BOLD activations and also lead to a more precise spatial localization of these activations. It appears, however, generally difficult to determine an appropriate voxel volume in a fMRI experiment, since sensitivity and spatial specificity issues counteractively affect the choice of voxel volume. The BOLD CNR simulation results indicated that the optimum voxel volume when determined by $V_E$ is a good compromise, as it balances the two opposing issues. This is because $V_E$ corresponds to the minimum voxel volume at which a sufficiently high BOLD CNR is warranted for a wide range of BOLD activation volumes. Thus, the suggested voxel volume, $V_E$ can be a useful parameter for choice of imaging volume for fMRI studies.

# Conclusion

In this article, we have described recent progress on the quantitative aspects of BOLD fMRI. In the context of qualitative fMRI for identifying activated areas in response to stimulation, the quantitative evaluation of BOLD CNR allows us to optimize imaging parameters for maximizing the detection of functional activations. In particular, it is suggested that the ratio of physiological noise to thermal noise is the key index to optimize the voxel volume, which is one of the most important variables affecting activation detection and specificity in fMRI. In the context of quantitative fMRI, there has recently been a noticeable trend towards quantitative measurements of the baseline states of the brain using MRI. This is ascribed to the fact that there have been arising some physiological questions to be answered using the quantitative BOLD fMRI approach as described here. Traditionally, studies on quantitative measurements of hemodynamic parameters such as OEF and $CMRO_2$ have been performed using PET imaging techniques. If such quantitative BOLD fMRI methods as described here are validated and widely applied, they will provide an extraordinary tool for deciphering the brain's baseline activity and physiology in health and disease.

# References


[1] Ogawa S, Lee TM, Nayak AS, Glynn P. Oxygenation-sensitive contrast in magnetic resonance image of rodent at high magnetic fields. *Magn. Reson. Med.* 1990; 14: 68-78.

[2] Ogawa S, Lee TM, Kay AR, Tank DW. Brain magnetic resonance imaging with contrast dependent on blood oxygenation. *Proc. Natl. Acad. Sci. USA.*1990; 87: 9868-9872.

[3] Parrish TB, Gitelman DR, LaBar KS, Mesulam MM. Impact of signal-to-noise on functional MRI. *Magn. Reson. Med.* 2000; 44: 925-932.

[4] Yoo SS, Guttmann CRG, Panych LP. Multiresolution data acquisition and detection in functional MRI. *NeuroImage* 2001; 14:1476-1485.

[5] Yablonskiy DA, Haacke EM. Theory of NMR signal behavior in magnetically inhomogeneous tissue; static dephasing regime. *Magn. Reson. Med.* 1994; 32: 749-763.

[6] An H, Lin W. Quantitative measurements of cerebral blood oxygenation saturation using magnetic resonance imaging. *J. Cereb. Blood Flow Metab.* 2000; 20: 1225-1236

[7] Fujita N, Shinohara M, Tanaka H, Yutani K, Nakamura H, Murase K. Quantitative mapping of cerebral deoxyhemoglobin content using MR imaging. *NeuroImage.* 2003; 20:2071-2083.

[8] Fujita N, Matsumoto K, Tanaka H, Watanabe Y, Murase K. Quantitative study of changes in oxidative metabolism during visual stimulation using absolute relaxation rates. *NMR Biomed.* 2006; 19:60-68

[9] He X, Yablonskiy DA. Quantitative BOLD: Mapping of human cerebral deoxygenated blood volume and oxygen extraction: Default state. *Magn. Reson. Med.* 2007; 57: 115-126.

[10] Wu G, Li S-J. Theoretical noise model for oxygenation-sensitive magnetic resonance imaging. *Magn. Reson. Med.* 2005; 53: 1046-1054.

[11] Bodurka J, Ye F, Petridou N, Murphy K, Bandettini PA. Mapping the MRI voxel volume in which thermal noise matches physiological noise-implications for fMRI. *NeuroImage* 2007; 34:542-549.

[12] Krueger G, Glover G H. Physiological noise in oxygenation-sensitive magnetic resonance imaging *Magn. Reson. Med.* 2001; 46 :631–637

[13] Krueger G, Kastrup A, Glover G H. Neuroimaging at 1.5T and 3.0T: comparison of oxygenation-sensitive magnetic resonance imaging *Magn. Reson. Med.* 2001;45 :595–604

[14] Triantafyllou C, Hoge R D, Krueger G, Wiggins C J, Potthast A, Wiggins G C, Wald L L. Comparison of physiological noise at 1.5 T, 3T, and 7T and optimization of fMRI acquisition parameters *NeuroImage.* 2005; 26: 243–250

[15] Ogawa S, Menon RS, Tank DW, Kim SG, Merkle H, Ellermann JM, Ugurbil K. Functional brain mapping by blood oxygenation level-dependent contrast magnetic resonance imaging: a comparison of signal characteristics with a biophysical model. *Biophys. J.* 1993; 64: 803–812.

[16] Boxerman JL, Hamberg LM, Rosen BR, Weisskoff RM. MR contrast due to intravascular susceptibility perturbations. *Magn. Reson. Med.* 1995; 34: 555-566.

[17] Boxerman JL, Bandettini PA, Kwong KK, Baker JR, Davis TL, Rosen BR, Weisskoff RM. The intravascular contribution to fMRI signal changes: Monte Carlo modeling and diffusion-weighted studies in vivo. *Magn. Reson. Med.* 1995; 34:4-10

[18] Kiselev VG, Posse S. Analytical model of susceptibility-induced MR signal dephasing: effect of diffusion in a mivrovascular network model. *Magn. Reson. Med.* 1999; 41:499-509

[19] Fujita N. Extravascular contribution of blood oxygenation level dependent signal changes: a numerical analysis based on a vascular network model. *Magn. Reson. Med.* 2001; 46: 723-734.

[20] Lu H, van Zijl PCM. Experimental measurement of extravascular parenchymal BOLD effects and tissue oxygen extraction fractions using multi-echo VASO fMRI at 1.5 T and 3.0T *Magn. Reson. Med.* 2005; 53:808-816

[21] Hoogenraad FGC, Pouwels PJW, Hofman MBM, Reichenbach JR, Sprenger M, Haacke EM. Quantitative differentiation between BOLD models in fMRI. *Magn. Reson. Med.* 2001; 45: 233–246.

[22] Yacoub E, Duong TQ, Van de Moortele PF, Lindquist M, Adriany G, Kim SG, Ugurbil K, Hu X. Spin-echo fMRI in humans using high spatial resolutions and high magnetic fields. *Magn. Reson. Med.* 2003; 49:655-664.

[23] Posse S, Kemna LJ, Elghahwagi B, Wiese S, Kiselev VG. Effect of graded hypo- and hypercapnia on fMRI contrast in visual cortex: quantification of $T_2$* changes by multiecho EPI. *Magn. Reson. Med.* 2001; 46: 264-271.

[24] Yablonskiy DA, Ackerman JJ, Raichle ME. Coupling between changes in human brain temperature and oxidative metabolism during prolonged visual stimulation. *Proc. Natl. Acad. Sci. USA.* 2000; 97: 7603–7608.

[25] Davis TL, Kwong KK, Weisskoff RM, Rosen BR. Calibrated functional MRI: mapping the dynamics of oxidative metabolism. *Proc. Natl. Acad. Sci. USA* 1998; 95: 1834–1839.

[26] Hoge RD, Atkinson J, Gill B, Crelier GR, Marrett S, Pike GB. Investigation of BOLD signal dependence on cerebral blood flow and oxygen consumption: the deoxyhemoglobin dilution model. *Magn. Reson. Med.* 1999; 42: 849–863.

[27] Kim SG, Rostrup E, Larsson HB, Ogawa S, Paulson OB. Determination of relative $CMRO_2$ from CBF and BOLD changes: significant increase of oxygen consumption rate during visual stimulation. *Magn. Reson. Med.* 1999; 41: 1152–1161.

[28] Grubb RL, Raichle ME, Eichling JO, Ter-Pogossian MM. The effects of changes in $PaCO_2$ on cerebral blood volume, blood flow, and vascular mean transit time. *Stroke.* 1974; 5: 630–639.

[29] Ito H, Takahashi K, Hatazawa J, Kim SG, Kanno I. Changes in human regional cerebral blood flow and cerebral blood volume during visual stimulation measured by positron emission tomography. *J Cereb. Blood Flow Metab.* 2001; 21: 608–612.

[30] Okazawa H, Yamauchi H, Sugimoto K, Toyoda H, Kishibe Y, Takahashi M. Effects of acetazolamide on cerebral blood flow, blood volume, and oxygen metabolism: a positron emission tomography study with healthy volunteers. *J. Cereb. Blood Flow Metab.* 2001; 21: 1472–1479.

[31] Lee SP, Duong TQ, Yang G, Iadecola C, Kim SG. Relative changes of cerebral arterial and venous blood volumes during increased cerebral blood flow: implications for BOLD fMRI. *Magn. Reson. Med.* 2001; 45: 791–800.

[32] Kastrup A, Krueger G, Glover GH, Moseley M. Assessment of cerebral oxidative metabolism with breath holding and fMRI. *Magn. Reson. Med.* 1999; 42: 608-611.

[33] Bock C, Schmitz B, Kerskens CM, Gyngell ML, Hossmann KA, Hohen-Berlage M. Functional MRI of somatosensory activation in rat: effect of hypercapnic up-regulation on perfusion- and BOLD-imaging. *Magn. Reson. Med.* 1998; 39;457-461.

[34] Dutka MV, Scanley BE, Does MD, Gore JC. Changes in CBF-BOLD coupling detected by MRI during and after repeated transient hypercapnia in rat. *Magn. Reson. Med.* 2002; 48;262-270.

[35] Ma J, Wehrli FW. Method for image-based measurement of the reversible and irreversible contribution to the transverse relaxation rate. *J. Magn. Reson. B* 1996; 111: 61–69.

[36] Yablonskiy, DA. Quantitation of intrinsic magnetic susceptibility-related effects in a tissue matrix. *Magn. Reson. Med.* 1998; 39:417-428

[37] Shulman RG, Rothman DL, Hyder F. A BOLD search for baseline. *NeuroImage.* 2007; 36:277-281

[38] Vincent JL, Patel GH, Fox MD, Snyder AZ, Baker JT, Van Essen DC, Zempel JM, Snyder LH, Corbetta M, Raichle ME. Intrinsic functional architecture in the anaesthetized monkey brain. *Nature.* 2007; 447:83-86

[39] D'Esposito M, Deouell LY, Gazzaley A (2003) Alterations in the BOLD fMRI signal with ageing and disease: a challenge for neuroimaging. *Nature Rev. Neurosci.* 2003; 4: 863–872.

[40] Pasley BN, Inglis BA, Freeman RD. Analysis of oxygen metabolism implies a neural origin for the negative BOLD response in human visual cortex. *NeuroImage.* 2007; 36: 269-76

[41] Tamura H, Hatazawa J, Toyoshima H, Shimosegawa E, Okudera T. Detection of deoxygenation-related signal change in acute ischemic stroke patients by T2*-weighte magnetic resonance imaging. *Stroke.* 2002; 33: 967-971

[42] Powers WJ. Cerebral hemodynamics in ischemic cerbrovascular disease. *Ann. Neurol.* 1991; 29:231-240

[43] Friedman L, Glover GH. Report on a multicenter fMRI quality assurance protocol. *J. Magn. Reson. Imag.* 2006; 23:827-839

[44] Weisskoff RM, Baker JR, Belliveau JW, Davis TL, Kwong KK, Cohen MS, Rosen BR. Power spectrum analysis of functionally-weighted MR data: what's in the noise? In: *Proceedings of the Society of Magnetic Resonance in Medicine,* New York, 1993. p 7.

[45] Edelstein WA, Glover GH, Hardy CJ, Redington RW. The intrinsic signal-to-noise ratio in NMR imaging. *Magn. Reson. Med.* 1986; 3: 604-618.

[46] Glover G H, Krueger G. Optimum voxel size in BOLD fMRI. In Proceedings of the 10th Annual Meeting of ISMRM, Honolulu, 2002. p.1395

[47] Ogawa S, Lee TM, Barrere R. The sensitivity of magnetic resonance image signals of a rat brain to changes in the cerebral venous blood oxygenation. *Magn. Reson. Med.* 1993; 29:205-210

[48] Hyde, J.S., Biswal, B.B., Jesmanowicz, A. High-resolution fMRI using mutislice partial k-space GR-EPI with cubic voxels. *Magn. Reson. Med.* 2001; 46:114-125.

In: Research Topics on Brain Mapping
Editor: Yuanzhu Liáng, pp. 153-173
ISBN: 978-1-60456-001-5


*Chapter VII*

# Advances in Neurosurgical Applications of Functional Magnetic Resonance Imaging

***M. Parsons*** *[*1,2], ***W. Boling*** [1,3], ***M. Moran*** [1,2], ***M. Kraszpulski*** [1], ***A. Puce*** [1], ***S. Lemieux*** [1], ***C. Rosen*** [3], ***J. Collins*** [3] ***and J. Bailes*** [3]
[1] West Virginia University Department of Radiology-Center for Advanced Imaging
[2] West Virginia University Department of Behavioral Medicine and Psychiatry
[3] West Virginia University Department of Neurosurgery

## Introduction

Modern neurosurgery is an arena in which advances in technology are applied to the care of patients. Neurosurgeons have been integral to the development and application of numerous methods for understanding brain-behavior relationships. Functional magnetic resonance imaging (FMRI) has been added to the neurosurgeons armamentarium over the past decade and is rapidly moving into place as established "standard of care" for surgeries involving cortical regions critical for a variety of motor, sensory, and cognitive functions. In this chapter, we will describe briefly the development of the FMRI technique and the history of its application to the neurosurgical theater. Technological challenges to the integration of FMRI data with other modalities of neuroimaging in the operating room are now being overcome, and the chapter provides examples of this integration as well as describing the future promise of this endeavor. The majority of this chapter is devoted to description and illustration of imaging paradigms that are used to study specific brain functions, along with case examples.

[*] Address correspondence to Michael W. Parsons, Ph.D. Department of Behavioral Medicine and Psychiatry Box 9137 West Virginia University School of Medicine, Morgantown, WV 26506, USA.

# Historical Background

Biological MRI was first introduced in the 1970's and quickly revolutionized medical diagnosis. By 1996, there were over 10,000 MRI machines in use around the world (Mallard 2003). Such wide access to MRI equipment intensified research into further development and wider use of this technique, and functional brain mapping become one of the major goals. FMRI refers to the detection of hemodynamic changes associated with neural activity, using the technology of MRI (Savoy 2001). The technique is possible due to differences between the magnetic properties of oxyhemoglobin and deoxyhemoglobin (Pauling and Coryell 1936). Using test tubes of blood, Thulborn et al. (1982) verified experimentally that the oxygenation based differences in the hemoglobin molecule produced changes in magnetic field properties and these changes could be detected by MRI. Similar experiments *in vivo* were performed by Ogawa and colleagues (Ogawa and Lee 1990, Ogawa et al. 1990) on anesthetized rodents, who demonstrated reduced MR signal in brain areas with increased concentration of deoxygenated hemoglobin. This phenomenon, later called Blood Oxygenation Level Dependent (BOLD) contrast, enables researchers to observe changes in the relative concentration of deoxyhemoglobin in the body.

The other piece of the FMRI puzzle is based on the principle of neurovascular coupling: increased neural activity results in increased concentration of oxyhemoglobin in the local vasculature (for review, see Raichle, 1998). The mechanism by which neural tissue induces this rapid change in blood supply are only partially understood. Nonetheless, it is known that within a few seconds of increased neural activity, regional increases in blood flow, glucose utilization, and oxyhemoglobin concentration can be observed. Based on the principle of neurovascular coupling and the capability of measuring BOLD contrast with MRI, the first FMRI experiments performed with humans were reported (Bandettini et al. 1992, Kwong et al. 1992, Ogawa et al. 1992). It is fair to say that the technique has had a profound impact on the study of human brain activity since it was first published. For example, FMRI was used as a keyword in 553 presentations made at the last (2004) meeting of the Society for Neuroscience. The potential clinical applications of FMRI began to be exploited shortly after its discovery (Jack et al., 1994; Puce, 1995) and have continued to develop to date.

## FMRI Methods

While a thorough discussion of the many paradigms used in FMRI experiments is beyond the scope of this chapter, a basic understanding of FMRI methodology is important to appreciate some of the strengths and weaknesses of the technique. The original FMRI experiments (e.g., Bandettini et al., 1992) were called "block-design" tasks. This means that subjects performed a task (e.g. simple hand movements) for a set period of time (a "block") and then rested for a set period of time. This simple on-off cycle between hand movements and rest alternated several times during the course of a single scan. Functional activation was detected using the cross-correlation method (Bandettini et al., 1992), which identified those image voxels with MR signal intensity changes that were temporally correlated with the subjects' activity (see figure 1). While the explosion of interest in FMRI has created many more complex and flexible task designs (e.g., single trial activation studies, sparse temporal sampling, and others), this basic design has proven to be the most fruitful for the application of FMRI to individual patients due to the relatively large signal change induced by such designs (e.g., Fitzgerald et al., 1997; Jack et al., 1994; Meuller et al., 1996).

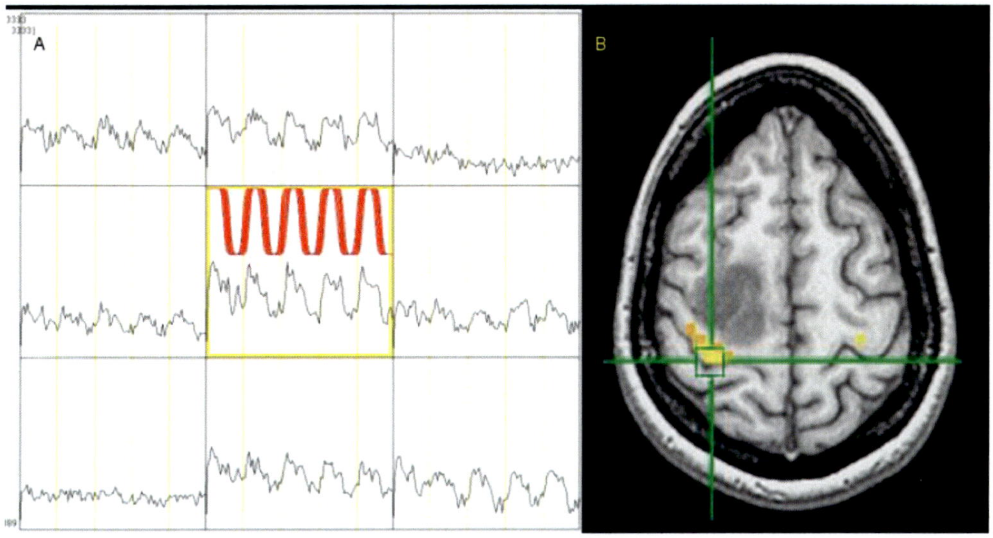


Figure 1. The 9 graphs in part A of the figure (left) show the actual MR signal intensity change (y axis) over time (x axis) in 9 contiguous voxels of the image in part B (inside the green square). Superimposed on the central graph is a representation of the timing of the finger tapping task performed by this subject (red line). The actual MR signal intensity in the central voxel is highly correlated with task performance. The strongest correlations are represented by the brightest shades of yellow, superimposed on structural brain image of this patient with a right frontal low grade glioma. Note, the image is shown in radiologic orientation.

## FMRI in the Neurosurgical Theater

The advances in neurosurgery over the past two to three decades have arisen primarily from the seemingly endless improvements in imaging capabilities that have led to modern image guided neurosurgery. The neurosurgeon is now able to identify lesions and normal anatomy with a clarity never seen previously using numerous imaging techniques. Image guided neurosurgery refers to the integration of multiple imaging modalities with the patient in the operating room. Image guided surgery requires brain images to be integrated in the operating room once the patient is present. A series of coregistration steps allows the images in the virtual space of the computer to be linked to the real space around the patient's head. The advantages of image guidance to the neurosurgeon are multiple. By using a pointer in real space the surgeon can navigate using the brain images. This gives the surgeon a virtual eye into the patient's brain, providing critical information for planning surgical approaches, calculating distance to targets, and comparing alternative surgical trajectories prior to beginning the surgery. Many tumors and lesions are better seen on imaging than under direct vision, and image guidance improves the ability to localize and define its boundaries. Multiple modalities of imaging can potentially be coregistered and utilized for brain navigation, including structural images such as MRI scans, functional activation data, such as functional MRI and positron emission tomography (PET), and even chemical imaging, such as magnetic resonance spectroscopy (MRS). These multiple modalities provide far more information than has been available previously. Any volumetric imaging data set can potentially be integrated into image guidance for navigation. At WVU, we have successfully integrated diverse imaging types such as MRI (i.e. anatomical MRI, MR Angiography, Diffusion Tensor Imaging, FMRI), CT, CTA, ultrasound, PET, and 3D angiography. Other imaging types are soon to be utilized (i.e. MRS, single photon emission tomography; SPECT).

FMRI presents unique challenges to image guidance, primarily because FMRI is not pure imaging data. Each voxel contains statistical information based on the BOLD response, as described above, and this information must be transformed into a volumetric image data set. Without an "image" to allow for feature based coregistration for FMRI with anatomical scans, accurate alignment of data has been challenging. Regardless of the technical hurdles for the integration of FMRI into image guidance, it has tremendous potential in neurosurgery to improve the surgical approach by identifying the relationship of a lesion to important functioning cortex, and localizing function on the cortex itself. Below, we describe several of the most reliably studied cortical regions in image guided neurosurgery.

## Central Area

The localization of the central sulcus has become standard in image guided neurosurgery. However, the localization of specific sensory and motor functions on the pre- and postcentral gyrus may be difficult to predict despite the well known top to bottom relationship represented by the homunculus. Activation studies to identify individual finger function using PET or FMRI can be used to identify the location of sensorimotor function on the precentral gyrus, and this approach has been reliably correlated with cortical stimulation (Meuller et al., 1996; Puce, 1995; Pujol et al., 1996; Vinas et al., 1997; Yousry et al., 1995). Recently, sulcal and gyral landmarks have been identified that reliably localize specific motor and sensory functions in the central area.

Motor hand activation on FMRI occurs in a characteristic Ω or knob - like structure seen on the axial MRI that extends posteriorly from the precentral gyrus (Gelderen et al., 1995; White et al., 1997; Yousry et al., 1997). The anatomical substratum for hand motor function is the *pli de passage moyen* (Boling et al., 2002). A structure found between the superior and middle frontal gyrus and at the apex of the posterior pointing middle bend of the central sulcus. The *pli de passage moyen* is a deep fold of cortex within the central sulcus. It elevates the floor of the sulcus and connects the pre- and postcentral gyri. Functional imaging (FMRI and PET) show hand motor function to lie within the precentral portion of the *pli de passage moyen*. Hand sensory function is localized to the postcentral gyrus' contribution to the *pli de passage moyen* (Boling, Olivier, et al., 2004; see figure 2).

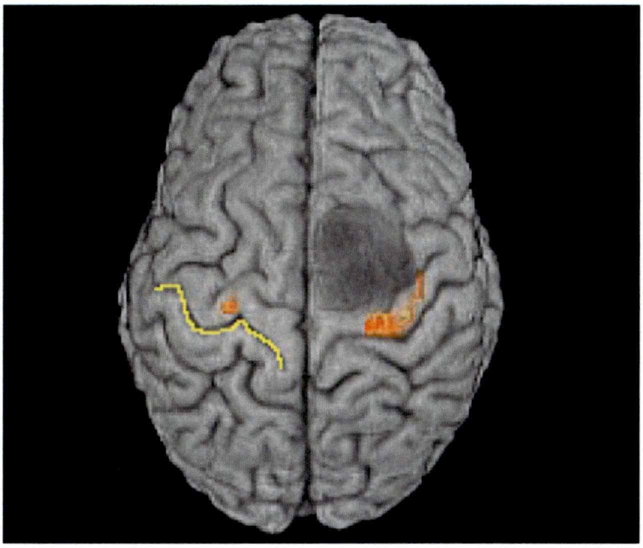

Figure 2. Activation in the precentral gyrus hand area induced by finger to thumb opposition movements in a patient with a right frontal glioma. The *pli de passage moyen* (anterior to the yellow line delineating the central sulcus) is visible in the left (dominant) hemisphere as described in the text.

Cortical landmarks in the inferior third of the central area are reliable guides to identification of the tongue (Picard and Olivier, 1983 ), and lips/lower face areas (Boling, Reutens, et al., 2002). The tongue sensory area is a triangle shaped region, the apex pointing superiorly, of the postcentral gyrus just superjacent to the Sylvian fissure. The broad inferior base subserves base of the tongue sensation and the top, apex, of the triangular shaped area of the postcentral gyrus is the tip of the tongue sensory region. The adjacent important functional region superior to the tongue area is the lower face and lips cortical sensory area. The lower face and lips sensory area is reliably the most narrow portion of the postcentral gyrus immediately superior to the tongue sensory area (see figure 3).

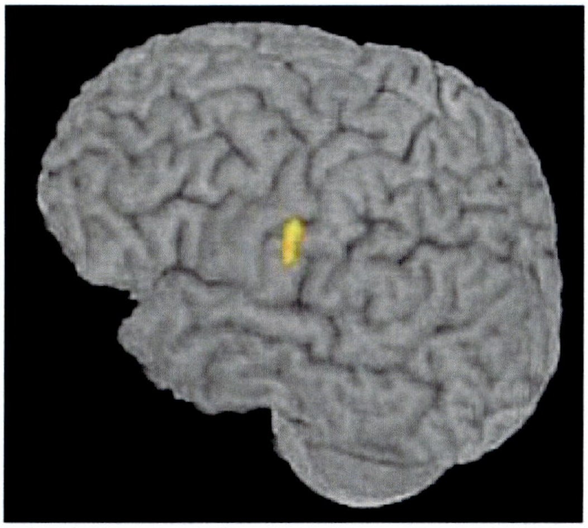

Figure 3. Activation of the face sensory area near the inferior reaches of the postcentral gyrus.

The gyral and sulcal landmarks localizing function in the primary sensorimotor area are best identified on the 3D reconstruction of the volumetric MRI, and that information transferred to the cortical surface at surgery using image guidance. The MRI allows definite identification of sulci and strips the pia/arachnoid and vessels that may obscure anatomical identification in vivo. However, the topographic landmarks are usually observable in vivo with attention to detail.

### *Motor Association Areas*

Once we leave the "hard-wired" confines of the central sulcus and its surrounding gyri, the somatotopy of the associative regions of motor and sensory related cortical areas becomes more plastic. Despite the variability inherent in these regions, an important functional relationship has been elucidated in a medial secondary motor area known as the supplementary motor area (SMA; see Rizzolatti, Luppino and Matelli, 1996 for an anatomical description). The SMA appears to play a role in the planning, initiation, and sequencing of complex motor behaviors (Eccles, 1982; Goldberg, 1985; Orgogozo and Larsen, 1979; Parsons et al., 2005). In the dominant hemisphere, the SMA also plays a role in speech and language, and seems to be particularly critical for the initiation of language output (Jonas, 1981; Krainik et al., 2003; Nelson et al., 2002; Ojemann et al, 1989). Surgical resections in the region of the SMA, particularly in the dominant hemisphere, may produce a transient syndrome characterized by hemiparesis of the contralateral body side, neglect of the contralateral body side and mutism (Rostomily et al., 1991). Fortunately, this SMA syndrome is most commonly a transient occurrence, resolving over a period of weeks to months with few residual deficits. Despite it's transient nature, the dramatic features of the syndrome make it imperative that it is properly understood and that patients and their families can be educated about the risk of the syndrome. Functional MRI has been shown to have a valuable role in predicting the likelihood of the SMA syndrome following surgery (Krainik et al., 2001 and 2003). In a series of studies, Krainik and colleagues have demonstrated that the proximity of the surgical boundary to FMRI activation in the SMA can be used to predict the syndrome. Specifically, when the authors had subjects perform a simple motor task in which they alternated opening and closing of the two hands synchronously with a rest period, activation in the SMA was observed. When the resection margin included this area of activation, subjects showed the SMA syndrome, which resolved over a period of weeks (Krainik et al., 2001). This study demonstrates the potential value of FMRI in patient education and outcome prediction.

### *Language Areas*

Broca's language area has been recognized since Broca's original description to lie in the posterior part of the inferior frontal gyrus (F3) in the dominant hemisphere (for a discussion see Joynt, 1964). Functional imaging also consistently localizes Broca's area to F3 and characteristically at the depth of a sulcus in the posterior and inferior part of F3. Numerous FMRI paradigms have been used to localize this brain area, but the most consistently utilized are tasks that involve cued word generation (Adcock et al., 2003; Rutten et al., 1999, Sabbah et al., 2003, Schlosser et al., 2002). In general, these paradigms tend to produce lateralized activation that indicates hemispheric dominance for language. Results of language FMRI using productive or general language tasks have been shown to correlate well with intraoperative mapping procedures (e.g., Ruge et al., 1999; Rutten et al, 1999) and the Wada test (e.g., Aldekamp et al, 2003; Binder et al., 1996; Ries et al, 2004; Sabbah et al., 2001; Spreer et al., 2002). In FMRI studies, activation in and around the posterior F3 region is quantified and a laterality index is calculated, which indicates the degree of lateralization of language functions in the patient. The laterality indices derived from FMRI studies typically correlate highly with other methods of language lateralization (e.g., in Binder et al., 1996, the correlation between the two tests was $r=0.96$; $p<0.0001$). The ability to lateralize and locate this frontal language area has been shown to be robust and readily detected in many patients with lesions affecting the frontal lobe (e.g., Schlosser et al., 2002).

In a recent study, we (Yamamoto et al., 2005) have studied the role of lateralized activation within the SMA as a predictor of language laterality. Based on indications in the literature that there is lateralized activation during word generation tasks in the SMA (e.g., Keihl et al., 2002; Seghier, et al., 2004) and our own observation of SMA activation during a word generation task used in our patients, we predicted that SMA activity would correlate with language lateralization as determined by other methods. The gold standard for determining language lateralization pre-operatively is the intracarotid amobarbital procedure (IAP), which is also known as the Wada test for it's originator. During the IAP, one hemisphere is briefly anesthetized and language is tested with the contralateral "awake" hemisphere, providing definitive lateralization of language function. The Wada test is frequently used to lateralize language in patients with epilepsy prior to surgery. In patients with brain tumors, the most commonly used method of verifying language localization and lateralization is intraoperative stimulation mapping. We studied eight patients undergoing presurgical FMRI for either brain tumor or epileptic focus resection. All subjects completed a visually cued block-design word generation task while undergoing FMRI, in which they silently generated words beginning with a specific letter or belonging to a semantic category alternating with rest. A cross correlation analysis was conducted and statistically active voxels above a probability threshold of $p<0.001$ were retained within a specified region of interest (ROI) in the SMA bilaterally (ROI defined according to the landmarks defined in Krainik, 2003; see figure 4).

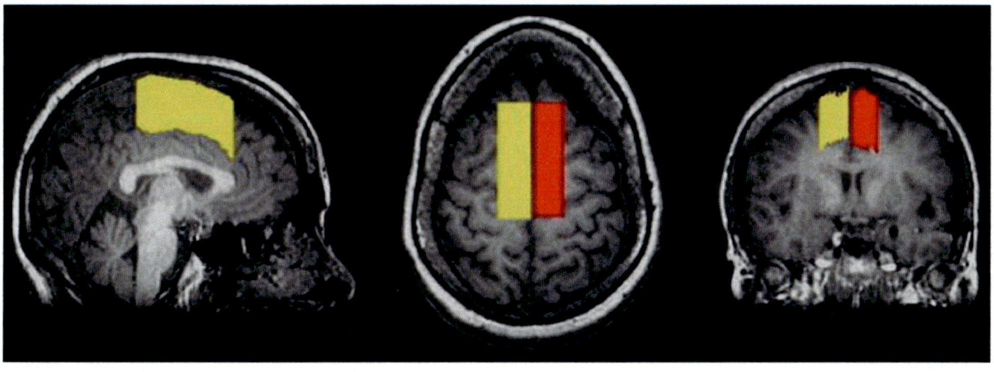

Figure 4. Example of ROI including the supplementary motor area.

The percent of voxels active in each ROI was determined and a laterality index was calculated for each subject using the % active voxels within the left (L) and right (R) hemispheres as follows: **LI = (L-R)/(L+R)**. Results for all 8 subjects are presented in table 1.

**Table 1. comparison of Laterality indices (LI) generated from FMRI activation within the SMA, with Wada test, or intraoperative mapping**

| Subj | LI | FMRI Dominance | Wada or Mapping? | Wada/Mapping Dominance | Agreement |
|---|---|---|---|---|---|
| 1 | .50 | Left | Mapping | Left | Yes |
| 2 | -.58 | Right | Wada | Right | Yes |
| 3 | .29 | Moderately Left | Wada | Left | Yes |
| 4 | -.02 | Mixed | Both | Left | - |
| 5 | .20 | Moderately Left | Both | Left | Yes |
| 6 | -.68 | Right | Wada | Mixed<br>Right = Productive<br>Left= Receptive | Yes |
| 7 | .18 | Weakly Left | Wada | Left | Yes |

Based on these findings, we concluded that FMRI activation of the SMA during word generation correlates well with other methods of mapping language function, even in the presence of anomalous language organization (e.g., subjects 2 and 6, above). These findings are consistent with the notion that the SMA plays a critical role in the generation of language, even when overt speech is not produced, as was the case in our FMRI paradigm. Furthermore, the findings are consistent with a study by Krainik et al. (2003) which demonstrates that surgical resections impinging on language related FMRI activation in the SMA produced the typical transient mutism seen in the SMA syndrome.

Wernicke's language area is not as precisely anatomically defined and with cortical stimulation may be localized in the posterior temporal or inferior parietal areas of the dominant hemisphere (Ojemann et al., 1989). That is to say, within the gyral continuum surrounding the posterior termination of the Sylvian fissure. FMRI activation of Wernicke's area can be seen with simple language tasks, such as listening to spoken language (e.g., as in Hirsch et al., 2000) or performing a complex language tasks that require semantic associations (e.g., Binder et al., 1996). However, a limitation of these methods is that they often include activation of many language related regions or large expanses of the dominant hemisphere, or they may be continuous with activation in auditory receptive regions (Carpentier et al., 2001). Because auditory cortex activation in these paradigms occurs bilaterally, the determination of lateralized dominance for receptive language can be difficult. Several studies have been conducted to attempt to improve the spatial resolution of FMRI in localization of receptive language structures. Most of these paradigms have attempted to use multiple modalities of stimulus input to activate receptive language cortex (e.g. Carpentier et al., 2001; Ashtari et al., 2005). Others have used clever "rest" conditions, in an attempt to subtract out the auditory activation. For example, Schlosser et al., 1999 conducted a block design FMRI task in which subjects heard blocks of English sentences alternating with blocks of sentences in Turkish (which they did not understand). The activation map resulting from the subtraction of the Turkish from English condition should theoretically remove the auditory commonalities to both conditions. This was effective in the majority of the subjects, though the extent of cortical tissue identified by FMRI did not always overlap completely with that identified by intraoperative mapping.

We have recently designed and piloted a receptive language task in our laboratory (Sollinger et al., submitted). We sought to design a protocol, simple and brief enough for easy use with patients, but able to reliably discriminate language comprehension from sensory perception. Eleven right-handed, healthy young adults completed two language comprehension tasks during fMRI: participants alternated between blocks of visually presented or auditorily presented yes/no questions (e.g., "Will a good pair of rubber boots keep water out?"). Subjects responded via a button press. A conjunction analysis identified common areas of activation across the visual and auditory tasks. At the group level, a large area of activation in the region of the left superior and middle temporal gyri (see figures 5 and 6) was identified and was used as a region of interest (ROI) to query individual subject FMRI data.

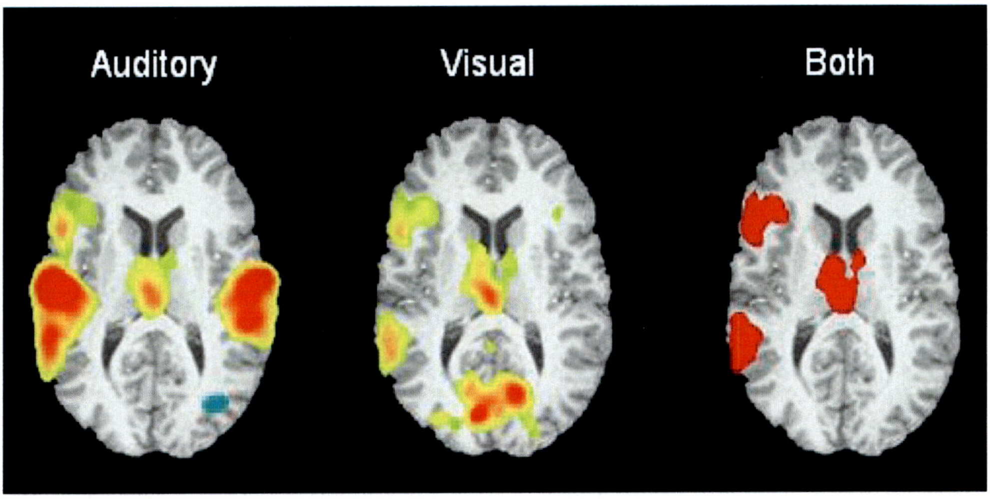


Figure 5. FMRI activation during a language comprehension task. Images show activation with auditory presentation of stimuli, visual presentation of stimuli, and finally, only brain regions activated by both tasks. The posterior temporal region on the left was used as an ROI in individual subject analyses.

At the individual subject level, nine of eleven subjects demonstrated clear activation in this ROI. Preliminary use of this task in patients with neurosurgical lesions has shown mixed results: some subjects have failed to show activation, whereas others have shown activation which was confirmed as language related by intraoperative mapping. Results suggest that this protocol offers promise as a means of reliable identification of language comprehension areas in individual subjects.

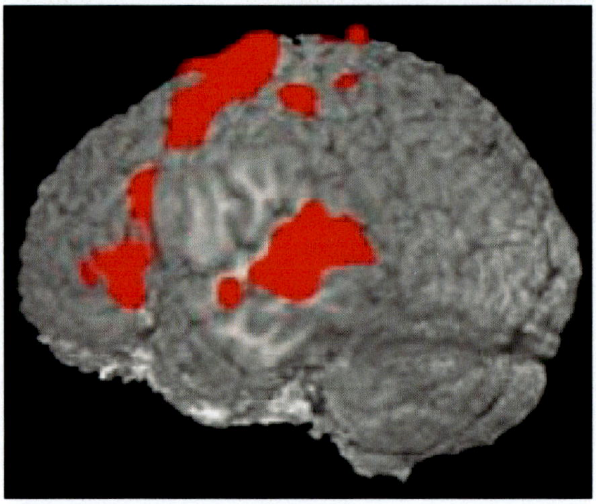

Figure 6. Left lateral view of the temporal lobe activation depicted in figure 5. This area was active during both auditorily and visually presented language comprehension tasks.

### *Medial Temporal Lobes*

Resection of temporal lobe structures is an effective treatment of intractable temporal lobe epilepsy (TLE; Wiebe, Blume, et al., 2001). Efficacy of the treatment in terms of seizure control and minimization of cognitive effects is improved with careful selection of patients. At the present time, patient selection includes examination of data from video EEG monitoring, structural MRI, neuropsychological evaluation, and other procedures. Patient selection considers both the lateralization/localization of the seizure focus, as well as the risk of significant cognitive decline following surgery. Currently, the best tool to predict memory deficits following medial temporal lobe resections for epilepsy is the Wada test (described above). In addition to its value for language lateralization, the Wada test can also determine lateralized memory dominance. Although widely used and effective in prediction of surgical outcome, the Wada test is invasive and not without risk. The development of non-invasive procedures that improve selection of patients for surgery and thereby improve seizure and cognitive outcome would potentially be of benefit. Functional neuroimaging techniques, including FMRI, offer promise in this regard.

FMRI has been productively used to study language laterality in surgical epilepsy patients using a variety of paradigms, with widely demonstrated concordance with Wada test results (see Baxendale, 2002 for review). Determination of laterality of memory ability in TLE using FMRI has been less frequently reported. Such investigations typically examine activation in medial temporal areas, often limiting analysis to a specific region of interest (ROI), that includes the hippocampus and parahippocampal areas (see Figure 7). Task-related activation in the ROI is measured and often compared between the hemispheres. Reduced activity in the ROI in one hemisphere relative to the other is considered to represent relatively poorer function of those structures. As confirmation, the FMRI-determined asymmetry is compared to a laterality ratio derived from the Wada test. In addition, the relationship between FMRI hemispheric asymmetry or activation in the ROI and memory performance may be examined.

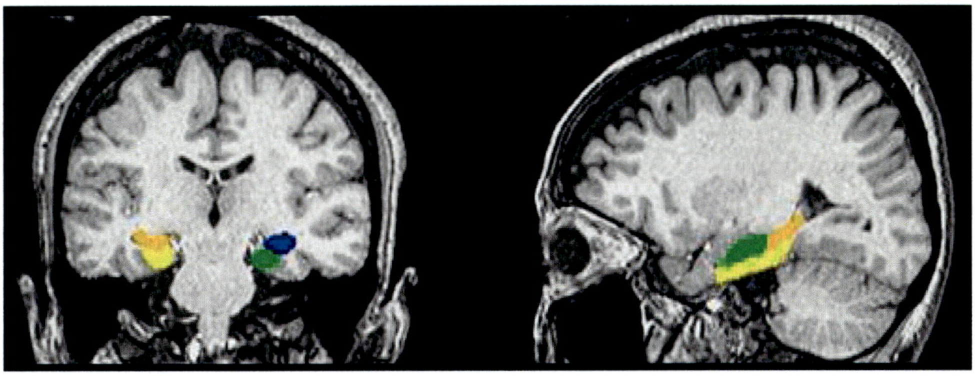

Figure 7. ROI's showing multiple subregions of the medial temporal lobes.

Studies have found an association between FMRI and Wada test performance using a variety of activation paradigms. Asymmetry of medial temporal lobe activation of individual patients with unilateral TLE was examined with a mental navigation and landmark recall task (Jokeit, Okujava, and Woermann, 2001). This procedure correctly classified 27/30 (90%) of TLE subjects by side of seizure focus. Additionally, left temporal lobe activation was significantly correlated with left hemisphere Wada test performance. Similarly, a complex scene encoding task revealed asymmetrical medial temporal lobe FMRI activation in individuals with TLE, but not in controls (Detre, Maccotta, et al., 1998). This asymmetry corresponded to the epileptogenic hemisphere and was in agreement with laterality findings from the Wada test in all nine patients. Notably, this agreement between FMRI activation and Wada test results was observed even for TLE patients in whom memory laterality by Wada test was discordant with seizure focus. FMRI activation during encoding of various stimuli (words, faces, scenes, and patterns) also demonstrated good concordance with Wada test results; FMRI and Wada test laterality agreed in eight of nine patients (Golby, Poldrack, et al., 2002).

More recently, attempts have been made to predict post-surgical memory outcome using pre-surgical FMRI. In 10 patients with left medial temporal lobe epilepsy, degree of hemispheric asymmetry in activation during a verbal encoding FMRI task predicted degree of post-surgical decline on the task (Richardson, Strange, et al., 2004). Rabin and colleagues (2004) also found a correlation between hemispheric asymmetry in FMRI activation on a scene encoding task and pre- to post-surgical change in performance on the task.

The scientific literature to date suggests that FMRI has the potential to lateralize memory ability and predict cognitive outcome in TLE. However, limitations remain. Activation tasks vary greatly and often do not represent memory functions typically examined clinically. The utility of such tasks in predicting memory morbidity following surgery and their applicability to real-world functioning remain to be determined. More critically, to be clinically useful the procedures must be validated as highly predictive in individual patients. At present, while highly correlated, FMRI and Wada test laterality do not agree in all patients. In addition, there is evidence that FMRI and the Wada test together provide better prediction, at least of post-surgical seizure control, than either procedure alone (Killgore, Glosser, et al., 1999).

# Role of FMRI in Surgical Planning

Our approach in patients undergoing surgery in the crucial language, cognitive, sensory or motor areas is to perform FMRI to plan preoperatively and assist in localizing function during surgery. Preoperatively, the FMRI activation tasks are tailored to identify the relationship of the lesion or surgical area to nearby important function. Several analysis steps are required to prepare the imaging data for image guidance. First, the FMRI BOLD response must be analyzed as described earlier and coregistered with the anatomical MRI. The resulting FMRI activation maps must then be converted to a volumetric data set that can be utilized in image guided surgery. Image guided FMRI provides a number of advantages to the surgeon. For surgery within an important functioning area, we always confirm function localization with cortical stimulation. However, the combination of FMRI localization of function using image guidance and cortical landmark functional localization provides the surgeon with an excellent guide to the location of function that can then be confirmed with cortical stimulation. Fewer stimulation attempts make the process of cortical stimulation safer, more efficient, and less stressful for the patient. Therefore, the surgery itself is shorter and fewer stimulation attempts are less likely to induce a seizure.

For surgery outside but near the crucial language or central areas, cortical stimulation may not be necessary. Landmark functional localization and image guided FMRI provide quite reliable assessments of function location. Nowadays, fewer awake craniotomies and cortical stimulation are performed due to the advances in image guided surgery. General anesthesia is more comfortable for the patient and the surgeon, and is desirable if it is an equally safe approach. The central sulcus is readily identified using image guidance, and FMRI for primary sensorimotor responses can be performed if there is a doubt. In the dominant hemisphere, sulcal and gyral landmarks can generally guide surgery to avoid eloquent regions. Surgery in the frontal lobe dorsal to the inferior frontal sulcus is considered safe. In the parietal lobe, the intraparietal sulcus is the key to defining the safe region in the dominant hemisphere. The superior parietal lobule (P1) can be approached safely at surgery, but P2 (the supramarginal and angular gyri) are considered eloquent in the dominant hemisphere. In the temporal lobe we maintain the corticectomy and resection in T1 anterior to the level of the precentral sulcus to avoid eloquent cortex, T2 – T6 resection can be carried a little more posterior. The occipital lobes are not considered eloquent but surgery always carries the risk of hemianopsia. For this reason, FMRI mapping of primary visual fields can provide additional useful information (e.g., as in Hirsch et al., 2000).

## Limitations and Challenges

### *Sensitivity vs. Specificity*

As noted above, we do not use FMRI as the sole method of identifying critical brain regions. Instead, we use FMRI as presurgical information and as a guide to reduce intraoperative mapping time. The critical difference between FMRI and stimulation mapping is that FMRI provides information about what brain structures are active during performance of a cognitive or motor task, but does not identify those areas that are truly *necessary* for task performance. This information must come from an ablative technique, such as cortical stimulation or the Wada test, which are capable of determining whether or not a given task can be performed without the participation of one of the critical active sites. While numerous studies have demonstrated correspondence between FMRI and intraoperative mapping, as described in the sections above, what many of the studies do not discuss is that there are multiple additional sites of activation around the brain that were not examined with intraoperative stimulation mapping. These findings illustrate the fact that most cognitive, sensory, and even motor tasks draw on multiple interconnected brain regions, only some of which may be critical for task performance. Therefore, using FMRI as an initial guide to surgical approach and then using intraoperative mapping to query suspicious active sites provides the best balance of the two techniques. We believe that FMRI is best utilized as one of many tools in the surgeons armamentarium for the elucidation of brain-behavior relationships.

### *FMRI Activation Paradigms*

The simple block design paradigm for FMRI activation described earlier is intuitive and appealing, but there are several important assumptions that underlie the method and principles that must be carefully examined in task construction. Specifically, the block design rationale assumes that brain function is organized hierarchically, meaning that the difference between task A and task B is assumed to reflect a simple linear subtraction between the two conditions. This assumption is reasonably accurate for simple motor tasks, but becomes more tenuous when applied to complex cognitive activities, such as memory, abstract reasoning, or emotional arousal. Another inherent assumption in these designs is that "rest" is an insignificant contributor to brain activity. Several studies have demonstrated that simply alternating a complex cognitive task with a nonspecific resting state provides limited information or even spurious information (Binder et al., 1999; Shulman et al., 1997). The limited value of the rest state is clear when one reflects on one's own internal cognitive processes when resting. For instance, consider what one might do when told to "just relax" while in an MRI scanner. The mental state is one that may involve subvocal language activity, retrieval of semantic or episodic memory information, or even rehearsal of the recently conducted FMRI task. This state, which has been termed Random Episodic Semantic Thought (Shulman et al., 1997) is clearly not the same as the kind of blank slate that might be assumed when one subtracts brain activity during rest from brain activity during some active state. Thus, the activity of the subjects during the rest phase of an FMRI activation task is of critical importance when trying to understand subtraction based activation maps. For this reason, FMRI tasks used in clinical applications should typically be designed by individuals with training in cognition, behavior, and statistical analysis, as well as an understanding of the imaging technology. Most centers that design these types of studies employ teams of professionals with diverse training backgrounds that support this activity.

### *Pathological Disruption of Blood Flow*

The neuropathological entity involved in these cases often disturbs local hemodynamics, particularly in cases of vascular malformations and highly vascularized brain tumors. Because FMRI is based on a hemodynamic response, any change in the relationship between neural activity and the vascular response to that neural activity (termed neurovascular coupling) may result in FMR images that are difficult to interpret. In particular, *neurovascular uncoupling* has been described as occurring in the region of highly vascularized tumors, such as glioblastoma multiformae (Holodny et al., 1999). There appear to be several factors that may contribute to neurovascular uncoupling, including a loss of the autoregulation capability of tumor related vasculature (Pronin et al., 1997). When autoregulation fails, vasculature in a region of interest that is near a brain tumor may not show the fluctuation in blood oxygen level that allows for the detection of signal change in FMRI. Under these circumstances, FMRI is likely to produce a false-negative result. In other words, it may fail to show activation in brain regions that are, in fact, neurally active. A thorough description of just this phenomenon is described by Ulmer et al. (2003), in which the absence of FMRI signal in a language areas has led to the (erroneous) assumption that language functions had been reorganized and were being subserved by alternate brain regions. This important limitation underscores the importance of using multiple methods to ascertain the functional role of eloquent brain regions.

### *Future Developments*

Now that the usefulness of FMRI in neurosurgical navigation is firmly established, the improvement of patient care with FMRI depends on resolving some of the above noted problems and developing new capabilities. Most significant to the enhanced widespread use of this technology are developments in the ability to integrate FMRI data with other brain images in the operating room. In our initial attempts to integrate FMRI maps in our surgical guidance system, we used a time consuming and computationally complex process to superimpose activation on an anatomical image and import that image into the neuronavigation system. Limitations of this method included the complexity, time consuming nature, and the potential for human error (e.g. image inversion or reversal). Additionally, because all images were in a DICOM format, there was no capability to display colored overlays on the grey scale brain image, leading to limited and potentially confusing display of activation maps (see figure 8).

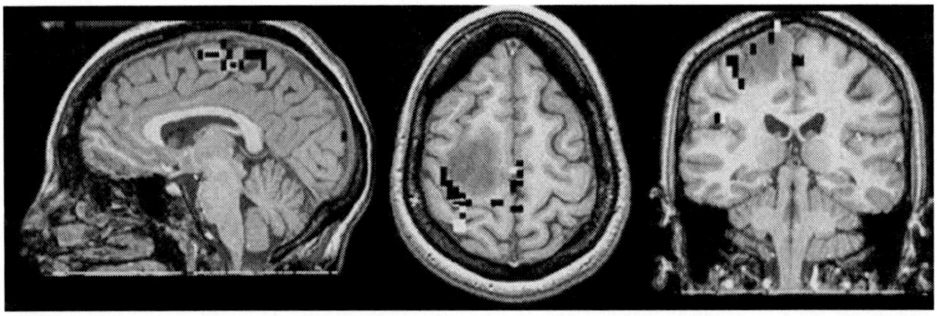

Figure 8. An example of early attempts to integrate FMRI activation into neuronavigational software. Voxels colored black indicate hand and foot motor activation, those colored white indicate hand sensory activation, and those with white borders and black centers indicate supplementary motor activation.

More recently, through a cooperative relationship with a manufacturer of neuronavigation equipment (BrainLab, Inc: Munich, Germany), we have participated in the development of more advanced software for the display of functional activation data. The current system allows for the integration of up to 8 functional activation maps, using distinct colors (see figure 9). It remains dependent on a separate analysis and is still somewhat vulnerable to human error. However, we are currently beta-testing new software developed by BrainLab, which will perform FMRI analysis with images taken directly from the scanner. The capability to analyze FMRI data in the same system used for neuronavigation will remove the potential for human error, because all brain images will contain information provided by the MRI scanner regarding image orientation, slice location, and geometry. Through this interactive partnership, our industry colleagues have developed their software based on the current scientific state of the art, and the potential for a dramatic increase in utilization of FMRI in neurosurgery is possible.

Technological advances have led to some exciting developments, most notably the capability for intraoperative FMRI. This has been accomplished for several years now, using specially designed operating rooms that contain an MRI scanner (Hadani et al., 2001). Functional MRI can be accomplished by these imaging systems, allowing the potential for surgical guidance to be aided by real-time FMRI activation maps, which can then be queried by intraoperative stimulation mapping (as in Schulder et al., 2003). One of the potential advantages of these systems is that they may be able to account for the fact that the brain moves once the skull is opened in neurosurgery. This "brain-shift" is not typically accounted for by most neuronavigation systems that use presurgical images.

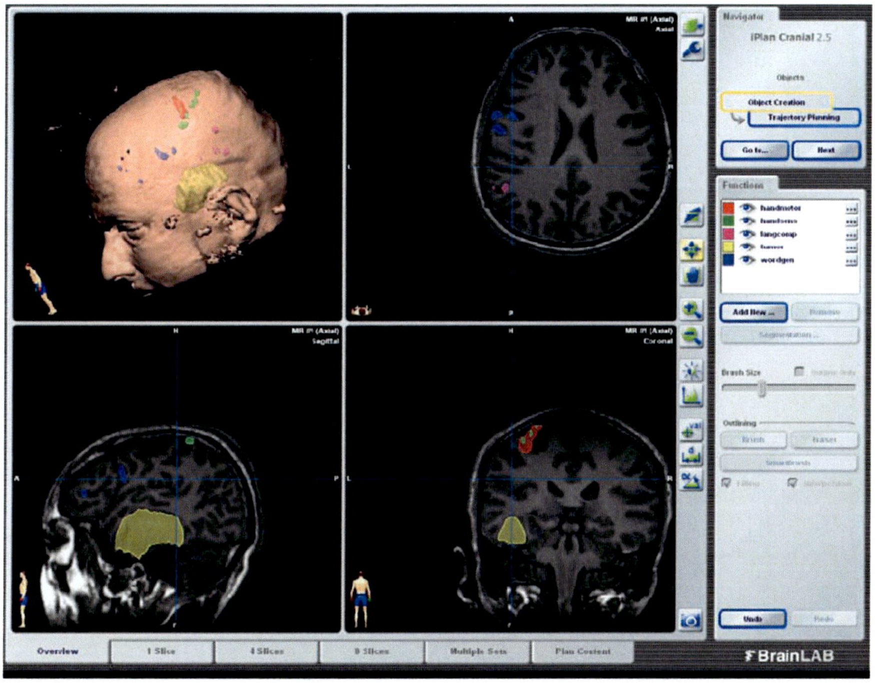


Figure 9. Example of a images created by the BrainLab neuronavigation software. The image shows the brain tumor (in yellow), as well as multiple FMRI modalities (reprinted by permission).

Integration with additional imaging modalities provides avenues for development as well. We are now beginning to incorporate chemical data from MRS studies, which may assist in identifying brain lesions that are not readily apparent on structural imaging studies or delineating the borders of infiltrative tumors. Most exciting, however, is the integration of diffusion tensor imaging (DTI), showing white matter fiber bundles (see figure 10).

In a recent study by Ulmer et al., (2004) DTI based tract tracing was added to FMRI results to identify critical brain regions. The addition of these tracts to the image produced improved correspondence between image-based identification of eloquent regions and intraoperative mapping. The improvement was due at least in part to the fact that DTI is not vulnerable to neurovascular uncoupling. It therefore allowed for increased sensitivity to detect functional brain assemblies in those regions that might be suffering reduced vascular autoregulation capabilities. In addition, the identification of fiber bundles allows surgeons to identify possible deformations in tracts emanating from eloquent regions, perhaps due to the local distorting effects of a tumor or other lesion. Ulmer et al. (2004) suggest that their very low complication rate (4%) is due in part to this factor.

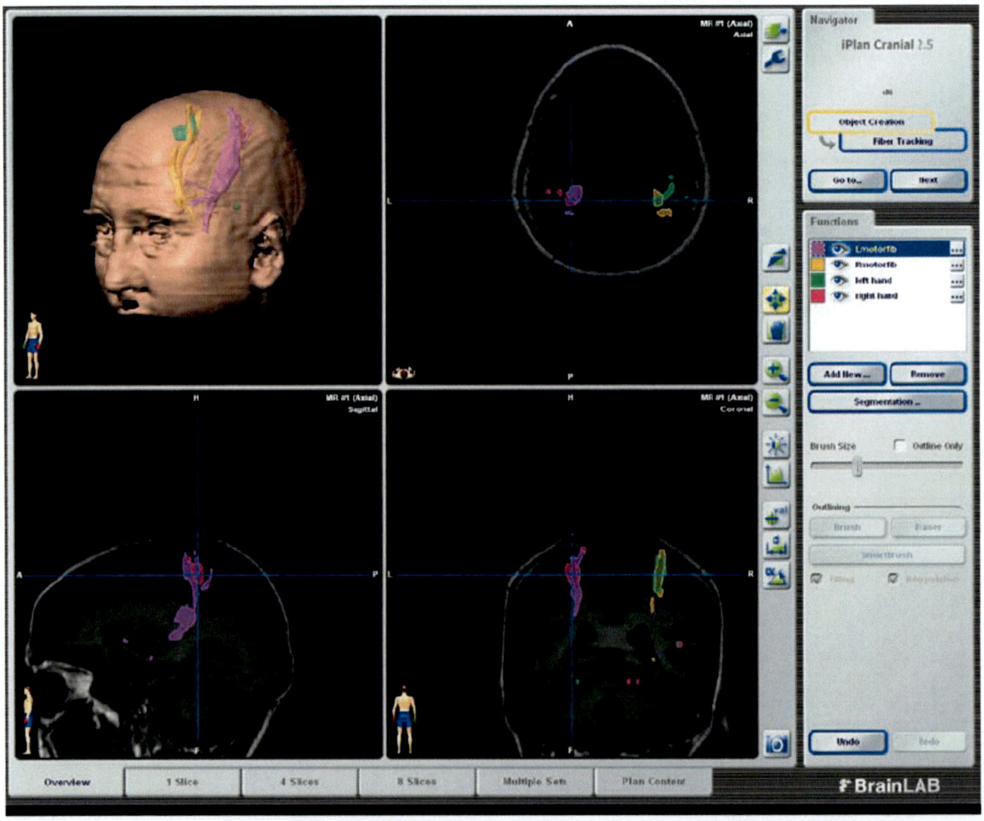


Figure 10. A combination of FMRI activation of hand motor area (shown in green – left hand, and pink- right hand) and the fiber tracts emanating from the regions of activation. In this healthy volunteer, the corticospinal tracts are readily demonstrated (reprinted by permission).

# Conclusion

FMRI provides potential advantages for the neurosurgeon during brain surgery. It supplies further evidence for the localization of function that may or may not require confirmation with cortical stimulation. When cortical stimulation is required, FMRI makes the procedure safer and more efficient. To fully utilize FMRI during surgery, it must be integrated into image guidance. This can be successfully done today, and the software and algorithms to accomplish this are improving rapidly. FMRI is an important tool available to neurosurgeons that improves the approach to surgery in and near important functioning cortical areas

# Acknowledgement

The authors gratefully acknowledge the support of the WVU School of Medicine Department of Radiology and the Center for Advanced Imaging. One of the authors on this chapter (MK) is supported by a contract awarded to the WVU Department of Neurosurgery from BrainLab Inc.

# References

Adcock JE, Wise RG, Oxbury JM, Oxbury SM, Matthews PM (2003) Quantitative fMRI assessment of the differences in lateralization of language-related brain activation in patients with temporal lobe epilepsy. *Neuroimage.* 18:423-438.

Aldenkamp AP, Boon PA, Deblaere K, Achten E, Backes WH, Boon P, Hofman P, Troost J, Vandemaele P, Vermeulen J, Vonck K, Wilmink J (2003) Usefulness of language and memory testing during intracarotid amobarbital testing: observations from an fMRI study. *Acta Neurol. Scand.* 108:147-152.

Ashtari M, Perrine K, Elbaz R, Syed U, Thaden E, McIlree C, Dolgoff-Kaspar R, Clarke T, Diamond A, Ettinger A (2005) Mapping the functional anatomy of sentence comprehension and application to presurgical evaluation of patients with brain tumor. AJNR *Am. J. Neuroradiol.* 26:1461-1468.

Bandettini PA, Wong EC, Hinks RS, Tikofsky RS, Hyde JS (1992) Time course EPI of human brain function during task activation. *Magn. Res. Med.* 25: 390-397.

Baxendale, S. (2002) The role of functional MRI in the presurgical investigation of temporal lobe epilepsy patients: A clinical perspective and review. *J. Clin. Exp. Neuropsychol.* 24: 664-676.

Benson RR, FitzGerald DB, LeSueur LL, Kennedy DN, Kwong KK, Buchbinder BR, Davis TL, Weisskoff RM, Talavage TM, Logan WJ, Cosgrove GR, Belliveau JW, Rosen BR (1999) Language dominance determined by whole brain functional MRI in patients with brain lesions. *Neurology.* 52:798-809.

Binder JR, Swanson SJ, Hammeke TA, Morris GL, Mueller WM, Fischer M, Benbadis S, Frost JA, Rao SM, Haughton VM (1996) Determination of language dominance using functional MRI: a comparison with the Wada test. *Neurology.* 46:978-984.

Binder J, Frost J, Hammeke T, Belgowan P, Rao S, Cox R. (1999) Conceptual processing during the conscious resting state: A functional MRI study. *J. Cog. Neuroscience.* 11: 80-93.

Boling W, Olivier A (2004) Localization of hand sensory function to the pli de passage of Broca. *J. Neurosurg.* 101:278-283.

Boling W, Reutens DC, Olivier A (2002) Functional topography of the low postcentral area. *J. Neurosurg.* 97:388-395.

Carpentier A, Pugh KR, Westerveld M, Studholme C, Skrinjar O, Thompson JL, Spencer DD, Constable RT (2001) Functional MRI of language processing: dependence on input modality and temporal lobe epilepsy. *Epilepsia.* 42:1241-1254.

Detre JA, Maccotta BS, King MD, Alsop DC, Glosser G, D'Esposito M, Zarahn E, Aguirre GK, French JA (1998) Functional MRI lateralization of memory in temporal lobe epilepsy. *Neurology.* 50: 926-932.

Eccles J. (1982) The initiation of voluntary movements by the supplementary motor area. *Arch. Psychiatr. Nervenkr.* 231: 423-441.

FitzGerald D, Cosgrove G, Ronner S (2997) Location of language in the cortex: a comparison between functional MR imaging and electrocortical stimulation. *AJNR.* 18: 1529-1539.

Golby AJ, Poldrack RA, Illes J, Chen D, Desmond JE, Gabrieli JDE (2002) Memory lateralization in medial temporal lobe epilepsy assessed by functional MRI. *Epilepsia.* 43: 855-863.

Goldberg G (1985) Supplementary motor area structure and function: review and hypotheses. *Behav. Brain Sci.* 8: 567-616.

Hadani M, Spiegelman R, Feldman z, Berkenstadt H, Ram Z (2001) Novel, compact, intraoperative magnetic resonance imaging-guided system for conventional neurosurgical operating rooms. *Neurosurg.* 48: 799-809.

Hirsch J, Ruge MI, Kim KHS, Correa DD, Victor JD, Relkin NR, Labar DR, Krol G, Bilsky MH, Souweidane MM, DeAngelis LM, Gutin PH (2000) An integrated functional magnetic resonance imaging procedure for preoperative mapping of cortical areas associated with tactile, motor, language, and visual functions. *Neurosurgery.* 47:711-722.

Holodny A, Schulder M, Liu W, Maldjian J, Kalnin A (1999) Decreased BOLD functional MR activation of the motor and sensory cortices adjacent to a glioblastoma multiforme: implications for image-guided neurosurgery. *AJNR.* 20: 609-612.

Jack C, Thompson R, Butts R (1994) Sensory motor cortex: correlation of presurgical mapping with functional MR imaging and invasive cortical mapping. *Radiology.* 190: 85-92.

Jokeit H, Okujava M, Woermann FG (2001) Memory fMRI lateralizes temporal lobe epilepsy. *Neurol.* 57: 1786-1793.

Jonas S (1981) The supplementary motor region and speech emission. *J. Commun. Disord.* 14: 349-373.

Joynt R (1964) Paul Pierre Broca: His contribution to the knowledge of aphasia. Cortex 1: 206-213.

Keihl (2002) Reading anomalous sentences: An event-related fMRI study of semantic processing. *Neuroimage.* 17: 842-850.

Killgore WDS, Glosser G, Casasanto DJ, French JA, Alsop DC, Detre JA (1999) Functional MRI and the Wada test provide complementary information for predicting post-operative seizure control. Seizure. 8: 450-455.

Krainik A, Lehericy S, Duffau H, et al. (2001) Role of the supplementary motor area in motor deficit following medial frontal lobe surgery. *Neurology.* 57: 871-878.

Krainik A, Lehericy S, Duffau H, et al. (2003) Postoperative speech disorder after medial frontal surgery: Role of the supplementary motor area. *Neurology.* 60: 587-594.

Kwong KK, Belliveau JW, Chesler DA, Goldberg IE, Weisskoff RM, Poncelet BP, Kennedy DN, Hoppel BE, Cohen MS, Turner R, Cheng HM, Brady TJ, Rosen BR (1992) Dynamic magnetic resonance imaging of human brain activity during primary sensory stimulation. *Proc. Natl. Acad. Sci. USA.* 89: 5675-5679.

Mallard JR (2003) The evolution of medical imaging from Geiger counters to MRI – a personal saga. *Perspectives Biol. Med. 46: 349-370.*

Mueller WM, Yetkin FZ, Hammeke TA, Morris GL 3rd, Swanson SJ, Reichert K, Cox R, Haughton VM (1996) Functional magnetic resonance imaging mapping of the motor cortex in patients with cerebral tumors. *Neurosurgery.* 39:515-521.

Nelson L, Lapsiwala S, Haughton V, et al. (2002) Preoperative mapping of the supplementary motor area in patients harboring tumors in the medial frontal lobe. *J. Neurosurg.* 97: 1108-1114.

Ogawa S, Lee TM (1990) Magnetic resonance imaging of blood vessels at high fields: *in vivo* and *in vitro* measurements and image stimulation. *Magn. Res. Med.* 16: 9-18.

Ogawa S, Lee TM, Nayak AS, Glynn P (1990) Oxygenation-sensitive contrast in magnetic resonance image of rodent brain at high magnetic fields. *Magn. Res. Med.* 14: 68-78.

Ogawa S, Tank DW, Menon R, Ellermann JM, Kim SG, Merkle H, Ugurbil K (1992) Intrinsic signal changes accompanying sensory stimulation: functional brain mapping with magnetic resonance imaging. *Proc. Natl. Acad. Sci. USA.* 89: 5951–5955.

Ojemann G, Ojemann J, Lettich E, et al., (1989) Cortical language localization in the left dominant hemisphere. An electrical stimulation mapping investigation in 117 patients. *J. Neurosurg.* 71: 316-326.

Orgogozo J, Larsen B (1979) Activation of the supplementary motor area during voluntary movement in man suggests it works as a supramotor area. *Science.* 206: 847-850.

Parsons M, Harrington D, Rao S (2005) Distinct Neural Systems Underlying Learning of Perceptual and Spatial Representations of Motor Skills. *Hum. Brain Mapping.* 24: 229-247.

Pauling L, Coryell CD (1936) The magnetic properties and structure of hemoglobin, oxygenated hemoglobin, and carbomonoxygenated hemoglobin. *Proc. Natl. Acad. Sci. USA.* 22: 210–236.

Picard C, Olivier A (1983) Sensory cortical tongue representation in man. *J. Neurosurg.* 59:781-789.

Puce A (1995) Comparative assessment of sensorimotor function using functional magnetic resonance imaging and electrophysiological methods. *J. Clin. Neurophysiol.* 12:450-459.

Pujol J, Conesa G, Deus J, Lopez-Obarrio L, Isamat F, Capdevila A (1996) Presurgical identification of the primary sensorimotor cortex by functional magnetic resonance imaging. *J. Neurosurg.* 84:7-13.

Rabin ML, Narayan VM, Kimberg DY, Casasanto DJ, Glosser G, Tracy JI, French JA, Sperling MR, Detre JA (2004) Functional MRI predicts post-surgical memory following temporal lobectomy. *Brain.* 127: 2286-2298.

Richardson MP, Strange BA, Thompson PJ, Baxendale SA, Duncan JS, Dolan RJ (2004) Pre-operative verbal memory fMRI predicts post-operative memory decline after left temporal lobe resection. *Brain.* 127: 2419-2426.

Ries ML, Boop FA, Griebel ML, Zou P, Phillips NS, Johnson SC, Williams JP, Helton KJ, Ogg RJ (2004) Functional MRI and Wada determination of language lateralization: a case of crossed dominance. *Epilepsia.* 45:85-89.

Rizzolatti G, Luppino G, Matelli M (1996) The classic supplementary motor area is formed by two independent areas. *Adv. Neurology.* 70: 45-56.

Ruge MI, Victor J, Hosain S, Correa DD, Relkin NR, Tabar V, Brennan C, Gutin PH, Hirsch J (1999) Concordance between functional magnetic resonance imaging and intraoperative language mapping. *Stereotact. Funct. Neurosurg.* 72:95-102.

Rutten GJM, Ramsey NF, van Rijen PC, Alpherts WC, van Veelen CWM (2002) fMRI-determined language lateralization in patients with unilateral or mixed language dominance according to the Wada test. *Neuroimage.* 17:447-460.

Rutten GJM, van Rijen PC, van Veelen CWM, Ramsey NF. Language area localization with three-dimensional functional magnetic resonance imaging matches intrasulcal electrostimulation in Broca's area. *Ann. Neurol.* 46:405-408.

Sabbah P, Chassoux F, Leveque C, Landre E, Baudoin-Chial S, Devaux B, Mann M, Godon-Hardy S, Nioche C, Aït-Ameur A, Sarrazin JL, Chodkiewicz JP, Cordoliani YS (2003) Functional MR imaging in assessment of language dominance in epileptic patients. *Neuroimage.* 18:460-467.

Savoy RL (2001) History and future directions of human brain mapping and functional neuroimaging. *Acta Psychol.* 107: 9-42.

Schlosser MJ, Luby M, Spencer DD, Awad IA, McCarthy G (1999) Comparative localization of auditory comprehension by using functional magnetic resonance imaging and cortical stimulation. *J. Neurosurg.* 91:626-635.

Schlösser R, Hunsche S, Gawehn J, Grunert P, Vucurevic G, Gesierich T, Kaufmann B, Rossbach W, Stoeter P(2002) Characterization of BOLD-fMRI signal during a verbal fluency paradigm in patients with intracerebral tumors affecting the frontal lobe. *Magn. Reson. Imaging.* 20:7-16.

Schulder M, Azmi H, Biswal B (2003) Functional magnetic resonance imaging in a low-field intraoperative scanner. *Stereotact. Funct. Neurosurg.* 80: 125-131.

Shulman G, Fiez J, Corbetta M, Buckner R, Meizin F, Raichle M, Petersen S (1997) Common blood flow changes across visual tasks: II. Decreases in cerebral cortex. *J. Cogn. Neuroscience.* 9: 648-663.

Seghier ML (2004) Variability of fMRI activation during a phonological and semantic language task in healthy subjects. *Hum. Brain Mapping.* 23: 140-155.

Sollinger A, Shaikh K, Parsons M. (in press) *Localization of Sensory-Independent Language Comprehension Cortex: A Functional Magnetic Resonance Imaging Protocol.* Presentation to be given at the 34th Annual Meeting of the International Neuropsychological Society.

Spreer J, Arnold S, Quiske A, Wohlfarth R, Ziyeh S, Altenmüller D, Herpers M, Kassubek J, Klisch J, Steinhoff BJ, Honegger J, Schulze-Bonhage A, Schumacher M (2002) Determination of hemisphere dominance for language: comparison of frontal and temporal fMRI activation with intracarotid amytal testing. Neuroradiology 44:467-474.

Thulborn KR, Waterton JC, Matthews PM, Radda GK (1982) Oxygenation dependence of the transverse relaxation time of water protons in whole blood at high field. *Biochim. Biophys. Acta.* 714:265-270.

Ulmer J, Krouwer H, Mueller W, Ugurel M, Kocak M, Mark L (2003) Pseudo-reorganization of language cortical function at FMR imaging: a consequence of tumor-induced neurovascular uncoupling. *AJNR.* 24: 213-217.

Van Gelderen P, Ramsey NF, Liu G, Duyn JH, Frank JA, Weinberger DR, Moonen CT (1995) Three-dimensional functional magnetic resonance imaging of human brain on a clinical 1.5-T scanner. *Proc. Natl. Acad. Sci. U.S.A.* 92:6906-6910.

Vinas FC, Zamorano L, Meuller RA, Jiang Z, Chugani H, Fuerst D, Muzik O, Manger TJ, Diaz FG (1997) [150]-water PET and intraoperative brain mapping: a comparison in the localization of eloquent cortex. *Neurol. Res.* 19:601-608.

Wiebe S, Blume WT, Girvin JP, Eliasziw M (2001) A randomized, controlled trial of surgery for temporal-lobe epilepsy. *N. Engl. J. Med.* 345: 311-318.

White LE, Andrews TJ, Hulette C, Richards A, Groelle M, Paydarfar J, Purves D (1997) Structure of the human sensorimotor system. I: Morphology and cytoarchitecture of the central sulcus. *Cereb. Cortex.* 7:18-30.

Yamamoto A, Shaikh K, Boling W, Bloomfield S, Parsons, M (2005) *Lateralized FMRI Activation of the Supplementary Motor Area During Productive Language Tasks:* Comparison with Wada and Intraoperative Mapping. Presentation at the 33rd Annual Meeting of the International Neuropsychological Society.

Yousry TA, Schmid UD, Alkadhi H, Schmidt D, Peraud A, Buettner A, Winkler P (1997) Localization of the motor hand area to a knob on the precentral gyrus. gyrus. A new landmark. *Brain.* 120:141-157.

Yousry TA, Schmid UD, Jassoy AG, Schmidt D, Eisner WE, Reulen HJ, Reiser MF, Lissner J (1995) Topography of the cortical motor hand area: prospective study with functional MR imaging and direct motor mapping at surgery. *Radiology.* 195:23-29.

In: Research Topics on Brain Mapping
Editor: Yuanzhu Liáng, pp. 175-194
ISBN: 978-1-60456-001-5


*Chapter VIII*

# Lost Without a Map: Pursuing Primate Homologies with Functional Imaging

***Christopher I. Petkov*[*], *Christoph Kayser and Nikos K. Logothetis***
Max Planck Institute for Biological Cybernetics,
Spemannstrasse 38, 72076 Tübingen, Germany.

## Abstract

Before we can begin to search for primate homologies, it is vital to first obtain accurate structural and functional maps of human brain areas and the related regions in nonhuman primates. Functional magnetic resonance imaging (fMRI) is an excellent tool for the balanced sampling of the brain at high resolutions, but for various technical reasons it has been less than ideal for imaging certain sensory systems in either monkeys or humans. It is only recently that developments in acquisition and analysis methods have made it possible to visualize the cortical representation of the senses in at least one of the species. In this chapter we pursue the question of how imaging in one of the species might be assisted by developments in another. We consider the advances that have been made in imaging the visual system to reveal the underlying functional organization of a number of different visual areas and compare their organization in humans and monkeys. As a result, more visual areas are now thought to have been evolutionarily conserved in these primates. We also summarize recent developments in the context of the auditory, somatosensory, vestibular, olfactory and gustatory systems. In these as well as in the visual system, numerous functional areas are thought to exist, but many more remain to be localized. In the context of this research, although most developments were done in the field of human neuroimaging, there are also areas where monkey functional mapping seems to be farther advanced. Comparative approaches will help to clarify further

[*] Author Information: The authors declare no competing financial interests. Correspondence and requests for materials should be addressed to C.I.P.(chris.petkov@tuebingen.mpg.de), phone: +49-7071-601-659.

primate evolutionary relationships by exploiting advances made in the imaging of individual species.

## Introduction

The homology of primate brain regions is of interest to evolutionary biologists, but it is also of great practical use to clinicians and scientists for understanding which invasive studies in animals can serve to model human neuronal function. However, the non-invasive techniques used to study the human brain are either indirect measures of neuronal activity -- such as positron emission tomography (PET) and functional magnetic resonance imaging (fMRI) -- or they sample large regions of the brain's electrical or magnetic potentials and suffer from poor localization of the actual activity sites. Differences across the species have been difficult to evaluate since it is difficult to relate results using a particular technique in one species to those obtained with another in a different species. Even with the same species, cross-technique comparisons require us to resolve complex issues such as how extracellular recordings from neurons compare to the hemodynamic response from functional imaging [1, 2]. The recently established PET and fMR imaging of nonhuman primates eliminates the immense methodological differences that have impeded our understanding of primate evolutionary relationships, e.g. [3-5]; for reviews see [6-9].

Functional MRI provides the relatively high spatial resolution needed for accurate maps of functional properties and is routinely used to investigate different areas in the human brain. The same technique is now being used to image the brains of nonhuman primates like the macaque monkeys (*Macaca*), but as we will see, it is seldom employed in a comparative context, i.e. with humans and monkeys in the same study. Imaging both humans and monkeys enables us to make a more direct comparison of the neuronal networks under study, with local electrophysiological recordings in monkeys providing the physiological detail needed for a scalable map of primate brain function. Here, we consider current developments in fMR imaging of the sensory systems and point out where further advances are possible, including where imaging of both monkeys and humans would be indispensable.

## Homology, Specialization or Something in between

A gross anatomical comparison makes it clear that human brains share the same lobular organization as the brains of many other mammals. However, even at the macroscopic level it is evident that the human brain is much more convoluted [10] and has regions that are proportionately smaller or larger than those of other animals, even of other primates [11]. These observations can be quantified, for example by using novel structural morphing techniques to register one primate brain to the scale of another, alleviating the problems stemming from comparing brains with different sizes [12, 13]. The process of morphing reveals how one brain needs to be deformed to register to another. A closer look at those areas with the most deformation shows that the primary visual cortex in humans is proportionately smaller than that of other primates [13]. Many other regions have expanded in humans, such as areas in associative sensory, parietal and prefrontal cortical regions [11, 14].

At the microscopic level we must acknowledge the foresight of Brodmann in characterizing not only architectonic differences across brain areas but also across species [15]. Brodmann histologically identified 46 regions in the human brain (that were distinctly different in their cytoarchitectonics) and about half that many in other primates. He also used the same numerical label for regions that were structurally similar across the species, or those that he felt might be homologous. Since then anatomists have refined and expanded Brodmann's taxonomy of brain areas. Depending on the criteria used, there are up to 40 areas in the macaque visual cortex alone [16, 17] and about 20 orbitofrontal areas [18, 19]; presumably there are even more in humans [11, 20]. Anatomical studies from other sensory regions also suggest that sensory processing is mediated by numerous functionally and structurally discrete areas, but not all anatomical parcellation schemes have found functional support; for a review see [21]. Although difficult to obtain, the more convincing areal borders are those that have been confirmed with both anatomical and functional techniques, or at least with multiple approaches, e.g., [22, 23]. Areal distinctions are still being updated, so the borders of many areas are in flux, but it is now clear that numerous functional areas exist in the sensory systems of humans and nonhuman primates. The question is which are homologous?

The problem in establishing homology is that similarity cannot ever be fully proven. It is much easier to detect differences across species. A subtle structural or functional difference in one species suffices to establish that a homology is not complete. It is commonly assumed that there are fundamental primate homologies at the initial processing stages of all of the sensory systems and that hierarchically-higher functional regions such as cognitive, speech and language areas are highly specialized in humans. However, as we will consider below in the case of the visual system, a system that has been more extensively studied than the others, this generalization holds but for only a few of the many areas [8, 9]. For other sensory systems, primate homologies are even less certain.

Comparative analyses of macaque and human brains need not be limited to MR imaging, as long as the methods are similar enough to allow a direct scrutiny of species-specific differences. However, MR-based maps are convenient for comparative purposes because they can incorporate detail from different datasets and methods (see the online SumsDB database: *http://brainmap.wustl.edu*). Cross-species maps that detail the organization of brain areas and their borders and relationship to other areas, including connectivity patterns, will help us to understand evolutionary relationships. Direct comparisons of accurate comparative maps could immediately reveal details such as 1) whether certain areas are bigger, 2) which areas have been lost or gained, 3) what rearrangements have occurred, and/or 4) if there is evidence of a functional divergence [11]. Structural and functional maps with accurate borders can reveal whether areas are proportionately larger when brains are registered to the same scale or if there is roughly the same quantity of neurons and supporting structures regardless of brain size. There is no *a priori* reason why an area should devote more neuronal machinery in a large animal to the same sensory process that is achievable with less in a smaller animal, given comparable sensitivity and scale of the peripheral input. For instance, human primary visual cortex (V1) is proportionately smaller than macaque V1 (3 compared to 10 percent relative to overall cortical surface area), but the general homology of this area is unquestioned. Accurate maps will also reveal which areas have been lost or even newly emerged if these can be observed in the map of one species but not in that of the other. Rearrangements would also be obvious, as similar functional areas that have been anatomically displaced. Lastly, functional divergence can be found by observing that areas have adopted species-specific functions but otherwise correspond structurally. In this regard, an indication of a functional divergence can be suggested by species-specific differences in connectivity patterns, including *in-vivo* connectivity patterns evaluated with MR.

While it is now feasible [6-9], the imaging of macaque monkeys is still at an early stage and the methods are not always identical to those used to image humans. On the other hand, one might think that in the time since the introduction of human PET [24, 25] and then fMRI [26, 27], all regions of the human brain have been 'activated' in one way or another. Until recently, however, accurate, high-resolution functional maps overlooked many of the senses even for humans, and there is little agreement as to how maps of the different sensory regions should be acquired and quantified. Let us now take a look at where we stand in our efforts to image the different senses in monkeys and humans.

## Lessons from Vision Studies

Of the several dozen visual sensory areas in the occipital, temporal and parietal lobes, only V1, V2 and MT/V5 can be considered largely homologous in humans and macaque monkeys [8, 9, 11, 28, 29]. The hesitance with which even these few homologies have been proposed underscores the caution with which these and other proposed homologies should be treated until the evidence is more complete.

As an example of the difficulties in establishing homologies, the presumed human homolog of the monkey area MT, which has neurons sensitive to translational motion, is thought to be within the human complex called hMT+ [30, 31]. This complex, however, contains areas that are difficult to resolve and localize since a number of surrounding regions are also sensitive to complex motion [9]. Neither is it clear where the presumed human homolog of monkey area MST lies; in monkeys MST is known to border area MT but it is sensitive to global motion. One study suggests that the human homolog of the monkey area MST is somewhat removed from the hMT+ complex [32], while another proposes that the area is well within the hMT+ complex [31]. A comparative study in both humans and monkeys using stimulation designed to selectively activate MT and MST could help resolve whether the human homolog of MST has separated from MT, possibly by a differentiation of other areas between the two, or whether it lies within the hMT+ complex. The comparative approach with carefully designed stimulation will also give us insights into the cross-species correspondence of the function of many other visual fields.

## Retinotopically Organized Areas

Ongoing visual work can rely on a strong foundation laid down in decades of detailed studies using electrophysiological and anatomical approaches, mainly in animal models. This large body of work in visual science was crucial for improving the stimulation and imaging methods used to determine fMRI borders between visual areas in humans [33, 34] and monkeys [35]; for a review see [29, 36]. Many visual areas are retinotopically organized, which means that the visual field is represented multiple times, one or more times in each such area ('area' V3 is an example of the latter [11, 29]). Thus, the visual field representations of many areas can be topographically mapped in the two orthogonal directions representing the visual field: eccentricity from the center of gaze and polar angle around this center. Mapping how visual areas represent the polar angle of stimulation, for instance, reveals mirror-reversing patterns between neighboring areas, like V1 and V2 [34, 35, 37]. These patterns can be used to quantify the gradient of a particular functional property, and the point at which the gradient reverses can be used to objectively delineate a border between areas. The adjacent borders of an area can then be mapped using stimuli that change their position in eccentricity rather than polar angle [33-35, 37]. However, in the case of the anatomically described area V3 which has multiple representations of the visual field, there can be discrepancies between functionally and anatomically defined areal borders [11, 29]. Studying homologies of areas such as V3 underscores the need to first eliminate gross methodological differences before approaching comparative analysis of human and monkey data.

## Limitations and Considerations

Retinotopic maps have also proved helpful in distinguishing visually sensitive areas in parietal and frontal cortex [38]. But retinotopic mapping is less successful where the neuronal representation of the visual field is not as strong, for example as a result of large neuronal receptive fields, such as with neurons from area MST [31]. Some parietal visual areas might also be mapped in head-centered rather than eye-centered (retinotopic) coordinates. Moving the head while imaging creates problems, but a clever paradigm could map such areas by having the subject move their eyes while the visual field is simultaneously moved so that the retinotopic representation does not change. In addition, many visual areas in occipital, temporal, parietal and frontal cortex are attentionally labile, so another challenge in assembling retinotopic maps of awake individuals, whether monkey or human is controlling the focus of attention [39, 40]. Otherwise, attentionally labile functional organization might at best be undetectable, or at worst suggest a false organization.

Unfortunately, even visual retinotopic maps are not always subjected to statistical analysis, calling into question the objectivity of any categorization of an observed pattern as an intrinsic property of an area versus noise. This is less of an issue for V1 and V2, especially when a strong retinotopic gradient reverses and can be statistically quantified. However, when one property merely fades into an area that has no related organization, or into an area that merely continues the organizational pattern, it is difficult to determine an objective measure by which we can reliably define a border [36].

Another concern is that human studies commonly scan multiple subjects and then evaluate reliability by group analysis or on the basis of the consistency with which the subjects show a similar functional pattern over the same brain region. Group analysis is preferable but tends to restrict the activation patterns to the strongest locus of the activity response across subjects, which could obscure accurate maps in individuals that have been morphed to a group template.

In monkey studies, on the other hand, reliability is determined across fewer subjects, in part because it is very time-consuming to train monkeys for imaging. Thus, it is difficult to conduct group statistics with the monkey data. On the other hand, the individual data in the monkey studies are more robust and better reveal the inter-individual variability in the location of activity patterns [41, 42]. Recent human studies show a trend toward using fewer subjects while carrying out more scans to increase statistical power (e.g. [31]), providing some convergence with the monkey studies.

Other imaging differences that complicate analyses, especially comparative analyses, are the differences in task difficulty used with humans and monkeys or the use of contrast agents in monkeys but not in humans [30, 43]. Some of these differences are difficult to mitigate. For instance, even if both humans and monkeys are given the same task, monkeys might find a particular task more immediately interesting because a motivating reward, such as water or juice, is frequently offered to them. Humans, on the other hand, commonly look forward to a monetary reward at the completion of the experiment. Also, an injectable contrast agent is problematic for human use but could be critical for obtaining monkey data, especially at lower scanning magnetic fields, [30, 43]; for a review see [9].

## Recent Visual Comparative Imaging Studies

At around the turn of the century, functional imaging in monkeys began with the monkey somatosensory [4] and visual systems [3]. Since those initial studies, comparative imaging has concentrated on vision, where many of the advances have been made. Some of the recent imaging performed in humans and monkeys focused on mapping the higher-level temporal lobe regions, such as face- and object-selective regions in the inferior temporal lobe and superior temporal sulcus [42]. Electrophysiological studies of these imaged regions in monkeys augment our understanding of their neuronal function [41]. Other comparative imaging studies in monkeys and humans concentrate not just on the temporal lobe but also in parietal cortex where additional higher-level visual areas reside [44-46]. The activation patterns resulting from different types of stimulation often differ in humans and monkeys with respect to anatomical location, number and activation strength, suggesting that many of the parietal visual areas differ considerably between monkeys and humans [9]. Van Essen and colleagues interpret the current evidence to mean that monkey and human areas might be largely conserved on a regional scale, while individual areas could have specialized extensively in both species [9, 11]. A systematic comparative effort is needed to focus on a few of the visual areas at a time in order to quantify how the different areas correspond across humans and monkeys in location, scale, detailed function and connectivity patterns. Such efforts, besides providing information on primate homologies, will yield important information that can be used to understand how the brain supports sensation, perception and behavior.

Visual comparative imaging has advanced farther than comparative work on the other sensory systems. At the same time, it is also clear that most visual areas require further comparative work with selective stimulation, so we still have far to go before the maps in both species will be detailed enough to allow the scrutiny of additional primate evolutionary relationships. However, visual studies have already established useful approaches and the analogous methods will facilitate progress in the other systems.

## Filling in the Gaps in Auditory and Somatosensory Regions

In contrast to the evidence of homologies in early visual areas in humans and monkeys, work on the auditory and somatosensory systems has not kept pace. It is difficult to image auditory cortex because of the loud noise caused by the switching gradients during MR scanning. Thus, optimal auditory activity is achieved with special "sparse-imaging" sequences designed to minimize the auditory response to the scanner noise and allow quiet periods for sound presentation [47-50]. The small size and close proximity of the neighboring sensory cortical areas in the auditory system have also required high-resolution imaging and high-fidelity, MR-compatible sound systems (e.g., [51]). Somatosensory studies, on the other hand, are less affected by scanner noise but have benefited from more precise and reliable MR compatible stimulation [52]. Solutions to a number of these problems open the way for further advances in comparative imaging.

### Auditory Cortical Mapping

In analogy to visual retinotopic organization, many auditory areas in the brain stem, auditory thalamus and auditory cortex show a spatial topography reflecting how the peripheral auditory organ (the cochlea) is stimulated by the frequencies in sounds. This auditory organization is called cochleotopy or tonotopy, and although animal electrophysiological work suggested that multiple auditory cortical areas are cochleotopically organized [53, 54], it took many years of work to establish this for human auditory cortex. Early noninvasive electroencephalography (EEG) and magnetoencephalography (MEG) work, while unable to spatially localize different regions, suggested that areas with different tonotopic organization existed in the human auditory cortex [55]. Since then, numerous studies have imaged a certain amount of tonotopic organization in the human auditory cortex [56-58]. Some of the work even suggests that a number of frequency-preferring regions exist, but has been unable to identify them [59].

It was not until recently that a high-resolution human study conducted at 7 Tesla was able to convincingly show that two auditory areas with mirror-reversed tonotopy existed side by side in the human primary auditory cortex [60]. The study by Formisano and colleagues [60] carefully quantified the frequency tuning of clusters of voxels, which helped identify the characteristic or 'best' frequency response of the spatially resolved regions on the human superior temporal plane, in Heschl's gyrus (the site of the human primary auditory cortex). The authors then quantified the direction of the observed tonotopic gradients, a method analogous to that used to delineate the retinotopically organized visual cortical areas [34]. This allowed them to define a border between areas hA1 and hR (see figure 1), the presumed homologs of the monkey primary auditory cortical areas A1 and R.

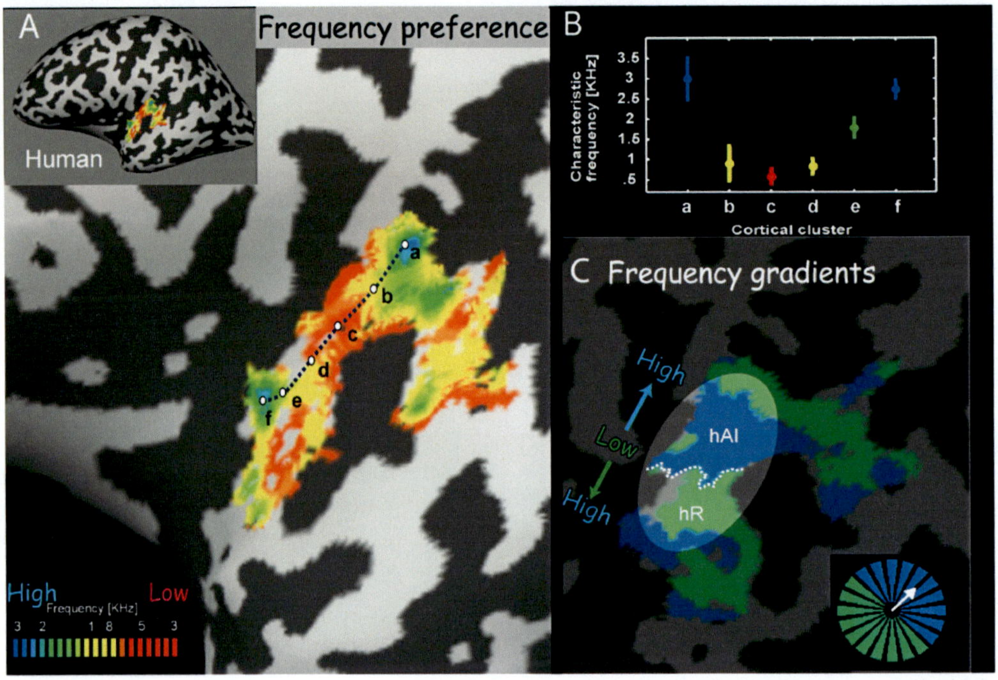


Figure 1. Mapping auditory cortical areas in humans. (A) A best frequency color map that is observed in primary auditory cortex is shown on an inflated representation of a human subject's cerebral cortex, sulci are shown in gray and gyri in white. (B) The characteristic frequency tuning of cortical clusters is shown caudal to rostral for the locations labeled with the letters (a) to (f). A progression from high to low frequencies can be observed from (a) to (c). The frequency representation is then reversed so that (d-f) mirrors the representation of (a-c). (C) A frequency gradient map quantifies the opposing frequency gradients. A border can be delineated where the blue and green colors meet (the gradient reversal point). This border lies between the two auditory cortical areas hA1 and hR, the presumed homologs to monkey areas A1 and R. Figure used with permission from [60].

This impressive study revealed two of the many expected auditory areas, begging the question whether functional imaging had reached its limit in auditory mapping. A subsequent study also carried out at 7 Tesla and one of the first fMRI studies of the monkey auditory cortex, seems to indicate that this is not the case [49]. The authors used an approach similar to that of Formisano and colleagues and quantified multiple mirror reversals (see figure 2). The pattern that they found in the rostro-caudal direction over A1 and R matched the gradient directions obtained in the human study for the presumed human homologs [49, 60]. The monkey study also identified another two areas caudal and rostral to A1 and R and many others lateral and medial to these, including approximating the regional boundary between the primary auditory cortex and the next stage of auditory cortical processing. Their data fit well with a model from the anatomical literature proposing that eleven areas exist within the primary and secondary auditory cortex [22] and with the electrophysiological data from seven of those [23, 54, 61]. In all, the functional imaging identified 3 areas in primary auditory cortex and 8 in the surrounding 'belt' cortex (figure 2C). The gradient patterns were also tested statistically in individual subjects, substantiating the proposed locations and positions of the observed monkey auditory areas.

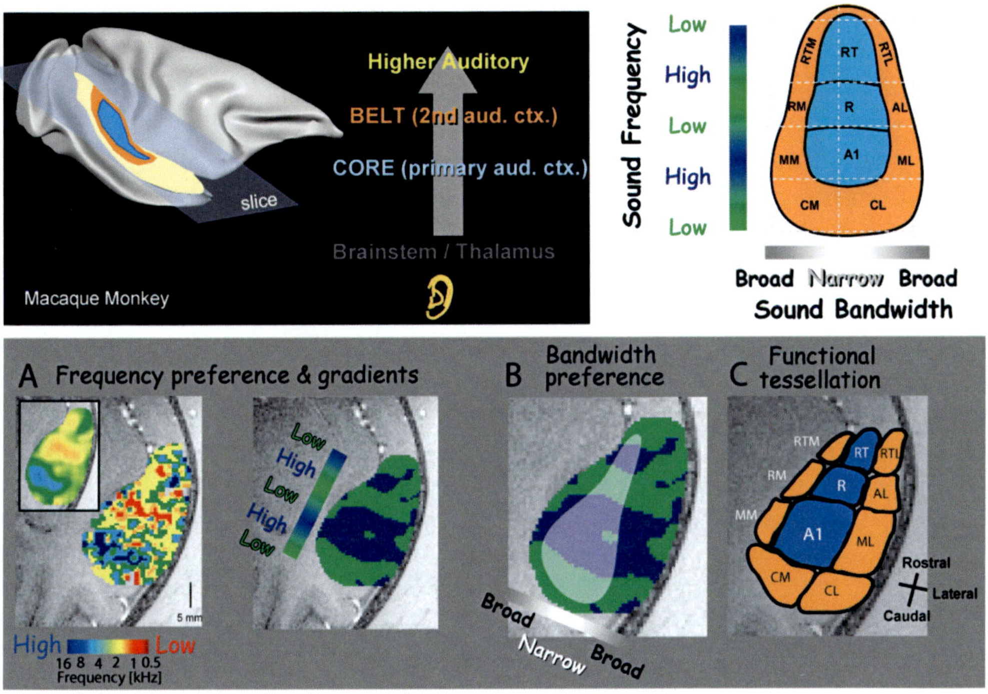


Figure 2. Mapping auditory cortical areas in the monkey. (Top left) An inflated representation of a monkey subject's cerebral cortex. The color scheme shows the cortical stages of processing from core (primary auditory cortex) and belt (secondary cortex) to higher auditory regions whose functional properties are poorly understood. (Top right) One proposed model of the monkey auditory cortical areas in the core and belt regions (adapted from [22]). (A) The best frequency response of individual voxels is shown on a slice from the auditory cortex of a monkey. Observe the multiple spatially alternating patters of frequency preference (from caudal to rostral: low-high-low-high-low), which is consistent with four mirror-reversing tonotopic representations. A gradient analysis reveals borders between areas, where the green and blue colors meet. (B) From medial to lateral the frequency patterns extend beyond the expected position of the primary auditory cortex: the 'core'. A bandwidth preference analysis in the medio-lateral dimension approximates the position of the centrally located core with its preference for single frequency tones (narrow-band stimulation). The surrounding belt areas prefer more complex sounds like band-passed noise. (C) The combined analyses help to localize 11 functional areas in auditory cortex of the monkey, see text. Figures used with permission from [49].

In light of the monkey imaging data, the recent human imaging studies can be interpreted to mean that we can expect to identify further human areas with functional properties similar to those in monkeys. A careful look at the data by Formisano *et al.* [60] shows that tonotopic patterns extend lateral to hA1 and hR into the presumed human 'belt' areas, although it was not possible for the authors to identify further areas or borders (see figure 1). Also, in one of their human subjects Seifritz and colleagues [62] observed a spatial pattern of multiple frequency selective regions similar to that reported in the monkey study (compare their figure 7A for Subject 3 in [62] with figure 3A in [49]). These findings suggest that additional human mapping is possible and will provide a basis for testing further possible auditory cortex homologies between humans and monkeys; if more human areas are identified it will be possible to at least make area size comparisons between the auditory areas in the different primate species.

Beyond tonotopic mapping, imaging work suggests that there is a pitch-sensitive region in human auditory cortex; for a review see [63]. Pitch is the perceived overall frequency of a sound and is not always related to the frequency composition of a sound, so not all frequency-sensitive or tonotopic areas will necessarily support pitch perception. A pitch-sensitive region had been identified in anterior portions of the human auditory cortex. Since there is no detailed functional map of these areas available for humans, it is not clear which of the human auditory areas is involved in pitch processing, but we can probably exclude hA1 [64, 65]. An electrophysiological study in monkeys recently identified a pitch region in the marmoset monkey that was also anterior but involved the secondary 'belt' cortex [61]. A comparative imaging study using marmosets, if possible, could bridge the results in humans and monkeys. Alternatively, if it is not possible to image the smaller marmosets with sufficient resolution, the electrophysiology might replicate in macaque monkeys and could then be followed by comparative imaging of pitch in humans and macaques. Although our example focuses on the auditory system, such an approach need not be limited even to the sensory modalities. We have presented it to underscore the need for comparative approaches to help bridge gaps between results obtained from different techniques that are difficult to relate across the species.

## Somatosensory Cortex Mapping

One of the first comparative fMR imaging studies of monkeys and humans showed evidence of a similar somatotopic organization across the two species. Disbrow and colleagues [4] stimulated the hand and face of their subjects, and the resulting somatotopy of these body regions emanated from primary somatosensory cortex (SI) in the central sulcus, which in animals seems to contain four somatotopic representations of the body in areas 3a, 3b, 1, and 2 [66, 67]. Other work in humans and animals has also revealed multiple body representations in the secondary somatosensory cortex (SII) in the upper bank of the lateral sulcus, which contains at least two somatotopic representations, and another one in a neighboring area PV [68, 69].

A recent study in humans has taken steps toward a detailed mapping of the many somatosensory cortical areas. Huang and Sereno [52] used the same approach that has succeeded for visual [34] and auditory mapping [49, 60]. The study also improved the precision and reliability of somatosensory stimulation by designing a system capable of stimulating around the face or lips. This stimulation capability allowed the authors to map the polar angle of the somatosensory stimulation. In doing so they observed multiple representations of the angle with which they stimulated the face or lips. One broad representation spanned the central sulcus (SI), another was located in SII and PV, as expected. Other areas were observed as well, such as area 7, posterior to PV. The authors also confirmed their previous observation that a human area possibly related to monkey area VIP was somatotopically organized [52, 70]. Their study used the observation of similar patterns across subjects as a measure of reliability.

Similarly detailed somatotopic mapping now remains to be done in monkeys, where the multiple somatotopic representations could be compared to the ones in humans with respect to functional organization, scale and location. A limitation of the human study, however, was its inability to map the second dimension of the somatosensory stimulation, which would have required a different organization of the stimulation apparatus or a denser somatosensory stimulation apparatus [52]. Without this capability, it is difficult to delineate the borders between many somatosensory areas such as the multiple side by side areas in SI, for example areas 3a, 3b, 1 and 2, which have similarly oriented somatotopic representations spanning the central sulcus.

# Beyond Sight, Sound and Touch

A complete functional mapping of the brain must include the remaining sensory modalities. The neuronal representations of different senses are well distributed throughout the primate brain but there is overlap, so that a comparative approach across the senses can provide both anchor points between difficult-to-map higher level processing areas [17] and a more detailed understanding of areas supporting multiple sensory functions. Many of the sensory functions and processing stages, including certain cortical areas, could be largely conserved in primates, but we can also expect to find interesting differences [71].

## Pain and Thermal Senses

The other primate somatosensory sensations besides touch and proprioception (mechanoception) also involve regions of SI, SII, the parietal operculum and the insula [72, 73]. Lesions involving SII affect pain and thermal sensations in humans, and fMRI work suggests that these sensations are largely restricted to SII rather than SI, which would be principally involved with low-intensity mechanical stimuli [74]. This is an interesting hypothesis which will benefit from comparative testing, especially since monkey SI neurons also respond strongly to intense mechanical stimulation like pain and to thermal stimulation [75]. The same seems to be true of neurons in SII and area 7 of the parietal operculum, which can support multiple somatosensations [76]. Comparative functional imaging will be useful in clarifying the different aspects of the somatosensory system. Also, the sense of touch, heat, pain and proprioception all have different perceptual qualities, sensitivities and acuities, so differences in their cortical representations would be expected, whether or not these representations also differ across primate species.

### Chemical Senses

The chemical senses have a cortical representation in olfactory and gustatory cortex in the ventral and anterior portions of the brain. There is a primary olfactory cortex (POC), and multiple olfactory areas in POC might be imageable in humans under certain conditions. Zelano and colleagues [77] used a clever olfactory attention paradigm to dissociate attentionally labile areas in POC versus those unmodulated by attention. Imaging studies of the gustatory (taste) sense have been able to activate primary and secondary gustatory regions in the human ventral frontal areas, e.g., [78]. Imaging these regions on the ventral portions of the brain has been difficult because of the dramatic signal loss on images of the brain near the air sinuses, but techniques are now available to improve imaging quality there [77, 79].

### Vestibular Sense

The vestibular sense has a strong cortical representation in primates, with recent evidence suggesting that the primary vestibular cortex has been identified in humans and monkeys [80]. Recent human fMRI using galvanic vestibular stimulation suggests that the human parietal operculum, rather that the posterior insula as suggested by previous studies, is the homolog of the monkey primary vestibular cortex [81]. That study observed strong vestibular responses to cytoarchitectonically localized human area OP2 on the upper bank of the lateral sulcus, in the parietal operculum. The corresponding monkey region could be the parieto-insular vestibular cortex (PIVC) which contains neurons strongly driven by vestibular stimulation [82]. The locations of the human OP2 and monkey PIVC regions seem to roughly correspond, but it is difficult to rule out the possibility that the human region might have repositioned away from the insular cortex [81-83]; this aspect could be addressed by a comparative imaging study. High-resolution fMRI could also determine whether there is a topography of vestibular stimulation, although currently available information suggests that this is not the case. Lastly, since the representation of the vestibular sense is observed in different multisensory parietal and frontal regions [80], it will be important to compare the different loci of vestibular activation observed in humans with data obtained from monkeys.

## Comparative Imaging of Multisensory Interactions

Our environment constantly bombards us with information for our different senses thus our perception is rarely restricted to a single sensory modality. Often the brain must form coherent percepts of environmental events across their many sensory representations. Some regions in the brain like the superior colliculus (a subcortical structure) and the superior temporal sulcus (a cortical region) have been the traditional sites of multisensory studies. But some authors are questioning if there are any strictly unisensory processing regions at least at the cortical level, for a review see [84, 85].

Certainly many more brain regions than had been originally considered are important for multisensory interactions. Some like the insular cortex, which has a number of subdivisions

[86], come up so often in individual sensory studies that they must certainly be multisensory regions. Further cross-sensory work will help us to understand if different neuronal populations in these regions process multisensory information in parallel or if the neurons integrate the sensory information. Currently, we are still at the stage of describing the extent of the multisensory influences in the brain before we can understand the nature of these influences on the processing in a given area. In this final section, we will consider two examples, one from the classical multisensory regions in the superior temporal sulcus, and another where visual stimulation modulates specific areas of the monkey *auditory* cortex.

The multisensory region in the superior temporal sulcus (STS) has been shown in macaques to have a 'patchy' organization. Some anatomical markers like cytochrome oxidase stain darker in patches [87]. A recent functional imaging study showed a patchy organization of spatially resolvable auditory, visual and combined functional regions in the human STS [88]. High-resolution functional imaging in the monkey might be able to resolve these patches and then directly relate, in the same animal, their function to specific histochemical markers in anatomical studies or to *in-vivo* structural data evaluated with MRI. Human and monkey fMRI can then establish cross-species relationships based on the functional properties of the unisensory and multisensory 'patches' across the species.

With this last example, we illustrate how fMRI studies need not conclude, but rather become more useful, following the spatial mapping or localization of brain areas. For example, by first mapping areas (e.g. by using a uni-sensory property like retinotopy) their other functional capabilities, such as multisensory interactions, can then be evaluated. Using this strategy, a recent monkey study localized the strength of the visual influence to specific *auditory* areas [50]. The authors aimed to evaluate and more precisely localize where cross-modal effects occur in the auditory cortical processing hierarchy. Cross-modal effects had already been suggested to occur even at the earliest sensory processing stages both in studies imaging the human brain with EEG, MEG and fMRI and in studies using electophysiological recordings in animals; for a review see [84, 85]. In their monkey fMRI study the authors first localized the multiple core and belt areas in the monkey auditory cortex, as described above and in [49], then evaluated the strength of the visual influence in specific auditory areas [50]. The visual influence is strongest in the caudal areas of the monkey auditory cortex, mainly in the second stage of auditory cortical processing (the auditory belt), but extends also into primary auditory cortex [50]. A study in humans using a similar approach is now needed but would first require a detailed map of auditory cortical areas which, as mentioned above, has not yet been produced. Once such a map becomes available, however, then the comparative maps would reveal whether the same auditory areas are equally modulated by visual stimuli or if there are quantifiable differences across the species. Without evidence from direct comparative approaches it is difficult to argue that multisensory influences in primates share homologous functional processes. The most that one could hope to show is that there is a similarity in the cross-modal influence on sensory processing.

# Conclusion

Additional comparative imaging of the senses will help us to understand the cortical representation of each sense and provide us with more complete functional maps of the monkey and human brains in order to evaluate under what circumstances the monkey brain can serve as an animal model of human neuronal function. Such maps together with in vivo connectivity studies are also likely to yield important information that can be used to understand the neuronal basis of sensation, perception and behavior. We have reviewed how human studies have made advances in imaging the different sensory systems. Monkey imaging is more advanced for vision than for the other senses, allowing more combined human and monkey imaging studies. For the auditory system, it seems that the monkey auditory mapping could be helpful in mapping the human auditory cortex. Areas that appear similar in humans and monkeys will need to be carefully scrutinized with respect to size, location, function and connectivity patterns. Beyond fMR imaging, the goal would be to incorporate data from various techniques and continuously update the maps to reflect the ongoing efforts across the senses and species. Brain maps are beginning to be available on the internet for comparative analyses (see the online surface visualization in the SumsDB database: *http://brainmap.wustl.edu*) which can well serve the need to bring together cross-species data. A more concerted comparative imaging effort on the sensory systems will also provide a stronger basis for mapping the functional areas of the brain which depend on sensory input, such as areas supporting motor and cognitive functions.

# References

[1] Logothetis, N.K., J. Pauls, M. Augath, T. Trinath, and A. Oeltermann, *Neurophysiological investigation of the basis of the fMRI signal. Nature,* 2001. 412(6843): p. 150-7.

[2] Mukamel, R., H. Gelbard, A. Arieli, U. Hasson, I. Fried, and R. Malach, *Coupling between neuronal firing, field potentials, and FMRI in human auditory cortex. Science,* 2005. 309(5736): p. 951-4.

[3] Logothetis, N.K., H. Guggenberger, S. Peled, and J. Pauls, *Functional imaging of the monkey brain. Nat. Neurosci,* 1999. 2(6): p. 555-62.

[4] Disbrow, E., T.P. Roberts, D. Slutsky, and L. Krubitzer, The use of fMRI for determining the topographic organization of cortical fields in human and nonhuman primates. Brain Res, 1999. 829(1-2): p. 167-73.

[5] Poremba, A., M. Malloy, R.C. Saunders, R.E. Carson, P. Herscovitch, and M. Mishkin, *Species-specific calls evoke asymmetric activity in the monkey's temporal poles. Nature,* 2004. 427(6973): p. 448-51.

[6] Logothetis, N.K., The underpinnings of the BOLD functional magnetic resonance imaging signal. *J. Neurosci*, 2003. 23(10): p. 3963-71.

[7] Logothetis, N.K., The neural basis of the blood-oxygen-level-dependent functional magnetic resonance imaging signal. Philos. *Trans. R. Soc. Lond. B. Biol. Sci*, 2002. 357(1424): p. 1003-37.

[8] Sereno, M.I. and R.B. Tootell, From monkeys to humans: what do we now know about brain homologies? *Curr. Opin. Neurobiol*, 2005. 15(2): p. 135-44.

[9] Orban, G.A., D. Van Essen, and W. Vanduffel, Comparative mapping of higher visual areas in monkeys and humans. Trends Cogn. Sci, 2004. 8(7): p. 315-24.

[10] Zilles, K., E. Armstrong, A. Schleicher, and H.J. Kretschmann, *The human pattern of gyrification in the cerebral cortex. Anat. Embryol.* (Berl), 1988. 179(2): p. 173-9.

[11] Van Essen, D.C., Surface-based comparisons of macaque and human cortical organization., in *From Monkey Brain To Human Brain.*, S. Dahaene, et al., Editors. 2005, MIT Press: Cambridge, MA. p. 1-19.

[12] Schormann, T. and K. Zilles, Three-dimensional linear and nonlinear transformations: an integration of light microscopical and MRI data. *Hum. Brain Mapp*, 1998. 6(5-6): p. 339-47.

[13] Van Essen, D.C., *Organization of visual areas in macaque and human cerebral cortex.*, in *The Visual Neurosciences*, L. Chalupa and J.S. Werner, Editors. 2004, MIT Press: Cambridge, MA. p. 507-521.

[14] Zilles, K., Evolution of the human brain and comparative cyto- and receptor architecture., in *From Monkey Brain To Human Brain.*, S. Dahaene, et al., Editors. 2005, MIT Press: Cambridge, MA. p. 41-56.

[15] Brodmann, K. and L.J. Garey, *Brodmann's Localisation in the Cerebral Cortex*. 1999, London: Imperial College Press.

[16] Lewis, J.W. and D.C. Van Essen, Mapping of architectonic subdivisions in the macaque monkey, with emphasis on parieto-occipital cortex. *J. Comp. Neurol*, 2000. 428(1): p. 79-111.

[17] Van Essen, D.C., Surface-based approaches to spatial localization and registration in primate cerebral cortex. *Neuroimage*, 2004. 23 Suppl 1: p. S97-107.

[18] Petrides, M. and D.N. Pandya, Comparative cytoarchitectonic analysis of the human and the macaque ventrolateral prefrontal cortex and corticocortical connection patterns in the monkey. *Eur. J. Neurosci*, 2002. 16(2): p. 291-310.

[19] Ongur, D. and J.L. Price, The organization of networks within the orbital and medial prefrontal cortex of rats, monkeys and humans. *Cereb. Cortex*, 2000. 10(3): p. 206-19.

[20] Ongur, D., A.T. Ferry, and J.L. Price, Architectonic subdivision of the human orbital and medial prefrontal cortex. *J. Comp. Neurol*, 2003. 460(3): p. 425-49.

[21] Kaas, J.H., The organization of neocortex in mammals: Implications for theories of brain function. *Annual Review of Psychology*, 1987. 38: p. 129-151.

[22] Kaas, J.H. and T.A. Hackett, Subdivisions of auditory cortex and processing streams in primates. *Proc. Natl. Acad. Sci. U S A*, 2000. 97(22): p. 11793-9.

[23] Rauschecker, J.P., B. Tian, and M. Hauser, Processing of complex sounds in the macaque nonprimary auditory cortex. *Science*, 1995. 268(5207): p. 111-4.

[24] Fox, P.T., M.A. Mintun, M.E. Raichle, F.M. Miezin, J.M. Allman, and D.C. Van Essen, Mapping human visual cortex with positron emission tomography. *Nature,* 1986. 323(6091): p. 806-9.

[25] Fox, P.T., M.E. Raichle, and W.T. Thach, Functional mapping of the human cerebellum with positron emission tomography. *Proc. Natl. Acad. Sci. U S A*, 1985. 82(21): p. 7462-6.

[26] Ogawa, S., T.M. Lee, A.S. Nayak, and P. Glynn, Oxygenation-sensitive contrast in magnetic resonance image of rodent brain at high magnetic fields. *Magn. Reson. Med*, 1990. 14(1): p. 68-78.

[27] Ogawa, S., D.W. Tank, R. Menon, J.M. Ellermann, S.G. Kim, H. Merkle, and K. Ugurbil, Intrinsic signal changes accompanying sensory stimulation: functional brain mapping with magnetic resonance imaging. *Proc. Natl. Acad. Sci. U S A*, 1992. 89(13): p. 5951-5.

[28] Tootell, R.B., D. Tsao, and W. Vanduffel, Neuroimaging weighs in: humans meet macaques in "primate" visual cortex. *J. Neurosci*, 2003. 23(10): p. 3981-9.

[29] Wandell, B.A., A.A. Brewer, and R.F. Dougherty, Visual field map clusters in human cortex. Philos. *Trans. R. Soc. Lond. B. Biol. Sci*, 2005. 360(1456): p. 693-707.

[30] Vanduffel, W., D. Fize, J.B. Mandeville, K. Nelissen, P. Van Hecke, B.R. Rosen, R.B. Tootell, and G.A. Orban, *Visual motion processing investigated using contrast agent-enhanced fMRI in awake behaving monkeys. Neuron,* 2001. 32(4): p. 565-77.

[31] Huk, A.C., R.F. Dougherty, and D.J. Heeger, Retinotopy and functional subdivision of human areas MT and MST. *J. Neurosc*i, 2002. 22(16): p. 7195-205.

[32] Morrone, M.C., M. Tosetti, D. Montanaro, A. Fiorentini, G. Cioni, and D.C. Burr, *A cortical area that responds specifically to optic flow, revealed by fMRI. Nat. Neurosci,* 2000. 3(12): p. 1322-8.

[33] Engel, S.A., D.E. Rumelhart, B.A. Wandell, A.T. Lee, G.H. Glover, E.J. Chichilnisky, and M.N. Shadlen, fMRI of human visual cortex. *Nature,* 1994. 369(6481): p. 525.

[34] Sereno, M.I., A.M. Dale, J.B. Reppas, K.K. Kwong, J.W. Belliveau, T.J. Brady, B.R. Rosen, and R.B. Tootell, Borders of multiple visual areas in humans revealed by functional magnetic resonance imaging. *Science,* 1995. 268: p. 889-93.

[35] Brewer, A.A., W.A. Press, N.K. Logothetis, and B.A. Wandell, Visual areas in macaque cortex measured using functional magnetic resonance imaging. *J. Neurosc*i, 2002. 22(23): p. 10416-26.

[36] Rosa, M.G.P. and R. Tweedale, Maps of the visual field in the cerebral cortex of primates: Functional organization and significance, in *The Primate Visual System.*, J. Kaas, Editor. 2004, CRC Press: Collins CE. p. 261-288.

[37] Engel, S.A., G.H. Glover, and B.A. Wandell, Retinotopic organization in human visual cortex and the spatial precision of functional MRI. *Cereb Cortex,* 1997. 7(2): p. 181-92.

[38] Hagler, D.J., Jr. and M.I. Sereno, Spatial maps in frontal and prefrontal cortex. *Neuroimage,* 2006. 29(2): p. 567-77.

[39] Schluppeck, D., P. Glimcher, and D.J. Heeger, Topographic organization for delayed saccades in human posterior parietal cortex. *J. Neurophysiol*, 2005. 94(2): p. 1372-84.

[40] Silver, M.A., D. Ress, and D.J. Heeger, Topographic maps of visual spatial attention in human parietal cortex. *J. Neurophysiol*, 2005. 94(2): p. 1358-71.

[41] Tsao, D.Y., W.A. Freiwald, R.B. Tootell, and M.S. Livingstone, A cortical region consisting entirely of face-selective cells. *Science,* 2006. 311(5761): p. 670-4.

[42] Tsao, D.Y., W.A. Freiwald, T.A. Knutsen, J.B. Mandeville, and R.B. Tootell, Faces and objects in macaque cerebral cortex. *Nat. Neurosci,* 2003. 6(9): p. 989-95.

[43] Smirnakis, S.M., M.C. Schmid, B. Weber, A.S. Tolias, M. Augath, and N.K. Logothetis, Spatial specificity of BOLD versus cerebral blood volume fMRI for mapping cortical organization. *J. Cereb. Blood Flow Metab*, 2007. 27(6): p. 1290.

[44] Vanduffel, W., D. Fize, H. Peuskens, K. Denys, S. Sunaert, J.T. Todd, and G.A. Orban, Extracting 3D from motion: differences in human and monkey intraparietal cortex. *Science,* 2002. 298(5592): p. 413-5.

[45] Tsao, D.Y., W. Vanduffel, Y. Sasaki, D. Fize, T.A. Knutsen, J.B. Mandeville, L.L. Wald, A.M. Dale, B.R. Rosen, D.C. Van Essen, M.S. Livingstone, G.A. Orban, and R.B. Tootell, Stereopsis activates V3A and caudal intraparietal areas in macaques and humans. *Neuron,* 2003. 39(3): p. 555-68.

[46] Denys, K., W. Vanduffel, D. Fize, K. Nelissen, H. Peuskens, D. Van Essen, and G.A. Orban, The processing of visual shape in the cerebral cortex of human and nonhuman primates: a functional magnetic resonance imaging study. *J. Neurosci*, 2004. 24(10): p. 2551-65.

[47] Hall, D.A., M.P. Haggard, M.A. Akeroyd, A.R. Palmer, A.Q. Summerfield, M.R. Elliott, E.M. Gurney, and R.W. Bowtell, *"Sparse" temporal sampling in auditory fMRI. Hum. Brain Mapp,* 1999. 7(3): p. 213-23.

[48] Schwarzbauer, C., M.H. Davis, J.M. Rodd, and I. Johnsrude, Interleaved silent steady state (ISSS) imaging: A new sparse imaging method applied to auditory fMRI. *Neuroimage*, 2005.

[49] Petkov, C.I., C. Kayser, M. Augath, and N.K. Logothetis, Functional imaging reveals numerous fields in the monkey auditory cortex. *PLoS. Biol*, 2006. 4(7): p. e215.

[50] Kayser, C., C.I. Petkov, M. Augath, and N.K. Logothetis, Functional imaging reveals visual modulation of specific fields in auditory cortex. *J. Neurosci*, 2007. 27(8): p. 1824-35.

[51] Baumgart, F., T. Kaulisch, C. Tempelmann, B. Gaschler-Markefski, C. Tegeler, F. Schindler, D. Stiller, and H. Scheich, Electrodynamic headphones and woofers for application in magnetic resonance imaging scanners. *Med. Phys,* 1998. 25(10): p. 2068-70.

[52] Huang, R.S. and M.I. Sereno, Dodecapus: An MR-compatible system for somatosensory stimulation. *Neuroimage,* 2007. 34(3): p. 1060-73.

[53] Merzenich, M.M., G.L. Knight, and G.L. Roth, Representation of cochlea within primary auditory cortex in the cat. *J. Neurophyisol.*, 1975. 38: p. 231-249.

[54] Merzenich, M.M. and J.F. Brugge, Representation of the cochlear partition of the superior temporal plane of the macaque monkey. *Brain Res*, 1973. 50(2): p. 275-96.

[55] Pantev, C., O. Bertrand, C. Eulitz, C. Verkindt, S. Hampson, G. Schuierer, and T. Elbert, Specific tonotopic organizations of different areas of the human auditory cortex revealed by simultaneous magnetic and electric recordings. *Electroencephalography and Clinical Neurophysiology*, 1995. 94: p. 26-40.

[56] Talavage, T.M., P.J. Ledden, R.R. Benson, B.R. Rosen, and J.R. Melcher, Frequency-dependent responses exhibited by multiple regions in human auditory cortex. *Hear Res,* 2000. 150(1-2): p. 225-44.

[57] Bilecen, D., K. Scheffler, N. Schmid, K. Tschopp, and J. Seelig, *Tonotopic organization of the human auditory cortex as detected by BOLD-FMRI. Hear Res,* 1998. 126(1-2): p. 19-27.

[58] Wessinger, C.M., M.H. Buonocore, C.L. Kussmaul, and G.R. Mangun, Tonotopy in human auditory cortex examined with functional magnetic resonance imaging. *Neuroimage*, 1997. 5: p. 18-25.

[59] Talavage, T.M., M.I. Sereno, J.R. Melcher, P.J. Ledden, B.R. Rosen, and A.M. Dale, Tonotopic organization in human auditory cortex revealed by progressions of frequency sensitivity. *J. Neurophysiol*, 2004. 91(3): p. 1282-96.

[60] Formisano, E., D.S. Kim, F. Di Salle, P.F. van de Moortele, K. Ugurbil, and R. Goebel, Mirror-symmetric tonotopic maps in human primary auditory cortex. *Neuron,* 2003. 40(4): p. 859-69.

[61] Bendor, D. and X. Wang, The neuronal representation of pitch in primate auditory cortex. *Nature*, 2005. 436(7054): p. 1161-5.

[62] Seifritz, E., F. Di Salle, F. Esposito, M. Herdener, J.G. Neuhoff, and K. Scheffler, Enhancing BOLD response in the auditory system by neurophysiologically tuned fMRI sequence. *Neuroimage,* 2006. 29(3): p. 1013-22.

[63] Bendor, D. and X. Wang, Cortical representations of pitch in monkeys and humans. *Curr Opin Neurobiol*, 2006. 16(4): p. 391-9.

[64] Patterson, R.D., S. Uppenkamp, I.S. Johnsrude, and T.D. Griffiths, The processing of temporal pitch and melody information in auditory cortex. *Neuron,* 2002. 36(4): p. 767-76.

[65] Schneider, P., V. Sluming, N. Roberts, M. Scherg, R. Goebel, H.J. Specht, H.G. Dosch, S. Bleeck, C. Stippich, and A. Rupp, *Structural and functional asymmetry of lateral Heschl's gyrus reflects pitch perception preference. Nat. Neurosci,* 2005. 8(9): p. 1241-7.

[66] Merzenich, M.M., J.H. Kaas, M. Sur, and C.S. Lin, Double representation of the body surface within cytoarchitectonic areas 3b and 1 in "SI" in the owl monkey (Aotus trivirgatus). J. Comp. Neurol, 1978. 181(1): p. 41-73.

[67] Kaas, J.H., R.J. Nelson, M. Sur, C.S. Lin, and M.M. Merzenich, Multiple representations of the body within the primary somatosensory cortex of primates. *Science*, 1979. 204(4392): p. 521-3.

[68] Disbrow, E., T. Roberts, and L. Krubitzer, Somatotopic organization of cortical fields in the lateral sulcus of Homo sapiens: evidence for SII and PV. *J. Comp. Neurol*, 2000. 418(1): p. 1-21.

[69] Krubitzer, L., J. Clarey, R. Tweedale, G. Elston, and M. Calford, A redefinition of somatosensory areas in the lateral sulcus of macaque monkeys. *J. Neurosci,* 1995. 15(5 Pt 2): p. 3821-39.

[70] Sereno, M.I. and R.S. Huang, A human parietal face area contains aligned head-centered visual and tactile maps. *Nat. Neurosci*, 2006. 9(10): p. 1337-43.

[71] Krubitzer, L., The organization of neocortex in mammals: are species differences really so different? Trends Neurosci, 1995. 18(9): p. 408-17.

[72] Price, D.D., Psychological and neural mechanisms of the affective dimension of pain. *Science*, 2000. 288(5472): p. 1769-72.

[73] Disbrow, E., M. Buonocore, J. Antognini, E. Carstens, and H.A. Rowley, Somatosensory cortex: a comparison of the response to noxious thermal, mechanical, and electrical stimuli using functional magnetic resonance imaging. *Hum. Brain Mapp*, 1998. 6(3): p. 150-9.

[74] Bowsher, D., J. Brooks, and P. Enevoldson, Central representation of somatic sensations in the parietal operculum (SII) and insula. *Eur. Neurol*, 2004. 52(4): p. 211-25.

[75] Kenshalo, D.R., Jr. and O. Isensee, Responses of primate SI cortical neurons to noxious stimuli. *J. Neurophysiol*, 1983. 50(6): p. 1479-96.

[76] Dong, W.K., L.D. Salonen, Y. Kawakami, T. Shiwaku, E.M. Kaukoranta, and R.F. Martin, Nociceptive responses of trigeminal neurons in SII-7b cortex of awake monkeys. *Brain Res,* 1989. 484(1-2): p. 314-24.

[77] Zelano, C., M. Bensafi, J. Porter, J. Mainland, B. Johnson, E. Bremner, C. Telles, R. Khan, and N. Sobel, Attentional modulation in human primary olfactory cortex. *Nat. Neurosci,* 2005. 8(1): p. 114-20.

[78] Smits, M., R.R. Peeters, P. van Hecke, and S. Sunaert, A 3 T event-related functional magnetic resonance imaging (fMRI) study of primary and secondary gustatory cortex localization using natural tastants. *Neuroradiology*, 2007. 49(1): p. 61-71.

[79] Tabert, M.H., J. Steffener, M.W. Albers, D.W. Kern, M. Michael, H. Tang, T.R. Brown, and D.P. Devanand, Validation and optimization of statistical approaches for modeling odorant-induced fMRI signal changes in olfactory-related brain areas. *Neuroimage*, 2007. 34(4): p. 1375-90.

[80] Gunny, R. and T.A. Yousry, Imaging anatomy of the vestibular and visual systems. *Curr. Opin. Neurol*, 2007. 20(1): p. 3-11.

[81] Eickhoff, S.B., P.H. Weiss, K. Amunts, G.R. Fink, and K. Zilles, Identifying human parieto-insular vestibular cortex using fMRI and cytoarchitectonic mapping. *Hum. Brain Mapp*, 2006. 27(7): p. 611-21.

[82] Akbarian, S., K. Berndl, O.J. Grusser, W. Guldin, M. Pause, and U. Schreiter, Responses of single neurons in the parietoinsular vestibular cortex of primates. *Ann. N. Y. Acad. Sci,* 1988. 545: p. 187-202.

[83] Stephan, T., A. Deutschlander, A. Nolte, E. Schneider, M. Wiesmann, T. Brandt, and M. Dieterich, Functional MRI *of galvanic vestibular stimulation with alternating currents at different frequencies. Neuroimage,* 2005. 26(3): p. 721-32.

[84] Ghazanfar, A.A. and C.E. Schroeder, Is neocortex essentially multisensory? *Trends Cogn. Sci,* 2006. 10(6): p. 278-85.

[85] Schroeder, C.E. and J. Foxe, Multisensory contributions to low-level, 'unisensory' processing. *Curr. Opin. Neurobiol*, 2005. 15(4): p. 454-8.

[86] Nagai, M., K. Kishi, and S. Kato, Insular cortex and neuropsychiatric disorders: A review of recent literature. *Eur. Psychiatry*, 2007.

[87] Padberg, J., B. Seltzer, and C.G. Cusick, Architectonics and cortical connections of the upper bank of the superior temporal sulcus in the rhesus monkey: an analysis in the tangential plane. *J. Comp. Neurol*, 2003. 467(3): p. 418-34.

[88] Beauchamp, M.S., B.D. Argall, J. Bodurka, J.H. Duyn, and A. Martin, Unraveling multisensory integration: patchy organization within human STS multisensory cortex. *Nat. Neurosci*, 2004. 7(11): p. 1190-2.

In: Research Topics on Brain Mapping
Editor: Yuanzhu Liáng, pp. 195-208
ISBN: 978-1-60456-001-5


*Chapter IX*

# Functional Brain Imaging of the Human Somatosensory System

***S.M. Golaszewski*[*1,3], *C.M. Siedentopf*[2,3] *and E. Gallasch*[4]**

[1] Department of Neurology, Paracelsus Medical University Salzburg, Austria
[2] Department of Neuroradiology, Medical University Innsbruck, Austria
[3] fMRI Lab, Department of Psychiatry, Medical University Innsbruck, Austria
[4] Institute of Physiology, Medical University Graz, Austria

## Abstract

Functional brain imaging of the somatosensory system has become an important tool in the planning of neurosurgical procedures for patients with brain tumor or cavernoma and for the discrimination of the motor cortex from the surrounding brain tissue in order to accurately define resection boundaries. Moreover, these studies are important for the monitoring of neurorehabilitation processes and the understanding of motor recovery, e.g. after stroke, in brain trauma, spinal cord injury, extrapyramidal diseases or extremity transplantations for the planning of individual neurorehabilitation strategies.

A close relationship of movement related cortical areas and areas related to somatosensory sensation is well documented in the literature and led to the concept of the sensorimotor cortex. Positron emission tomography (PET) and functional magnetic resonance imaging (fMRI) studies have shown that somatosensory paradigms can activate somatosensory as well as motor areas of the cerebral cortex. Moreover, somatosensory stimulation for probing the nature and function of the sensorimotor cortex does not require the collaboration of the subject under examination and is therefore feasible in patients with hemiparesis or hemiplegia, which holds promise for a wide clinical applicability.

---

* Address for correspondence: Stefan Golaszewski, MD, PhD; Tel:+43-662-4483-56035; Department of Neurology; Fax: +43-662-4483-3004; Paracelsus Medical University Salzburg; Email: S.Golaszewski@salk.at; Ignaz-Harrer-Strasse 79; 5020 Salzburg - A U S T R I A

Somatosensory paradigms in fMRI also revealed a positive correlation between the intensity of phantom limb pain in amputees and the amount of reorganization of the sensorimotor cortex and thus led to a deeper understanding of the mechanisms of phantom limb pain.

For the purpose of somatosensory stimulation for the investigation of the sensorimotor cortex several MR compatible devices have been developed. These devices are based on pneumatic approaches, piezoelectric or magneto-mechanical principles. Pneumatic systems have the disadvantage of limited vibration frequencies, have shown to cause somatosensory without motorcortex activation and are difficult to control. Piezoelectric systems provide a wide range of frequencies but only small displacement amplitudes (smaller than 0.5 mm), which limits its application to the skin receptors and elicit only somatosensory without motorcortex activation, too. Magnetomechanical devices succeeded in the combined activation of the somatosensory as well as the motorcortex and are controllable.

In the paper a review of the whole area of somatosensory stimulation in functional brain imaging the past decades, advantages and disadvantages, optimal stimulation protocols and corresponding brain maps of different approaches of somatosensory stimulation in functional brain imaging and clinical and neurophysilogical applications are discussed.

## Introduction

Functional brain imaging of the somatosensory system has evolved since two decades and it has become an important tool in the preoperative planning in neurosurgery, in the monitoring in neurorehabilitation and for the understanding of motor recovery after brain damage for the planning and optimization of neurorehabilitation strategies.

Mapping of movement related cortical areas and areas that are related to sensation was initially performed during neurosurgical procedures using direct cortical stimulation (Penfield, 1937). Several functional brain mapping techniques have evolved subsequently (2000). During the eighties of the past century the era of functional brain imaging began with the implementation of the Positron Emission Tomography (PET) by measurements of the regional cerebral blood flow. Since the nineties of the last century functional brain imaging is dominated by the upcoming fMRI based on the blood oxygenation level dependant (BOLD) effect that was discovered in 1990 by Ogawa et al. (Ogawa et al., 1990;Ogawa et al., 1992). Then continuous evolution and progress of fMRI as well as its increasing popularity and spreading clinical use as a highly sensitive diagnostic neuroimaging instrument suitable for the assessment of a large variety of neurological and neurosurgical indications made fMRI to the leading functional neuroimaging modality. In the following the area of somatosensory stimulation in PET and BOLD fMRI the past decades, advantages and disadvantages, optimal stimulation protocols and corresponding brain maps of different approaches of somatosensory stimulation in functional brain imaging and clinical and neurophysilogical applications will be discussed.

# PET

In the eighties of the last century, PET was used for the first time to detect focal neuronal activation in the first somatosensory cortex (SI) of humans induced by cutaneous vibratory stimulation with a vibration frequency of 50 Hz and an amplitude of 1 mm (Fox et al., 1987). Water labeled with H2(15)O was used as a blood flow tracer. The cutaneous surfaces of lips, fingers, and toes were tested. Intense and highly focal distinct SI responses with a medial-to-lateral homunculus were seen in every subject. The study suggested that eliciting regional cerebral blood flow responses within the somatosensory cortex by cutaneous vibration provides a safe, rapid, and reproducible tool for locating and assessing its functional status and for the localization of the central sulcus that is crucial in preoperative neurosurgical planning. The study has established normative values for future applications of the vibration paradigm in functional brain imaging. 1990 Tempel and Perlmutter studied regional cerebral blood flow responses to vibrotactile stimulation in patients with predominantly unilateral idiopathic focal dystonia and normal subjects using H2(15)O PET (Tempel and Perlmutter, 1990). The somatosensory stimulation produced a consistently localized and robust peak response in the primary sensorimotor cortex contralateral to hand vibration in normal subjects. The sensorimotor response in dystonic patients was also consistently localized to the same area, but significantly reduced in magnitude whether vibrating the affected or unaffected hand. Furthermore, vibration induced a dystonic cramp in the stimulated arm/hand in some patients, but not in any normal subjects. This abnormal sensorimotor response had important implications for understanding of the pathophysiology of idiopathic dystonia. Two years later, Tempel and Perlmutter performed another interesting H2(15)O PET study with vibration-induced regional cerebral blood flow responses in healthy older subjects to investigate whether vibration-induced CBF responses change with advancing age in normals (Tempel and Perlmutter, 1992). Left and right hand vibration produced consistent responses in contralateral primary sensorimotor (SM1) and supplementary motor area (SMA) with no change with normal aging. In the same year, Seitz et al. could demonstrate with a vibratory stimulus to the right hand palm of healthy volunteers and H2(15)O PET that activation of some cerebral structures is accompanied by deactivations of corresponding other structures elsewhere in the brain (Pons et al., 1992). Regional cerebral blood flow (rCBF) increases were localized in the left primary somatosensory area (SI), the left secondary somatosensory area (SII), the left retroinsular field (RI), the left anterior parietal cortex, the left primary motor area (MI), and the left supplementary motor area (SMA). The decreases occurred bilaterally within the superior parietal cortex, paralimbic association areas, and the left globus pallidus. The mean global cerebral blood flow did not change compared with rest. The decreases of the cerebral oxidative metabolism was interpreted as regional depressions of synaptic activity. In a H2(15)O PET study by Drevets et al. changes in the human primary and secondary somatosensory cortices during the period when somatosensory stimuli were expected were investigated (Drevets et al., 1995). In anticipation of either focal or innocuous touching, or localized, painful shocks, blood flow decreased in parts of the primary somatosensory cortex map located outside the representation of the skin area that was the target of the expected stimulus. Specifically, attending to an impending stimulus to the fingers produced a significant decrease in blood flow in the somatosensory zones for the face, whereas attending to stimulation of the toe produced decreases in the zones for the fingers and face. Decreases were more prominent in the side ipsilateral to the location of the expected stimulus. No significant changes in blood flow occurred in the region of the cortex representing the skin locus of the awaited stimulation. These results were concurrent with a model of spatial attention in which potential signal enhancement may rely on generalized suppression of background activity. In the same year Ibanez et al. demonstrated in a PET study that there is no evidence that the primary motor and supplementary motor area are involved in the generation of the P22 and N30 components of somatosensory evoked potentials (SSEPs) evoked by electrical stimulation of the median nerve at the wrist (Ibanez et al., 1995). PET was performed in normal subjects to study the cerebral areas activated by median nerve electrical stimulation at frequencies of up to 20 Hz. Stimulation evoked a single focus of activation in the primary somatosensory area SI. An increase of rCBF in this area was linearly correlated with stimulus frequencies of up to 4 Hz and then reached a plateau. The SMA was not significantly activated by stimulation at any of the frequencies tested. In contrast to the SI, the SMA showed no trend toward a correlation between the rCBF changes and the stimulus repetition rate. These results suggested that a contribution of the primary motor cortex and the SMA to the generation of the P22 and N30 components of SSEPs is unlikely. H2(15)O PET studies with different forms and intensities of innocuous and noxious thermal stimuli were performed 1996 by Casey et. al. (Casey et al., 1994;Casey et al., 1996). To identify the forebrain and brain stem structures that are active during the perception of acute heat pain in humans. Healthy subjects received repetitive noxious (50°C) and innocuous (40°C) heat pulses with a duration of 5s to the forearm and each subject rated the subjective intensity of each stimulation series. Significant CBF increases to 50°C stimuli were found in the contralateral thalamus, cingulate cortex, S2 and S1 cortex, insula, ipsilateral S2 cortex and thalamus, the medial dorsal midbrain and cerebellar vermis. In the second study noxious and innocuous heat and cold thermal stimuli to the nondominant arm of healthy subjects were applied. A detailed analysis of somatosensory representations within parietal postcentral gyral (S1) and lateral sulcal-opercular cortex (S2) in a H2(15)O PET study was performed by Burton et al. (Burton et al., 1997). To address the issue of possible multiple activation foci in these regions and possible differences due to stimulating skin directly or through an imposed tool, changes in CBF during passive tactile stimulation of one or two fingertips were studied. Restrained fingers were rubbed with embossed gratings using a rotating drum stimulator. For different scans, gratings touched the skin directly for optimal stimulation of cutaneous receptors (skin mode stimulation) or indirectly through an imposed guitar plectrum snugly fitted to the same fingers (tool mode stimulation). The latter was expected to stimulate deep receptors better. Subjects estimated roughness after each scan. Direct skin contact activated statistically validated foci in both hemispheres. On the contralateral side these foci occurred in the anterior and posterior limbs of the postcentral gyrus and on the ipsilateral side only in the posterior limb. Tool mode stimulation activated one contralateral focus that was in the posterior limb of the postcentral gyrus. These results suggested at least two maps for distal fingertips in S1 with the anterior and posterior foci corresponding, respectively, to activations in area 3b and the junction between areas 1 and 2. In contralateral S2, skin mode stimulation activated a peak that was anterior and medial to a focus associated with tool mode stimulation. The magnitude of PET counts contralateral to stimulation was greater in the anterior S1 and the S2 regions during initial scans but reversed to more activation in the posterior S1 during later scans. These short-term practice effects suggested changes in neural activity with stimulus novelty. Xu et al. elucidated the functional localization and somatotopic organization of pain perception in the human cerebral cortex with PET during selective painful stimulation. Response to painful stimuli to the hand and foot were elicited using a special CO2 laser, which selectively activates nociceptive receptors (Xu et al., 1997). Multiple brain areas, including bilateral secondary somatosensory cortices (S2) and insula, and the frontal lobe and thalamus contralateral to the stimulus side, were found to be involved in the response to painful stimulation. While the data indicate that the bilateral S2 play an important role in pain perception, they also indicate that there is no pain-related somatotopic organization in the human S2 or insula. Pain processing during three levels of noxious stimulation that produced differential patterns of central activity was investigated by (Derbyshire et al., 1997). Bittar et al. investigated with H2(15)O PET presurgical mapping of primary somatosensory cortex compared with intraoperative cortical stimulation (ICS) (Bittar et al., 1999a;Bittar et al., 1999b). PET scanning with vibrotactile stimulation (of the face, hand, or foot) to localize the primary somatosensory cortex before surgical resection of mass lesions or epileptogenic foci affecting the central area was performed in patients with brain tumor. With the aid of image-guided surgical systems, the locations of significant activation foci on PET scanning were compared with those of positive ICS performed at craniotomy. In 95% PET activation foci were spatially concordant with ICS and ICS was positive in 40% of the PET activation studies that did not result in statistically significant activation and it was concluded that PET is an accurate method for mapping the primary somatosensory cortex before surgery. Boecker et al. investigated the functional anatomy of sensory processing in two clinical conditions characterized by basal ganglia dysfunction in Parkinson's and Huntington's disease (Boecker et al., 1999) in a H2(15)O PET study. Continuous unilateral high-frequency vibratory stimulation was applied to the immobilized metacarpal joint of the index finger. In the controls, the activation pattern was lateralized to the side opposite to stimulus presentation, including primary and secondary somatosensory cortex S1 and subcortical (globus pallidus, ventrolateral thalamus) regional cerebral blood flow (rCBF) increases. Between-group comparisons of the vibration-induced rCBF changes between patients and controls revealed differences in central somatosensory processing. In Parkinson's disease, decreased activation of contralateral sensorimotor (SM1) and lateral premotor (PM) cortex, contralateral S2, contralateral posterior cingulate, bilateral prefrontal cortex (Brodmann area 10) and contralateral basal ganglia. In Huntington's disease, decreased activation of contralateral S2, parietal areas 39 and 40, and lingual gyrus, bilateral prefrontal cortex (Brodmann areas 8, 9, 10 and 44), S1 and contralateral basal ganglia was found. In both clinical conditions relative enhanced activation of ipsilateral somatosensory cortical areas, notably caudal S1, S2 and insular cortex could be detected, too. The data show that Parkinson's and Huntington's disease, beyond well-established deficits in central motor control, are characterized by abnormal cortical and subcortical activation on passive sensory stimulation. Furthermore, the finding that activation increases in ipsilateral somatosensory cortical areas may be interpreted as an indication of either altered central focusing and gating of somatosensory impulses, or enhanced compensatory recruitment of somatosensory areas. A 18F-fluorodeoxyglucose PET study with somatosensory stimulation and spinal cord injuries was performed by Roelcke et al. (Roelcke et al., 1997) to assess the effect of a transverse spinal cord lesion on cerebral energy metabolism in view of sensorimotor reorganisation. PET was used to study resting cerebral glucose metabolism in patients with complete paraplegia or tetraplegia after spinal cord injury and healthy subjects. The global absolute glucose metabolism rate was lower in spinal cord injury than in controls. A relatively increased glucose metabolism particularly in the supplementary motor area, anterior cingulate, and putamen was discovered. Relatively reduced glucose metabolism in patients with spinal cord injury was found in the midbrain, cerebellar hemispheres, and temporal cortex. It was concluded that cerebral deafferentation due to reduction or loss of sensorimotor function results in the low level of absolute global glucose metabolism rate found in patients with spinal cord injury. Relatively increased glucose metabolism in brain regions involved in attention and initiation of movement may be related to secondary disinhibition of these regions.

## BOLD-fMRI

In many fMRI studies somatosensory stimuli were applied. Especially light touch with air puffs (Stippich et al., 1999a) or other tactile stimuli (Hodge et al., 1998;Moore et al., 2000;Rausch et al., 1998;Servos et al., 1998), scratching of the hand palm (Hoeller et al., 2002), vibration (Gelnar et al., 1998a;Golaszewski et al., 2002;Golaszewski et al., 2006;Golaszewski et al., 2002;Hodge et al., 1998), electrical stimulation (Arthurs et al., 2000;Backes et al., 2000;Korvenoja et al., 1999;Krause et al., 2001;Kurth et al., 1998;Takanashi et al., 2001), noxious stimuli (Apkarian et al., 2000;Peyron et al., 2000), and proprioception induced by passive joint movement (Rausch et al., 1998) were used. Usually the primary somatosensory cortex in the postcentral gyrus and the secondary somatosensory cortex in the parietal operculum, insula, and more posterior ventral parietal areas (PV) are activated. A clear somatotopic organization in the primary somatosensory cortex could be demonstrated, whereas this somatotopic organization could not be clearly shown in S2 (Disbrow et al., 2000;Gelnar et al., 1998a;Hodge et al., 1998;Krause et al., 2001;Kurth et al., 1998;Servos et al., 1998). An evident somatotopy also in S2. was demonstrated in a study by Gelnar et al.. A vibratory stimulus was applied to an individual digit tip (digit 1, 2, or 5) on the right hand of healthy adults which led to a BOLD response in cortical regions located on the upper bank of the Sylvian fissure, the insula, and the posterior parietal cortices. Multiple digit representations were observed in the primary somatosensory cortex, corresponding to the four anatomic subdivisions areas 3a, 3b, 1, and 2. There was no simple medial to lateral somatotopic representation in individual fMRI maps but a clear spatial distance between digit 1 and digit 5 on the cortex was seen in both the S1 and the S2 region. Kurth et al. could demonstrate a somatotopy in S1 cortex by electrical finger stimulation (Kurth et al., 2000). Using electrical finger nerve stimulation in normal human subjects, fMRI detected separate representations for all 5 fingers in the primary somatosensory cortex. Responses were located in the posterior wall of the deep central sulcus (corresponding to Brodmann area BA 3b), and the anterior (BA 1) or posterior crown of the postcentral gyrus (BA 2) with rare activations in BA 3a and 4. In BA 3b a regular somatotopic mediolateral digit arrangement for fingers 5 to

1 with a mean Euclidean distance of 16 mm between fingers 1 and 5 was found. In contrast, BA 1/2 showed a greater number of adjacent activation foci with significantly more overlap and partly even reversed ordering of neighboring fingers. This paradigm can properly be used to localize the central sulcus preoperatively (Kurth et al., 1998) and it is applicable even in patients with severe hemiparesis without severe hemianesthesia.

In many studies from the primary somatosensory cortex only a contralateral BOLD response could be elicited whereas the secondary somatosensory areas were activated bilaterally (Backes et al., 2000;Disbrow et al., 2001;Korvenoja et al., 1999). It is still uncertain what stimulus leads to the most robust BOLD response within the somatosensory cortex. There is evidence that pain stimuli are less reliable for evoking S1 activation than vibrotactile or electrical stimuli. (Backes et al., 2000;Disbrow et al., 2001;Korvenoja et al., 1999;Peyron et al., 2000). Activation magnitude in S1 depends on the intensity of stimulation (Arthurs et al., 2000;Krause et al., 2001), the size of the stimulated body surface (Apkarian et al., 2000;Peyron et al., 2000), and the rate of stimulation (Apkarian et al., 2000;Peyron et al., 2000;Takanashi et al., 2001). Nelson et al. demonstrated an increasing stimulus-response relationship between the amplitude of vibrotactile stimuli delivered to the volar surface of the right index finger and BOLD activity in S1 that persisted during an attention-demanding tactile tracking task (Nelson et al., 2004). Secondary somatosensory cortex did not reveal any clear relationship with vibration amplitude but was more often activated during the attention demanding tracking task compared with passive vibration. Responses in secondary areas seem to be less influenced by these variables but probably more dependant on the level of attention directed to the stimulus (Apkarian et al., 2000;Backes et al., 2000;Peyron et al., 2000;Takanashi et al., 2001) and on whether stimulation is delivered uni- or bilaterally (Apkarian et al., 2000;Backes et al., 2000;Disbrow et al., 2001;Peyron et al., 2000;Takanashi et al., 2001). With regard to attentional phenomena interfering with somatosensory processing, tactile processing while varying the focus of attention was studied. Activations were contrasted between attend and ignore conditions, both of which employed identical stimulation characteristics and an active task. Random effects analysis revealed significant attention effects in area SI (primary somatosensory cortex) in that the blood oxygenation level-dependent response was greater for attended than for ignored stimuli. Modulations were further found in the secondary somatosensory cortex and the middle temporal gyrus. These findings suggest that stimulus processing at the level of primary representations in area S1 is modulated by attention (Sterr et al., 2007).

Somatosensory stimulation has also the advantage of not requiring movement that could cause artifacts. With somatosensory stimulation (repetitive brushing of the hand palm) in brain tumor patients a lower incidence of severe movement artifacts compared to an active motor paradigm (finger-to-thumb-tapping) was found but the motor paradigm elicited a significantly higher percentage of signal increases. (Apkarian et al., 2000;Backes et al., 2000;Disbrow et al., 2001;Hoeller et al., 2002;Peyron et al., 2000;Takanashi et al., 2001). Several fMRI studies discovered a similar functional localisation comparing somatosensory stimulation and active motor paradigms (Golaszewski et al., 2002;Golaszewski et al., 2006;Golaszewski et al., 2002;Lee et al., 1998). Lee et al. proved in an fMRI study largely equivalent results with active and passive activation tasks by comparing palm-finger brushing with sponge-squeezing and active finger movements with regard to their functional localisation. The sensorimotor and somatosensory BOLD responses were located to a large extent in the postcentral gyrus, and their spatial locations were not significantly different. Golaszewski et al. proved largely identical functional maps by active finger-to-thumb tapping and vibration of the hand palm (Golaszewski et al., 2002;Golaszewski et al., 2002), which can be regarded as a proper paradigm in presurgical fMRI mapping of the sensorimotor hand area in patients who are physically unable to perform active finger-to- thumb tapping, hand-squeezing or fist clenching as sensorimotor activation tasks.

Francis et al. discovered in an fMRI study a frequency dependence of S1 and S2 (Francis et al., 2000) with a piezoelectric vibration device. An increase in vibrotactile frequency from 30 to 80 Hz, with both frequencies applied to digit 2 during the same scanning session showed a significant increase of BOLD response within both S2 and the posterior insula, while the number of pixels activated in S1 declined. No significant change in signal intensity with frequencies was found in any of the activated areas.

Moreover, functional imaging studies are important for the monitoring of rehabilitation and the understanding of motor recovery after cortical strokes (Cramer et al., 2000). Functional MRI was used to compare sensory and motor maps obtained in normal controls with functional map from 2 patients with good recovery 6 months after a cortical stroke. Cortical map reorganization along the infarct rim was seen that might be an important contributor to recovery of motor and sensory function after stroke. Moreover, functional imaging studies with somatosensory stimulation are also important for the monitoring of the rehabilitation after extremity transplantations (Piza, 2000). A close relationship between the intensity of phantom limb pain in amputees and the amount of reorganization of the somatosensory cortex was reported in fMRI studies (Flor et al., 2001;Hamzei et al., 2001;Koppelstaetter et al., 2007).

FMRI was also used to investigate brain activations underlying menthol-induced cold allodynia. Healthy volunteers were investigated using a block-design fMRI approach. Brain activity was measured during application of innocuous cold stimuli (5°C above cold pain threshold) and noxious cold stimuli (5°C below cold pain threshold) to normal skin of the forearm using a peltier- driven thermostimulator. The stimuli were adjusted to the individual cold pain threshold. Then cold allodynia was induced by topical menthol and cortical activations were measured during previously innocuous cold stimulation (5°C) that was then perceived as painful. On a numeric rating scale for pain (0-10) innocuous cold, cold pain and cold allodynia were rated. Sensory and affective components of allodynia and cold pain were equal in the McGill pain questionnaire. All tested conditions (innocuous cold, noxious cold and cold allodynia) led to significant activations of bilateral insular cortices, bilateral frontal cortices and the anterior cingulate cortex. When noxious cold and innocuous cold were compared, noxious cold contributed significantly more to activations of the posterior insula and innocuous cold contributed more to activations of ipsilateral anterior insular cortex. Comparing cold allodynia and equally intense cold pain conditions, significantly increased activations in bilateral dorsolateral prefrontal cortices and brainstem (ipsilateral parabrachial nucleus) were found during cold allodynia. Cold allodynia contributed significantly more to activations of the bilateral anterior insula, whereas the contribution to activation of the contralateral posterior insula was equal. It was concluded that cold allodynia activates a network similar to that of normal cold pain but additionally recruits bilateral dorsolateral prefrontal cortex and the midbrain, suggesting that these brain areas are involved in central nociceptive sensitization processes.

# Devices for Somatosensory Stimulation

## Mechanical Stimuli

Several vibration devices were implemented within the MR environment. Mechanical (Golaszewski et al., 2002) and pneumatically driven (Golaszewski et al., 2002) devices were designed. Previously reported MR compatible vibration devices are based on piezoceramic vibrotactile stimulators (Harrington et al., 2000), vibrotactile devices powered by air puffs (Stippich et al., 1999b) or magnetomechanical principles (Graham et al., 2001). The main problem is that the vibration device does not interfere with the fMRI scanning procedure and provides vibration stimuli with defined frequency and amplitude. Pneumatic systems have the disadvantage of limited vibration frequencies. Such devices have been shown to cause somatosensory activations, but failed to activate motor cortical areas. In the fMRI study of Gelnar et al. (Gelnar et al., 1998b), a pneumatic vibratory stimulus was applied to the fingertips with 100% activation of the postcentral gyrus and no motor cortex activation. Piezoelectric systems provide a wide range of frequencies but provide only small displacement amplitudes (< 0.5 mm), which limits its application to the skin receptors. Moreover, fMRI with piezoelectric vibrators showed activations of the somatosensory but not of the motor cortical areas (Harrington et al., 2000). In an fMRI study with a mechanical device with an eccentric mass, a frequency range between 1–130 Hz and displacement amplitudes up to 4 mm BOLD response within the somatosensory as well as the motor cortical areas could be shown. In the study of Harrington and Stippich and Gelnar et al., brain activation within the postcentral gyrus, the superior and inferior parietal lobule has been found (Gelnar et al., 1998b;Harrington et al., 2000;Stippich et al., 1999b). Further brain activation within BA 3a was detected due to somatosensory stimulation (Geyer et al., 1999;Geyer et al., 2000;Kurth et al., 2000), which can be explained by the fact that area 3a receives input from deep and proprioceptive receptors (Ibanez et al., 1989;Iwamura et al., 1993;Kaas et al., 1979;Maldjian et al., 1999;Recanzone et al., 1992;Tharin and Golby, 2007). The BOLD response in the primary motor cortex due to vibrotactile stimulation is an important finding because the stimulation does not require the collaboration of the subject under examination. In an fMRI study with vibration of Golaszewski et al. (Golaszewski et al., 2002) BOLD response with the primary sensorimotor cortex SM1 was found in 100%. The cortical activation of motor areas during vibration is presumably based on the simultaneous stimulation of cutaneous receptors and muscle spindles, which requires sufficient displacement amplitudes and vibration frequencies. Similar to the finger-to-thumb-tapping paradigm, vibration led to contralateral brain activity in the postcentral gyrus in all subjects. Vibration did not consistently activate the supplementary motor are and the cingular gyrus since it represents a passive paradigm which does not involve motor cortical areas for the planning of volitional movements. The vibratory stimulus is transmitted via the large afferents of the dorsal column to the thalamus and the brain cortex. This "information" originates from the extra personnel space and might be an explanation, why BA 9 in the superior frontal gyrus has been activated in some cases. Vibratory stimulation of the hand palm involves the whole sensorimotor cortex why there can be several clinical applications for the vibration paradigm in fMRI. Vibration can be used for preoperative functional brain mapping of the sensorimotor cortex in patients with perirolandic lesions. Further applications include the investigation of brain plasticity and reorganization (Pons et al., 1992) and investigation of patients in comatous and vegetative state (Kampfl et al., 1998).

Gallasch and Golaszewski [Gallasch et al., 2006; Golaszewski et al., 2006] presented a stationary moving magnet actuator as a noncommutated device which produces no high frequency emissions during operation. It therefore does not interfere with the imaging apparatus. A main feature of the system is the independent control of indentation force, vibration amplitude and vibration frequency which allowed to elucidate potential differences in somatosensory brain activation produced by different classes of superficial and deep skin receptors or proprioceptors. In contrast to previous vibration devices [Stippich et al., 1999; Golaszewski et al., 2002a; Maldijan et al., 1999; Harrington et al., 2000; Golaszewski et al., 2002b; Graham et al., 2001] an active motor component to contact the vibrating source, which is a source for systematic errors, is not needed. Such errors are further reduced by feedback control. The skin surface of the human foot cannot be completely immobilized. There are continuous fluctuations related to cardiac and respiratory events. The amplitudes of these movements and the thresholds of the cutaneous mechanoreceptors may introduce considerable variability in effective stimulus amplitude and indentation force. To overcome this difficulty the vibration stimulator was constructed with the facility to present the desired amplitude and indentation force of the vibration stimulus while controlling for the movements of the skin surface relative to the stimulator [Westling et al. 1976]. The vibration amplitude can be conserved against responding tissue forces and therefore, it is constant throughout the measurement. The vibrotactile stimuli were applied with a constant preload. Therefore, the presented system has the capability to deliver precisely controlled, exactly reproducible vibrotactile stimuli with frequencies between 0 - 100 Hz and displacement amplitudes between 0 - 4 mm. Thus, variability in time series data can be reduced which improves fMRI brain mapping using correlation or fitting methods that make a priori assumptions about the idealized hemodynamic response produced by neuronal activation during fMRI experiments. At least, it is also possible to quantify plantar stiffness by measurement of the indentation depth at a given force. This feature, therefore, is very important to establish quantitative stimulus-response relationships as a reference for diagnostic procedures.

# References

Apkarian, AV, P A Gelnar, B R Krauss, N M Szeverenyi, 2000, Cortical responses to thermal pain depend on stimulus size: a functional MRI study: *J. Neurophysiol,* v. 83, p. 3113-22.

Arthurs, OJ, E J Williams, T A Carpenter, J D Pickard, S J Boniface, 2000, Linear coupling between functional magnetic resonance imaging and evoked potential amplitude in human somatosensory cortex: *Neuroscience,* v. 101, p. 803-6.

Backes, WH, W H Mess, V van Kranen-Mastenbroek, J P Reulen, 2000, Somatosensory cortex responses to median nerve stimulation: fMRI effects of current amplitude and selective attention: *Clin. Neurophysiol,* v. 111, p. 1738-44.

Bittar, RG, A Olivier, A F Sadikot, F Andermann, R M Comeau, M Cyr, T M Peters, D C Reutens, 1999a, Localization of somatosensory function by using positron emission tomography scanning: a comparison with intraoperative cortical stimulation: *J. Neurosurg,* v. 90, p. 478-83.

Bittar, RG, A Olivier, A F Sadikot, F Andermann, G B Pike, D C Reutens, 1999b, Presurgical motor and somatosensory cortex mapping with functional magnetic resonance imaging and positron emission tomography: *J. Neurosurg,* v. 91, p. 915-21.

Boecker, H, A Ceballos-Baumann, P Bartenstein, A Weindl, H R Siebner, T Fassbender, F Munz, M Schwaiger, B Conrad, 1999, Sensory processing in Parkinson's and Huntington's disease: investigations with 3D H(2)(15)O-PET: *Brain,* v. 122 ( Pt 9), p. 1651-65.

Burton, H, A M MacLeod, T O Videen, M E Raichle, 1997, Multiple foci in parietal and frontal cortex activated by rubbing embossed grating patterns across fingerpads: a positron emission tomography study in humans: *Cereb Cortex,* v. 7, p. 3-17.

Casey, KL, S Minoshima, K L Berger, R A Koeppe, T J Morrow, K A Frey, 1994, Positron emission tomographic analysis of cerebral structures activated specifically by repetitive noxious heat stimuli: *J. Neurophysiol,* v. 71, p. 802-7.

Casey, KL, S Minoshima, T J Morrow, R A Koeppe, 1996, Comparison of human cerebral activation pattern during cutaneous warmth, heat pain, and deep cold pain: *J. Neurophysiol,* v. 76, p. 571-81.

Cramer, SC, C I Moore, S P Finklestein, B R Rosen, 2000, A pilot study of somatotopic mapping after cortical infarct: *Stroke,* v. 31, p. 668-71.

Derbyshire, SW, A K Jones, F Gyulai, S Clark, D Townsend, L L Firestone, 1997, Pain processing during three levels of noxious stimulation produces differential patterns of central activity: *Pain,* v. 73, p. 431-45.

Disbrow, E, T Roberts, L Krubitzer, 2000, Somatotopic organization of cortical fields in the lateral sulcus of Homo sapiens: evidence for SII and PV: *J. Comp. Neurol,* v. 418, p. 1-21.

Disbrow, E, T Roberts, D Poeppel, L Krubitzer, 2001, Evidence for interhemispheric processing of inputs from the hands in human S2 and PV: *J. Neurophysiol,* v. 85, p. 2236-44.

Drevets, WC, H Burton, T O Videen, A Z Snyder, J R Simpson Jr, M E Raichle, 1995, Blood flow changes in human somatosensory cortex during anticipated stimulation: *Nature,* v. 373, p. 249-52.

Flor, H, C Denke, M Schaefer, S Grusser, 2001, Effect of sensory discrimination training on cortical reorganisation and phantom limb pain: *Lancet,* v. 357, p. 1763-4.

Fox, PT, H Burton, M E Raichle, 1987, Mapping human somatosensory cortex with positron emission tomography: *J. Neurosurg,* v. 67, p. 34-43.

Francis, ST, E F Kelly, R Bowtell, W J Dunseath, S E Folger, F McGlone, 2000, fMRI of the responses to vibratory stimulation of digit tips: *Neuroimage,* v. 11, p. 188-202.

Gelnar, PA, B R Krauss, N M Szeverenyi, A V Apkarian, 1998a, Fingertip representation in the human somatosensory cortex: an fMRI study: *Neuroimage,* v. 7, p. 261-83.

Gelnar, PA, B R Krauss, N M Szeverenyi, A V Apkarian, 1998b, Fingertip representation in the human somatosensory cortex: an fMRI study: *Neuroimage,* v. 7, p. 261-83.

Geyer, S, A Schleicher, K Zilles, 1999, Areas 3a, 3b, and 1 of human primary somatosensory cortex: *Neuroimage,* v. 10, p. 63-83.

Geyer, S, T Schormann, H Mohlberg, K Zilles, 2000, Areas 3a, 3b, and 1 of human primary somatosensory cortex. Part 2. Spatial normalization to standard anatomical space: *Neuroimage,* v. 11, p. 684-96.

Golaszewski, SM, C M Siedentopf, E Baldauf, F Koppelstaetter, W Eisner, J Unterrainer, G M Guendisch, F M Mottaghy, S R Felber, 2002, Functional magnetic resonance imaging of the human sensorimotor cortex using a novel vibrotactile stimulator: *Neuroimage,* v. 17, p. 421-30.

Golaszewski, SM, C M Siedentopf, F Koppelstaetter, M Fend, A Ischebeck, V Gonzalez-Felipe, I Haala, W Struhal, F M Mottaghy, E Gallasch, S R Felber, F Gerstenbrand, 2006, Human brain structures related to plantar vibrotactile stimulation: a functional magnetic resonance imaging study:. v. 29, p. 923-9.

Golaszewski, SM, F Zschiegner, C M Siedentopf, J Unterrainer, R A Sweeney, W Eisner, S Lechner-Steinleitner, F M Mottaghy, S Felber, 2002, A new pneumatic vibrator for functional magnetic resonance imaging of the human sensorimotor cortex: *Neurosci. Lett,* v. 324, p. 125-8.

Graham, SJ, W R Staines, A Nelson, D B Plewes, W E McIlroy, 2001, New devices to deliver somatosensory stimuli during functional MRI: *Magn. Reson. Med,* v. 46, p. 436-42.

Hamzei, F, J Liepert, C Dettmers, T Adler, S Kiebel, M Rijntjes, C Weiller, 2001, Structural and functional cortical abnormalities after upper limb amputation during childhood: *Neuroreport,* v. 12, p. 957-62.

Harrington, GS, C T Wright, J H Downs 3rd, 2000, A new vibrotactile stimulator for functional MRI: Hum Brain Mapp, v. 10, p. 140-5.

Hodge, CJ Jr, S C Huckins, N M Szeverenyi, M M Fonte, J G Dubroff, K Davuluri, 1998, Patterns of lateral sensory cortical activation determined using functional magnetic resonance imaging: *J. Neurosurg,* v. 89, p. 769-79.

Hoeller, M, T Krings, M H Reinges, F J Hans, J M Gilsbach, A Thron, 2002, Movement artefacts and MR BOLD signal increase during different paradigms for mapping the sensorimotor cortex: *Acta Neurochir.* (Wien), v. 144, p. 279-84; discussion 284.

Ibanez, V, M P Deiber, F Mauguiere, 1989, Interference of vibrations with input transmission in dorsal horn and cuneate nucleus in man: a study of somatosensory evoked potentials (SEPs) to electrical stimulation of median nerve and fingers: *Exp. Brain Res,* v. 75, p. 599-610.

Ibanez, V, M P Deiber, N Sadato, C Toro, J Grissom, R P Woods, J C Mazziotta, M Hallett, 1995, Effects of stimulus rate on regional cerebral blood flow after median nerve stimulation: *Brain,* v. 118 ( Pt 5), p. 1339-51.

Iwamura, Y, M Tanaka, M Sakamoto, O Hikosaka, 1993, Rostrocaudal gradients in the neuronal receptive field complexity in the finger region of the alert monkey's postcentral gyrus: *Exp. Brain Res,* v. 92, p. 360-8.

Kaas, JH, R J Nelson, M Sur, C S Lin, M M Merzenich, 1979, Multiple representations of the body within the primary somatosensory cortex of primates: Science, v. 204, p. 521-3.

Kampfl, A, E Schmutzhard, G Franz, B Pfausler, H P Haring, H Ulmer, S Felber, S Golaszewski, F Aichner, 1998, Prediction of recovery from post-traumatic vegetative state with cerebral magnetic-resonance imaging: *Lancet,* v. 351, p. 1763-7.

Koppelstaetter, F, C M Siedentopf, P Rhomberg, S Lechner-Steinleitner, W Eisner, S M Golaszewski, 2007, *FMRT vor Motorkortexstimulation bei Phantomschmerz: Ein Fallbericht: Nervenarzt.*

Korvenoja, A, J Huttunen, E Salli, H Pohjonen, S Martinkauppi, J M Palva, L Lauronen, J Virtanen, R J Ilmoniemi, H J Aronen, 1999, Activation of multiple cortical areas in response to somatosensory stimulation: combined magnetoencephalographic and functional magnetic resonance imaging: *Hum. Brain Mapp,* v. 8, p. 13-27.

Krause, T, R Kurth, J Ruben, J Schwiemann, K Villringer, M Deuchert, M Moosmann, S Brandt, K Wolf, G Curio, A Villringer, 2001, Representational overlap of adjacent fingers in multiple areas of human primary somatosensory cortex depends on electrical stimulus intensity: an fMRI study: *Brain Res,* v. 899, p. 36-46.

Kurth, R, K Villringer, G Curio, K J Wolf, T Krause, J Repenthin, J Schwiemann, M Deuchert, A Villringer, 2000, fMRI shows multiple somatotopic digit representations in human primary somatosensory cortex: *Neuroreport,* v. 11, p. 1487-91.

Kurth, R, K Villringer, B M Mackert, J Schwiemann, J Braun, G Curio, A Villringer, K J Wolf, 1998, fMRI assessment of somatotopy in human Brodmann area 3b by electrical finger stimulation: *Neuroreport,* v. 9, p. 207-12.

Lee, CC, C R Jack Jr, S J Riederer, 1998, Mapping of the central sulcus with functional MR: active versus passive activation tasks: AJNR Am J Neuroradiol, v. 19, p. 847-52.

Maldjian, JA, A Gottschalk, R S Patel, J A Detre, D C Alsop, 1999, The sensory somatotopic map of the human hand demonstrated at 4 Tesla: *Neuroimage,* v. 10, p. 55-62.

Mazziotta, JCaTAW, 2000, *Brain Mapping: The methods,* Academic Press.

Moore, CI, C E Stern, S Corkin, B Fischl, A C Gray, B R Rosen, A M Dale, 2000, Segregation of somatosensory activation in the human rolandic cortex using fMRI: *J. Neurophysiol,* v. 84, p. 558-69.

Nelson, AJ, W R Staines, S J Graham, W E McIlroy, 2004, Activation in SI and SII: the influence of vibrotactile amplitude during passive and task-relevant stimulation: *Brain Res. Cogn. Brain Res,* v. 19, p. 174-84.

Ogawa, S, T M Lee, A R Kay, D W Tank, 1990, Brain magnetic resonance imaging with contrast dependent on blood oxygenation: *Proc. Natl. Acad. Sci. U S A,* v. 87, p. 9868-72.

Ogawa, S, D W Tank, R Menon, J M Ellermann, S G Kim, H Merkle, K Ugurbil, 1992, Intrinsic signal changes accompanying sensory stimulation: functional brain mapping with magnetic resonance imaging: *Proc. Natl. Acad. Sci. U S A,* v. 89, p. 5951-5.

Penfield, WaBE, 1937, Somatic motor and sensory representation in the cerebral cortex of man as studied by electrical stimulation.: *Brain,* v. 60, p. 389-443.

Peyron, R, B Laurent, L Garcia-Larrea, 2000, Functional imaging of brain responses to pain. A review and meta-analysis (2000): *Neurophysiol. Clin,* v. 30, p. 263-88.

Piza, H, 2000, [Transplantation of hands in Innsbruck]: Wien Klin Wochenschr, v. 112, p. 563-5.

Pons, TP, P E Garraghty, M Mishkin, 1992, Serial and parallel processing of tactual information in somatosensory cortex of rhesus monkeys: *J. Neurophysiol,* v. 68, p. 518-27.

Rausch, M, F Spengler, U T Eysel, 1998, Proprioception acts as the main source of input in human S-I activation experiments: a functional MRI study: *Neuroreport,* v. 9, p. 2865-8.

Recanzone, GH, M M Merzenich, W M Jenkins, 1992, Frequency discrimination training engaging a restricted skin surface results in an emergence of a cutaneous response zone in cortical area 3a: *J. Neurophysiol,* v. 67, p. 1057-70.

Roelcke, U, A Curt, A Otte, J Missimer, R P Maguire, V Dietz, K L Leenders, 1997, Influence of spinal cord injury on cerebral sensorimotor systems: a PET study: *J. Neurol. Neurosurg. Psychiatry,* v. 62, p. 61-5.

Servos, P, J Zacks, D E Rumelhart, G H Glover, 1998, Somatotopy of the human arm using fMRI: *Neuroreport,* v. 9, p. 605-9.

Sterr, A, S Shen, A Zaman, N Roberts, A Szameitat, 2007, Activation of SI is modulated by attention: a random effects fMRI study using mechanical stimuli: *Neuroreport,* v. 18, p. 607-11.

Stippich, C, R Hofmann, D Kapfer, E Hempel, S Heiland, O Jansen, K Sartor, 1999a, Somatotopic mapping of the human primary somatosensory cortex by fully automated tactile stimulation using functional magnetic resonance imaging: *Neurosci. Lett,* v. 277, p. 25-8.

Stippich, C, R Hofmann, D Kapfer, E Hempel, S Heiland, O Jansen, K Sartor, 1999b, Somatotopic mapping of the human primary somatosensory cortex by fully automated tactile stimulation using functional magnetic resonance imaging: *Neurosci. Lett,* v. 277, p. 25-8.

Takanashi, M, K Abe, T Yanagihara, Y Oshiro, Y Watanabe, H Tanaka, N Hirabuki, H Nakamura, N Fujita, 2001, Effects of stimulus presentation rate on the activity of primary somatosensory cortex: a functional magnetic resonance imaging study in humans: *Brain Res. Bull,* v. 54, p. 125-9.

Tempel, LW, J S Perlmutter, 1990, Abnormal vibration-induced cerebral blood flow responses in idiopathic dystonia: *Brain,* v. 113 ( Pt 3), p. 691-707.

Tempel, LW, J S Perlmutter, 1992, Vibration-induced regional cerebral blood flow responses in normal aging: *J. Cereb. Blood Flow Metab,* v. 12, p. 554-61.

Tharin, S, A Golby, 2007, Functional brain mapping and its applications to neurosurgery: *Neurosurgery,* v. 60, p. 185-201*; discussion.* 201-2.

Xu, X, H Fukuyama, S Yazawa, T Mima, T Hanakawa, Y Magata, M Kanda, N Fujiwara, K Shindo, T Nagamine, H Shibasaki, 1997, Functional localization of pain perception in the human brain studied by PET: *Neuroreport,* v. 8, p. 555-9.

In: Research Topics on Brain Mapping
Editor: Yuanzhu Liáng, pp. 209-220
ISBN: 978-1-60456-001-5


*Chapter X*

# Optical Imaging of Brainstem Autonomic Circuits Using Voltage-Sensitive Dyes

***Jeffrey T. Potts*[*1] and Julian F.R. Paton*[2]**
[1] Department of Biomedical Science, College of Veterinary Medicine, Dalton Cardiovascular Research Center, University of Missouri, 134 Research Park Dr., Columbia, Missouri 65211
[2] Department of Physiology and Pharmacology, Bristol Heart Institute, School of Medical Sciences, University of Bristol, Bristol, England BS8 1TD

## Abstract

The study of the central nervous system requires an understanding of structural and functional relationships amongst neurons. Recent advances in optical imaging techniques and fast voltage-sensitive dyes now provide a powerful tool for understanding neuronal function in the relatively intact environment of the living brain. Optical imaging provides a means to non-invasively measure changes in membrane potential using dyes that emit fluorescent signals related to changes in membrane potential. One obvious advantage of this technology is the possibility to obtain simultaneous measurements of neuronal activity from many locations, as well as offering the ability to record from processes which are too small or fragile for typical electrophysiological approaches. Optical recording also permits monitoring spatial and temporal features of information processing in complex neural networks composed of synaptically-connected populations of neurons. One potential limitation is the rather small focal penetration depth of these systems. A variety of experimental preparations (*in vitro, in situ* and *in vivo*) have been used to optically measure activity in the living brain. In this chapter, we will provide an overview of the recent applications of optical imaging to investigate autonomic neural networks. Autonomic circuits in the brainstem coordinate and shape motor patterns

[*] Correspondence: Jeffrey T. Potts, Ph.D. Department of Integrative Physiology, University of North Texas Health Science Center, 3500 Camp Bowie Blvd., Fort Worth, TX 76107; PHONE: 817-735-2075; FAX: 817-735-5084; EMAIL: jepotts@hsc.unt.edu

which target and control the heart, blood vessels, diaphragm and the upper airway that regulate cardiovascular and respiratory functions. With an emphasis on brainstem circuitry, we will discuss how optical imaging has been applied to study centrally-generated breathing activity and how spatial and temporal resolution monitoring of neuronal network activity has provided novel insights into the functional organization of brainstem autonomic circuits that are critical to overall systems homeostasis.

## Introduction

Spatiotemporal features of information processing in complex neural networks require the simultaneous monitoring and analysis of neuronal activity in populations of neurons. Over the years, a number of indirect approaches have been developed to assess neural network activity including the 2-deoxyglucose method (Sokoloff, 1977), immediate early gene activation assays such as c-fos (Sokoloff et al., 1977), magnetic encephalographic techniques (Kaufman and Williamson, 1982) and magnetic resonance imaging (Ogawa et al., 1990). Traditional electrophysiological techniques, including intracellular and extracellular recording, have also provided important insights into the function of neural circuits and revealed intrinsic membrane properties of single neurons. However, there remain important limitations with all of these approaches. Namely, the inability to record electrical activity from multiple neurons simultaneously. One approach has been to use microelectrode arrays (Lindsey et al., 2000). However, the advent of voltage-sensitive dyes (VSD) and optical imaging techniques (Cohen et al., 1978;Grinvald et al., 1988;Salzberg, 1989) has provided a powerful tool to measure mass activity of many neurons simultaneously and has permitted the detailed study of spatial and temporal patterns of neuronal activation in the intact environment of the living brain. Fast VSDs are amphipatic molecules that bind to membranes with potential-dependent fluorescence and/or absorption changes that linearly track membrane potential (Cohen et al., 1974). The response time for VSDs is less than a millisecond giving them excellent time resolution that enables them to function as molecular transducers that convert membrane potential into optical signals (Ebner and Chen, 1995). Determination of changes in membrane potential with VSD requires the optical detection of either a change in absorption or the emitted fluorescence. Absorbance measurements may be advantageous when deep tissue penetration is needed, such as in thick tissue section preparations, since the signal-to-noise ratio for epi-fluorescence measurements is reduced due to light loss (Grinvald et al., 1988). Non-specific background fluorescence also will reduce the signal size. The amplitude of the optical signal obtained using VSD also depends heavily on the optical recording technique. Two general approaches are used to record VSDs: photodiodes and charged-coupled device (CCD). Today multiple photodiodes or photodiode arrays consisting of 10 x 10 or 12 x 12 photodiodes have been successfully used (Nakashima et al., 1992;Sato and Momose-Sato, 2004). CCD technology has advanced considerably and is a popular option for optical imaging applications. CCD cameras offer low noise, wide dynamic range, excellent linearity and sensitivity to low light (Ebner and Chen, 1995), thus, making the CCD ideal to detect small changes in light intensity against a large background (Takashima et al., 1999). Finally, to measure optical signals requires the appropriate optics and illumination source. Details regarding the recording systems and optics used for VSD recording have previously reviewed and will not be covered here (Grinvald et al., 1988; Salzberg, 1989). The continued development of optical dyes and imaging technologies has recently provided excellent spatial resolution at the single cell level (also Barness et al., 2007 and Funke et al., 2007) and sufficient temporal resolution to track action potential and synaptic potential trajectories. This chapter concentrates on the use of fast VSDs and optical imaging as a tool to study the activity of a central autonomic neuronal network that is essential for the generation of breathing rhythms.

## Medullary Autonomic Circuits and Respiratory Rhythmogenesis

Breathing is an involuntary motor pattern consisting of periodic contractions of the diaphragm and abductors/adductors controlling the upper airway via spinal and cranial motor neurons respectively that together produce ventilation. This rhythmic activity is generated by a bilateral column of neurons in the ventrolateral medulla (VLM) of the mammalian brainstem known as the Ventral Respiratory Column (VRC) and pontine circuitry (Dutschmann and Herbert, 2006;Rybak et al., 2004;St-John and Paton, 2004). The rhythmic pattern of motor discharge is characterized by a coordinated alternation of inspiratory, post-inspiratory and expiratory neuronal activities (Richter and Spyer, 2001). The coordination of these activities is important not only to breathing but to other basic physiological functions such as swallowing and vocalization. The VRC lies just ventral to the nucleus ambiguus and extends caudally from the caudal pole of the facial nucleus to the level of the lateral reticular nucleus in the caudal VLM. Respiratory neurons in the VRC complex form a distributed network that include propriobulbar inspiratory and expiratory neurons, as well as bulbospinal inspiratory premotor neurons (Bianchi et al., 1995;Duffin, 2004;Feldman and Del Negro, 2006;Schwarzacher et al., 1995). A sub-population of propriobulbar inspiratory neurons located in the pre-Bötzinger complex (pre-BötC) can also exhibit endogenous bursting (Bianchi et al., 1995;Schwarzacher et al., 1995;Smith et al., 1991) which may be released under conditions of gasping (Paton et al., 2006).

The role of respiratory neurons in the VRC has been studied using the *in vitro* brainstem slice, *en bloc, in situ* perfused brainstem and *in vivo* preparations. Each has its own unique advantages and disadvantages and these have been detailed elsewhere (Feldman et al., 1990;Paton, 1996b;Ramirez et al., 1997). Using these approaches, a number of the intrinsic and synaptic properties of respiratory neurons have been identified. However, information describing the temporal and spatial propagation of synaptic activity within the VRC during respiratory rhythmogenesis cannot be described solely using electrophysiological approaches. The remainder of this chapter will discuss how the application of optical imaging with fast voltage-sensitive dyes has revelaed new insights into mammalian respiratory rhythmogenesis.

## Optical Imaging of Medullary Respiratory Circuits: *In Vitro* and *En Bloc* Preparations from Neonatal Rats

It is now becoming accepted that respiratory rhythm is generated by interactions between the pons and medulla (St. John and Paton, 2004;Rybak et al., 2004; Dutschmann and Herbert, 2006; (Dutschmann et al., 2000) and that the pre-BötC is a critical locus for rhythm generation in mammals (Koshiya and Smith, 1999). Although the importance of pre-BötC neurons has been demonstrated in reduced *in vitro* preparations, a number of questions remain regarding their contribution to respiratory rhythm generation during embryonic and post-natal development. To address the embryonic and post-natal development issue, the *in vitro* brainstem slice or *en bloc* preparations from neonatal animals (ie. rats or mice) have typically been employed. Although differences in neural connectivity exist, the pre-BötC is retained in both the *in vitro* and *en bloc* preparations and both models generate spontaneous respiratory-like motor output as measured from the hypoglossal nerve or the C4 ventral rootlet, respectively. The first study to use an optical approach to image central respiratory activity performed electrical stimulation of the nucleus tractus solitarii (NTS) to track excitatory propagation and subsequent inspiratory burst activity in the ventrolateral medulla (VLM) of the isolated medullary en bloc preparation of neonatal rat (Onimaru et al., 1996). Using a 128x128 photodiode array and the voltage-sensitive dye - RH795, changes in fluorescence activity corresponding to inspiratory burst discharge were observed in regions of the VLM that contain known populations of respiratory neurons (Arata et al., 1990). Subsequently, this group conducted a series of studies to identify mechanisms underlying centrally-generated respiratory rhythms (Onimaru and Homma, 2003;Onimaru et al., 2004;Onimaru and Homma, 2005b;Onimaru and Homma, 2005a;Tokumasu et al., 2001). Of these studies, Tokumasu et al. (2001) was the first to visualize the spatiotemporal distribution of mass neuronal activity that was produced spontaneously by the ventral medullary respiratory network in neonatal rats. The recorded optical signals corresponded with inspiratory motor activity recorded from the spinal C4 level and likely reflected the depolarizing drive potentials of the somata of inspiratory neurons. A surprising finding was the absence of optical signals corresponding to membrane hyperpolarization which would have been produced by expiratory neurons known to exist in this region. This result may have been due to the masking effects of depolarization related fluorescence. Nonetheless, these results demonstrate that the optical recording method can be used to track spontaneous neuronal activity in the medullary respiratory network.

A fundamental question that has puzzled respiratory physiologists is where does the start of inspiration originate in the medulla? There still is a lack of consensus regarding which part(s) of the medulla are essential for primary rhythm generation (Ballanyi et al., 1999;Richter and Spyer, 2001). In a landmark study, Onimaru and Homma (2003) identified a novel functional group of neurons (coined the para-facial respiratory group, pFRG) which they suggested may be the initiation site for respiratory rhythmogenesis. Using the en bloc preparation of neonatal rats, they reported that fluorescence activity in a small region of the medulla ventrolateral to the facial nucleus preceded the onset of inspiratory motor bursts recorded from the C4 rootlet. Further, they found that the changes in fluorescence which occurred during the pre-inspiratory (pre-I) phase correlated very well with the average membrane trajectory of recorded pre-I neurons using whole cell patch-clamp. Together, these results showed for the first time that respiratory activity in the VLM extends more rostrally and laterally with respect to the pre-BötC then previously described. Although these findings do not provide definitive proof that the pFRG initiates respiratory rhythm, respiratory rate and the spatiotemporal pattern of respiratory related fluorescent activity was significantly reduced when partial lesions of the pFRG were performed. These findings suggest that the pFRG was involved in the generation of respiratory rhythm and pFRG activation preceded pre-BötC activity. However, this highlights a serious limitation of the optical imaging technique, that of focal depth. It is unclear where within the z-axis the signals were detected. Since the pFRG lies more superficial than the pre-BötC caution needs to be aired as to whether it is reasonable to conclude temporal differences if deeper structures are not being imaged. A related issue and major caveat regards the dye loading technique employed by Onimaru and colleagues. In their studies this was by bath incubation of the section which will likely not load all depths equally.

## What about Citing More Recent Papers from Onimaru

Respiration-related rhythmic activity in the rostral medulla of newborn rats. J Neurophysiol. 2006 Jul;96(1):55-61. Epub 2006 Feb 22.

Spontaneous oscillatory burst activity in the piriform-amygdala region and its relation to in vitro respiratory activity in newborn rats. Neuroscience. 2007 Jan 5;144(1):387-94. Epub 2006 Oct 30.

The non-invasive nature of optical imaging has also been exploited to study the developmental patterns of neuronal activity in respiratory circuits (Eugenin et al., 2006;Onimaru and Homma, 2005a)). A fundamental question related to respiratory development is the spatial distribution of inspiratory and expiratory neurons in the fetal brainstem and whether fetal rhythms are produced by a single group of pacemaker neurons or by inhibitory reciprocal synaptic connections? Using optical approaches contrasting findings have been reported. Onimaru and Homma (2005a) measured the spatiotemporal pattern of respiratory related neuronal activity in the VLM during late fetal development of the rat. They found that pre-I activity in pFRG preceded fluorescence activity in pre-BötC by several hundred milliseconds in E20 – E21 animals and that this respiratory pattern was identical to that seen in neonatal rats. In contrast, they failed to record pre-I activity at the level of the facial nucleus in E17-E18 specimens and reported that neuronal activity was first observed in the pre-BötC region. From these findings they suggested that there is a developmental shift in the site of generation of respiratory rhythm from the pre-BötC to the pFRG that occurs around E19. In contrast, Eugenin et al. (2006) failed to observe a discrete region of the fetal brainstem that consistently generated respiratory related activity. Instead, they reported that there was no discrete region that initiated the respiratory rhythm and suggested instead that fetal respiratory-like rhythms were produced by a distributed network of interacting clusters of neurons that comprise a respiratory oscillator. It should be noted, however, that a major difference between these two studies was the optical dyes used. Whereas Eugenin and colleagues used a fluorescent calcium-sensitive dye (Oregon Green 488 Bapta-1, AM) that provided excellent signal-to-noise ratio and permitted analysis of respiratory activity frame-to-frame, Onimaru and Homma used voltage-sensitive dyes (Di-2-ANEPEQ and Di-4-ANEPPS) and typically required the averaging of 20 – 30 respiratory-triggered cycles to obtain a single fluorescent image. Therefore, it is possible that the intermittent discharge of respiratory neurons may have been masked by frame-to-frame averaging. In addition, these dyes may have resulted in differential depth loading that may have affected the focal depths in these studies. Despite these discrepancies, these study results demonstrate that optical imaging with fluorescent dyes provides a unique opportunity to examine the activity of respiratory neurons in the generation of central respiratory rhythms.

## Optical Imaging of Medullary Respiratory Circuits: *In Situ* Perfused Brainstem Preparations of Mature Rats

As mentioned above respiratory-related motor rhythms can be generated when the respiratory network is reduced, such as when using the transverse medullary slice or *en bloc* preparations. These approaches have provided new information showing that a small group of respiratory neurons are capable of generating respiratory-like rhythms in neonatal animals. However, the respiratory patterns of these *in vitro* preparations differ considerably from those generated *in vivo* and *in situ* preparations both of which contain an intact ponto-medullary circuit (St John, 1990). As such, the spatiotemporal patterns reported *in vitro* may be different compared to functionally intact brainstem preparations (ie. *in situ* and *in vivo*). In addition, most *in vitro* approaches are generally not applicable to study the role of sensory feedback in modulating respiratory rhythm. To address these questions requires a preparation that retains most, if not all, sensory input to medullary respiratory circuits. Our group (Potts and Paton, 2006) and one other (Fisher et al., 2006) has modified the *in situ* arterially-perfused brainstem preparation (Paton, 1996a) of the rat to enable optical imaging of brainstem respiratory circuits. This approach capitalizes on the mechanical stability of the brainstem which results from pump perfusion with the neural integrity of the pontomedullary axis. Moreover, the preparation retains a number of sensory inputs to the VRC that play a known role in modulating respiratory rhythm. It should be noted that these studies used a different approach of dye loading. Potts and Paton delivered the dye directly to the deep structures of the ventrolateral medulla via pressurized microinjection that was guided by extracellular recording of mixed inspiratory and expiratory activity in the pre-BötC (Schwarzacher et al., 1995). In contrast, Fisher and colleagues added the dye directly to the perfusate which may have resulted in more even loading throughout the brainstem.

Since respiratory neurons are spatially organized within the VLM, it is difficult to study the spatial organization of this network using convential electrophysiology. In 2005, Fisher and colleagues used optical imaging techniques with the *in situ* prefused preparation to simultaneously monitor the spatiotemporal activity patterns of populations of respiratory neurons in the pre-BötC. They reported that functionally distinct, respiratory related fluorescent signals were spatially distributed within the pre-BötC and that these regions

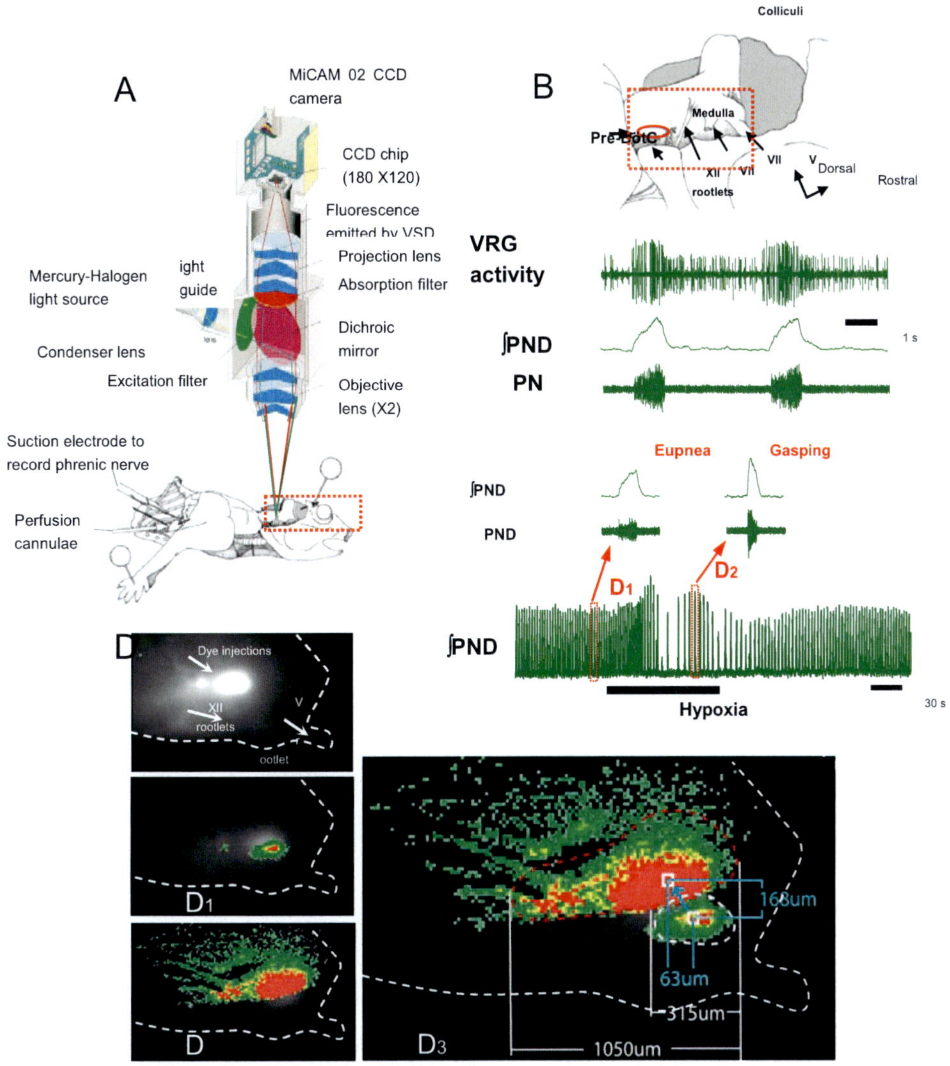


Schematic of the experimental and optical setup for fluorescence measurements of respiratory activity in the ventrolateral medulla of the *in situ* arterially perfused preparation. Panel A – The *in situ* preparation is pump-perfused via the aorta with a Ringer's solution that was oxygenated, heated and filtered. Respiratory motor activity generated by the central respiratory network is recorded from the phrenic nerve via a suction electrode. The imaging system consisted of a commercially available optical imaging system (SciMedia, Inc). The CCD camera (180x120 pixel) had high dynamic range (>66db) high quantal efficiency (75% @ 550nm, 55% @ 700 nm) and a time resolution of 3.5ms per frame (285 Hz). The voltage sensitive dye (Di-2-ANEPEQ) was excited using a 150W tungsten-halogen lamp and fluorescence was visualized using an excitation (510nm) / emission (590nm) filter, and a dichroic mirror. In order to visualize the ventrolateral medulla, the rats head was rotated 90° from horizontal and stabilized. Fluorescent images were triggered off the onset of inspiratory activity (as measured from the phrenic nerve) using a 2X objective. Panel B – Cartoon showing exposure of the ventrolateral medulla for optical imaging. The dye was delivered directly into the region containing the pre-Bötzinger Complex (pre-BötC) based on extracellular recording of mixed inspiratory and expiratory neuronal activity (lower portion of panel B). Panel C – Original tracing showing changes in phrenic nerve discharge (PND) during the transition from eupnea to gasping produced by hypoxia. Note, the pattern of PND changed from a ramp-like incremental pattern to a decrementing pattern, while breathing frequency exhibited a biphasic pattern characterized by initial excitation followed by depression. Panel D – Spatial pattern of optical activity recorded from the ventrolateral medulla during eupnea and hypoxic-induced gasping. The upper panel is an image of the ventrolateral surface of the medulla showing the location of the dye injection sites. Note, dye was localized in a region containing the pre-BötC. Panel D1 is a pseudocolored image showing the distribution of activated neurons during eupnea. The image was obtained during peak inspiratory activity (at the end of inspiration). Panel D2 shows peak fluorescence during gasping. Note, the spatial pattern of activity covered a substantially larger area of the medulla compared to that during eupnea. Panel D3 is an overlay of the peak inspiratory fluorescence activity during eupnea and gasping. The center of peak fluorescence shifted dorsally and caudally away from the pre-BötC region during gasping. We also found that there was minimal spatial overlap of the activated regions during eupnea and gasping. Some of these data were modified from Potts and Paton, *Eur. J. Neurosci.* 23, 3025-3033, 2006.

received widespread hyperpolarization directly following inspiratory termination. This latter result differs significantly from early studies that performed optical imaging in neonatal animals (Onimaru and Homma, 2003; 2005a; Onimaru et al., 2004) where inhibitory activity was absent or not reported. This suggests that inhibitory activity plays a more prominent role in the in situ preparation although a developmental difference cannot be ruled out as neonatal rats were used by Onimaru and juvenile rats by Fischer. This inhibitory synaptic activity is critical for rhythm generation in neonatal and juvenile rats with a functional pontomedullary circuit and depends on glycinergic and GABAergic mechanisms (Busselberg et al., 2001;Dutschmann and Paton, 2002;Ezure et al., 2003;Hayashi and Lipski, 1992;Paton and Richter, 1995;Rybak et al., 2004;St-John and Paton, 2004).

## State-Dependence of the Respiratory Network Revealed by Optical Imaging

The generation of respiratory activity is altered under different behavioral states. For instances, hypoxia substantially changes respiratory pattern and rhythm (St. John, 1990). However, the underlying mechanism(s) for these changes remain unknown (Lieske et al., 2001). Using optical imaging techniques and the *in situ* perfused brainstem preparation in juvenile rats, we recently reported that there was a marked shift in the spatial pattern of optical activity when gasping was produced by hypoxia (Potts and Paton, 2006). We found that optical activity in a discrete region of the VLM containing the pre-BötC dramatically increased during gasping and that the core of peak optical activity shifted dorsally and caudally (168 μm dorsal x 63 μm caudal) away from the pre-BötC (this is illustrated in the figure on the following page). This gasping-related region was similar to a region described previously by (Huang et al., 1997) that when lesioned eliminated gasping but not eupnea. Importantly, the medullary region lesioned by Huang and colleagues was also caudal and dorsal of the pre-BötC. Since eupnea activated a region that corresponded to the pre-BötC in our study, these results suggest that this region was involved in the generation of hypoxic-induced gasping in this experimental model. Furthermore, given the magnitude of the spatial shift of optical activity during hypoxia, it is unlikely that the same population of respiratory neurons initiated inspiratory drive during gasping.

## Summary

This review chapter has summarized the application of optical imaging techniques with voltage-sensitive dyes to visualize neuronal activity in medullary respiratory circuits. The ability of optical techniques to obtain real-time images with high spatial and temporal resolution has provided a means to efficiently map the spatiotemporal activity of respiratory neurons to better understand how this patterned activity is altered during different behavioral states. While there has been rapid progress in optical imaging, further developments will help to optimize this process. Advances such as imaging with two-photon excitation laser scanning microscopy, the use of genetically encoded indicators such as GFP-based voltage sensors, new fluorophores and automated analysis techniques to extract all of the useful information from live imaging will permit us to peer deeper into the living brain. Although this technology is unique in its ability to characterize the activity of a neuronal network comprised of hundreds of individual neurons, electrophysiology remains the gold standard to obtain high fidelity recordings of membrane events (ie. changes in membrane potential and ionic currents). With continued development of new optical dyes, imaging chips and optics the combination of optical imaging with modern electrophysiology represents powerful tools for continued investigation of the synaptic and cellular mechanisms of respiratory rhythmogenesis.

## Acknowledgements

Financial support from the National Institutes of Health (HL059167, JTP) and the British Heart Foundation (JFRP) is greatly appreciated. JFRP was in receipt of a Royal Society Wolfson Research merit award.

## References

Arata A, Onimaru H, Homma I (1990) Respiration-related neurons in the ventral medulla of newborn rats in vitro. *Brain Res. Bull.* 24:599-604.

Barnes BJ, Tuong CM, Mellen NM. (2007) Functional imaging reveals respiratory network activity during hypoxic and opioid challenge in the neonate rat tilted sagittal slab preparation. *J Neurophysiol.* 97:2283-92.

Ballanyi K, Onimaru H, Homma I (1999) Respiratory network function in the isolated brainstem-spinal cord of newborn rats. *Prog. Neurobiol.* 59:583-634.

Bianchi AL, avit-Saubie M, Champagnat J (1995) Central control of breathing in mammals: neuronal circuitry, membrane properties, and neurotransmitters. *Physiol. Rev.* 75:1-45.

Busselberg D, Bischoff AM, Paton JF, Richter DW (2001) Reorganisation of respiratory network activity after loss of glycinergic inhibition. *Pflugers. Arch.* 441:444-449.

Cohen LB, Salzberg BM, Davila HV, Ross WN, Landowne D, Waggoner AS, Wang CH (1974) Changes in axon fluorescence during activity: molecular probes of membrane potential. *J. Membr. Biol.* 19:1-36.

Cohen LB, Salzberg BM, Grinvald A (1978) Optical methods for monitoring neuron activity. *Annu. Rev. Neurosci.* 1:171-182.

Duffin J (2004) Functional organization of respiratory neurones: a brief review of current questions and speculations. *Exp. Physiol.* 89:517-529.

Dutschmann M, Herbert H (2006) The Kolliker-Fuse nucleus gates the postinspiratory phase of the respiratory cycle to control inspiratory off-switch and upper airway resistance in rat. *Eur. J. Neurosci.* 24:1071-1084.

Dutschmann M, Paton JF (2002) Inhibitory synaptic mechanisms regulating upper airway patency. Respir. *Physiol. Neurobiol.* 131:57-63.

Dutschmann M, Wilson RJ, Paton JF (2000) Respiratory activity in neonatal rats. *Auton. Neurosci.* 84:19-29.

Ebner TJ, Chen G (1995) Use of voltage-sensitive dyes and optical recordings in the central nervous system. *Prog. Neurobiol.* 46:463-506.

Eugenin J, Nicholls JG, Cohen LB, Muller KJ (2006) Optical recording from respiratory pattern generator of fetal mouse brainstem reveals a distributed network. *Neuroscience.* 137:1221-1227.

Ezure K, Tanaka I, Kondo M (2003) Glycine is used as a transmitter by decrementing expiratory neurons of the ventrolateral medulla in the rat. *J. Neurosci.* 23:8941-8948.

Feldman JL, Del Negro CA (2006) Looking for inspiration: new perspectives on respiratory rhythm. *Nat. Rev. Neurosci.* 7:232-242.

Feldman JL, Smith JC, Ellenberger HH, Connelly CA, Liu GS, Greer JJ, Lindsay AD, Otto MR (1990) Neurogenesis of respiratory rhythm and pattern: emerging concepts. *Am. J. Physiol.* 259:R879-R886.

Fisher JA, Marchenko VA, Yodh AG, Rogers RF (2006) Spatiotemporal activity patterns during respiratory rhythmogenesis in the rat ventrolateral medulla. *J. Neurophysiol.* 95:1982-1991.

Funke F, Dutschmann M, Muller M (2007) Imaging of respiratory-related population activity with single-cell resolution. *Am. J. Physiol. Cell Physiol.* 292:C508-C516.

Grinvald A, Frostig RD, Lieke E, Hildesheim R (1988) Optical imaging of neuronal activity. *Physiol. Rev.* 68:1285-1366.

Hayashi F, Lipski J (1992) The role of inhibitory amino acids in control of respiratory motor output in an arterially perfused rat. *Respir. Physiol.* 89:47-63.

Huang Q, Zhou D, St John WM (1997) Lesions of regions for in vitro ventilatory genesis eliminate gasping but not eupnea. *Respir. Physiol.* 107:111-123.

Kaufman L, Williamson SJ (1982) Magnetic location of cortical activity. *Ann. N. Y. Acad. Sci.* 388:197-213.

Koshiya N, Smith JC (1999) Neuronal pacemaker for breathing visualized in vitro. *Nature.* 400:360-363.

Lieske SP, Thoby-Brisson M, Ramirez JM (2001) Reconfiguration of the central respiratory network under normoxic and hypoxic conditions. *Adv. Exp. Med. Biol.* 499:171-178.

Lindsey BG, Morris KF, Segers LS, Shannon R (2000) Respiratory neuronal assemblies. *Respir. Physiol.* 122:183-196.

Nakashima M, Yamada S, Shiono S, Maeda M, Satoh F (1992) 448-detector optical recording system: development and application to Aplysia gill-withdrawal reflex. *IEEE Trans Biomed. Eng.* 39:26-36.

Ogawa S, Lee TM, Kay AR, Tank DW (1990) Brain magnetic resonance imaging with contrast dependent on blood oxygenation. *Proc. Natl. Acad. Sci. U S A.* 87:9868-9872.

Onimaru H, Arata A, Arata S, Shirasawa S, Cleary ML (2004) In vitro visualization of respiratory neuron activity in the newborn mouse ventral medulla. *Brain Res. Dev. Brain Res.* 153:275-279.

Onimaru H, Homma I (2003) A novel functional neuron group for respiratory rhythm generation in the ventral medulla. *J. Neurosci.* 23:1478-1486.

Onimaru H, Homma I (2005a) Developmental changes in the spatio-temporal pattern of respiratory neuron activity in the medulla of late fetal rat. *Neuroscience.* 131:969-977.

Onimaru H, Homma I (2005b) Optical imaging of respiratory neuron activity from the dorsal view of the lower brainstem. *Clin. Exp. Pharmacol. Physiol.* 32:297-301.

Onimaru H, Kanamaru A, Homma I (1996) Optical imaging of respiratory burst activity in newborn rat medullary block preparations. *Neurosci. Res.* 25:183-190.

Paton JF (1996a) A working heart-brainstem preparation of the mouse. *J. Neurosci. Methods.* 65:63-68.

Paton JF (1996b) The ventral medullary respiratory network of the mature mouse studied in a working heart-brainstem preparation. *J. Physiol.* 493 ( Pt 3):819-831.

Paton JF, Abdala AP, Koizumi H, Smith JC, St-John WM (2006) Respiratory rhythm generation during gasping depends on persistent sodium current. *Nat. Neurosci.* 9:311-313.

Paton JF, Richter DW (1995) Role of fast inhibitory synaptic mechanisms in respiratory rhythm generation in the maturing mouse. *J. Physiol.* 484 ( Pt 2):505-521.

Potts JT, Paton JF (2006) Optical imaging of medullary ventral respiratory network during eupnea and gasping in situ. *Eur. J. Neurosci.* 23:3025-3033.

Ramirez JM, Telgkamp P, Elsen FP, Quellmalz UJ, Richter DW (1997) Respiratory rhythm generation in mammals: synaptic and membrane properties. *Respir. Physiol.* 110:71-85.

Richter DW, Spyer KM (2001) Studying rhythmogenesis of breathing: comparison of in vivo and in vitro models. *Trends Neurosci.* 24:464-472.

Rybak IA, Shevtsova NA, Paton JF, Dick TE, St-John WM, Morschel M, Dutschmann M (2004) Modeling the ponto-medullary respiratory network. *Respir. Physiol. Neurobiol.* 143:307-319.

Salzberg BM (1989) Optical recording of voltage changes in nerve terminals and in fine neuronal processes. *Annu. Rev. Physiol.* 51:507-526.

Sato K, Momose-Sato Y (2004) Optical detection of convergent projections in the embryonic chick NTS. *Neurosci. Lett.* 371:97-101.

Schwarzacher SW, Smith JC, Richter DW (1995) Pre-Botzinger complex in the cat. *J. Neurophysiol.* 73:1452-1461.

Smith JC, Ellenberger HH, Ballanyi K, Richter DW, Feldman JL (1991) Pre-Botzinger complex: a brainstem region that may generate respiratory rhythm in mammals. *Science.* 254:726-729.

Smith JC, Abdala AA, Koizumi H, Rybak IA, Paton JF. Spatial and Functional Architecture of the Mammalian Brainstem Respiratory Network: A Hierarchy of Three Oscillatory Mechanisms (2007) J Neurophysiol. [Epub ahead of print]

Sokoloff L, Reivich M, Kennedy C, Des Rosiers MH, Patlak CS, Pettigrew KD, Sakurada O, Shinohara M (1977) The [14C]deoxyglucose method for the measurement of local cerebral glucose utilization: theory, procedure, and normal values in the conscious and anesthetized albino rat. *J. Neurochem.* 28:897-916.

St John WM (1990) Neurogenesis, control, and functional significance of gasping. *J. Appl. Physiol.* 68:1305-1315.

St-John WM, Paton JF (2004) Role of pontile mechanisms in the neurogenesis of eupnea. *Respir. Physiol. Neurobiol.* 143:321-332.

Takashima I, Ichikawa M, Iijima T (1999) High-speed CCD imaging system for monitoring neural activity in vivo and in vitro, using a voltage-sensitive dye. *J. Neurosci. Methods.* 91:147-159.

Tokumasu M, Nakazono Y, Ide H, Akagawa K, Onimaru H (2001) Optical recording of spontaneous respiratory neuron activity in the rat brain stem. *Jpn. J. Physiol.* 51:613-619.

In: Research Topics on Brain Mapping
Editor: Yuanzhu Liáng, pp. 221-232
ISBN: 978-1-60456-001-5


*Chapter XI*

# The Use of Nonlinear Analysis to Evaluate CNS Dysfunctions

***A. Kotini* and P. Anninos***
Lab of Medical Physics, Medical School, Democritus University of Thrace,
University Campus, Alex/polis, Greece

## Abstract

**Aim**: The aim of this study is to investigate the presence of any non-linearity in the magnetoencephalographic recordings (MEG) from the temporal lobe of epileptic, Parkinson diseased and schizophrenic patients in comparison with controls, in order to find out the differences underlying their brain waves. We calculated the correlation dimension, which is a measure of the complexity of the dynamic system, as well as the first Lyapunov exponent that indicates the system's unpredictability.

**Methods**: The epileptic group comprised with 10 patients aged 20-50 years (mean: 37.5 +/- 12.8) whereas 10 subjects within the same age range served as controls. The Parkinson diseased group comprised with 10 patients aged 50 to 80 years (mean=65.1+/-10.5), whereas the controls consisted of 10 subjects within the same age range. The schizophrenic group comprised with 10 patients aged 20-30 years (mean 23.2 +/- 2.8) whereas 10 subjects within the same age range served as controls. Biomagnetic measurements were performed using a second order gradiometer SQUID (model 601 of the Biomagnetic Technologies Inc.), which was located in an electrically shielded room of low magnetic noise. For each subject the magnetic activity was recorded from a total of 64 points of the skull (32 points from each temporal lobe) as defined by a recording reference system, which is based on the 10-20 Electrode Placement System.

* Corresponding author: Dr. A.Kotini, Asst. Professor ; Lab of Medical Physics, Medical School; Democritus University of Thrace; University Campus, Alex/polis, Greece; Tel/fax:+302551030519; E-mail: akotin@axd.forthnet.gr

**Results**: The non-linear analysis of the MEG activity in epileptic, Parkinson diseased and schizophrenic groups showed lower dimension complexity and lower values of the first Lyapunov exponent compared with controls.

**Conclusion**: The application of non-linear analysis on MEG activity may offer important perspectives to better evaluate the brain function in patients with CNS disorders.

**Keywords:** *MEG, non-linear analysis, Epilepsy, Parkinson, Schizophrenia.*

# Introduction

An important new approach of describing dynamical systems is the non-linear dynamics, called chaos theory, which allow us to determine changes in the dynamics of the system over time. Higher dimensionality or a higher rate of phase state transitions characterizes more complex systems. Such approaches have been shown to be useful in characterizing a variety of processes, including physiology (*Elbert et al., 1992*) and motor behaviors (*Haken et al., 1985*).

For the non-linear analysis of biological signals, the parameters most commonly studied are the correlation dimension (D) that shows the complexity of the system (*Grassberger and Procaccia, 1983a,b*) and the Lyapunov exponents (LE) that show the reactivity of the system to the deterministic external stimuli (*Rosenstein et al., 1993*).

Many investigations have revealed possible medical applications for non-linear analysis and have given rise to the possibility that it might be a useful tool in differentiating pathological and physiological brain states (*Babloyantz and Destexhe 1986, Babloyantz et al., 1985; Stam et al., 1995,1996, Stam, 2005; Frank et al., 1990; Pijn et al., 1991; Lutzenberger et al., 1992; Fell et al., 1993; Roschke and Aldenhoff, 1993; Toro et al., 1999; Lehnertz, 1999; Kowalik et al., 2001; Keshavana et al., 2004; Yambe et al., 2005*). According to these reports, the brain activity has a finite non-integer D and a positive LE. Pathologic conditions revealed decreased chaotic activities in the EEG, whereas normal states revealed increased chaotic activities by estimating the D. *Yambe et al.* (*2005*) shown that the EEG wave pattern was significantly modified before the seizure attack. Particularly, the EEG wave before the epileptic attack was analyzed by the chaos theory. As a result, the simplification of an attractor is observed before an epileptic attack. The simplification of an attractor was quantified based on the LE and D. EEG signals were influenced by the nonlinear dynamical behavior of the central nervous system. It is very interesting when we consider the modifications of the nonlinear dynamics before the seizure attack. Based on these results, it may be possible to predict an epileptic attack by the chaos analysis of EEG. Furthermore, it may also be possible to determine the excision range of a brain surgery by the chaotic analysis of EEG. Many nonlinear EEG/MEG studies use the notion of "complexity", usually to estimate the D. Dynamical complexity is the randomness or lack of interactions between the elements of a dynamical system. The higher level of synchronization between functional sources in a functional network is associated with lower dynamical complexity ( *Stam, 2005*).

Computational models aid in the quantitative understanding of cell signaling networks. One important goal is to ascertain how multiple network components work together to govern cellular responses, that is, to determine cell 'signal-response' relationships. Several methods exist to study steady-state signals in the context of differential equation-based models. However, many biological networks influence cell behavior through time-varying signals operating during a transient activated state that ultimately returns to a basal steady-state (*Aldridge et al., 2006*).

The brain is a complex dynamical system, so multi-channel measurements are necessary to gain a detailed understanding of its behavior. Such multi-channel measurements include optical brain images, multi-electrode recordings, functional magnetic resonance imaging (fMRI), MEG, etc (*Hamalainen et al. 1993; Grinvald et al. 1992; Kwong et al. 1992; Tonoike et al., 1998, Anninos et al., 1991;1999;2000;2003;2006*). In MEG, weak magnetic fields of the order of tens of ft/√Hz generated by electric currents in the brain are measured using superconducting quantum interferometric detector arrays positioned on the skull. The MEG is a noninvasive imaging technique, applicable to the human brain with temporal resolution approximately ~ 1 ms (*Mitra and Pesaran 1999*). Several authors have demonstrated the importance of the MEG in the investigation of normal and pathological brain conditions during the last decade (*Anninos et al., 1991; 1999; 2000;2003;2006;Timmermann et al. 2003; Volkmann et al. 1996; Tonoike et al.1998; Halgren et al. 2002; Marinkovic et al. 2003; Makela 1996*). The major advantage of MEG over EEG is that MEG has higher localization accuracy. This is due to the fact that the different structures of the head (brain, liquor cerebrospinalis, skull and scalp) influence the magnetic fields less than the volume current flow that causes the EEG. Additionally, the MEG is reference free, so that the localization of sources with a given precision is easier for MEG than it is for EEG (*Kristeva-Feige et al. 1997*). In addition, the MEG offers functional mapping information and measurement of brain activity in real time, unlike CT, MRI and fMRI which only provide structural, anatomical and metabolic information. With the MEG the brain is seen in 'action' rather than viewed as a still image. Finally, the MEG has far more superior ability to resolve millisecond temporal activity associated with the processing of information which is the main task of the brain.

The aim of this study is to investigate the complexity of brain activity using MEG measurements in 3 different study populations, (epileptic, Parkinson diseased (PD) and schizophrenic patients) in comparison with controls in order to determine if non-linear MEG dynamics measured by D and first LE could be able to find out changes in these groups.

## Material and Methods

The epileptic group comprised with 10 patients aged 20-50 years (mean: 37.5 +/- 12.8) whereas 10 subjects within the same age range served as controls. All epileptic patients have been diagnosed independently to suffer from idiopathic epilepsy and had normal routine serum biochemical studies. The PD group comprised with 10 patients aged 50 - 80 years (mean=65.1 +/-10.5), whereas the controls consisted of 10 subjects within the same age range. All PD patients have diagnosed to suffer from idiopathic PD on the basis of clinical observations and routine EEG recordings. None of them had a history of other neurological disease other than PD and all had normal routine serum biochemical studies. The schizophrenic group comprised with 10 patients aged 20-30 years (mean 23.2 +/- 2.8) having no medication histories whereas 10 subjects within the same age range served as controls. Informed consent for the methodology and the aim of the study was obtained from all the subjects prior to the procedure.

Biomagnetic measurements were performed using a second order gradiometer SQUID model 601 of the Biomagnetic Technologies Inc., which was located in an electrically shielded room. The noise level of the environment was of the order of 50 fT/√Hz. During the recording procedure the patients were relaxed lying on a wooden bed, with closed eyes, in order to avoid artifacts from eye flickering. The MEG recordings were performed after positioning the SQUID sensor 3 mm above the scalp of each subject at specified points as defined by a recording reference system. This reference system that is based on the International 10-20 Electrode Placement System (*Jasper, 1958*) uses any one of the standard EEG recording positions as its origin (*Anninos et al., 1991, 1999, 2000, 2003; 2006*). In this study we used the P3, P4, T3, T4, F3, and F4 recording positions. The reference system was devised to retrieve maximal information from a specified area of the skull given that the gradiometer coil is theoretically equally sensitive to all magnetic flux lines perpendicular to a circular area of the brain. In our case, this circle has been an effective diameter of 2.36 cm, i.e. the diameter of the SQUID sensor coil. Around the origin (T3 or T4 for temporal lobes) a rectangular 32-point matrix was used (4 rows x 8 columns, equidistantly spaced in a 4.5 cm x 10.5 cm rectangle) for positioning of the SQUID (*Anninos et al., 1991, 1999, 2000,2003; 2006*).

The MEG was recorded from each cerebral hemisphere at each of the 32 matrix points on the scalp for 32 consecutive epochs. Each epoch was of 1 sec duration and was digitized with a sampling frequency of 256 Hz (frequency resolution of the power spectrum being 1 Hz). The MEG signal was band-pass filtered with cut-off frequencies of 0.1 and 60 Hz. The MEG recordings were digitized using a 12 bit precision analog to digital converter with a sampling frequency of 256 Hz, and stored in a PC peripheral memory for off-line Fourier statistical analysis. The method, by its nature (i.e. temporal and spatial averaging), eliminates short-term abnormal artifacts in any cortical area, while it retains long lasting localized activation phenomena.

# Theory and Algorithm

We applied nonlinear analysis in order to investigate the difference in the complexity underlying the dynamics characterizing the MEG activity of all the participants. For the estimation of the dimension of the strange attractor we have considered the method proposed by *Grassberger and Procaccia* (*1983a,b*), which is based on the theorem introduced by *Takens* (*1981*). According to their method, the dynamics of the system can experimentally reconstructed from the observed MEG time series $B_i=B(t_i)$ (i=1,2...N). Then, the vector construction of $V_i$ is given by the following equation:

$$V_i=\{B_i,B_{i+\tau},\ldots,B_{i+(m-1)\tau}\} \qquad (1)$$

This equation gives a smooth embedding of the dynamics in a m-dimensional phase space. The evolution of the system in the phase space settles on a submanifold, which is a fractal set, the strange attractor. The concept of strange attractors is of great importance in chaotic dynamics, since its existence or absence is related to the behavior of the system as chaotic or deterministic. The strange attractor can be described by a geometrical parameter, the D. This parameter is related to the number of variables required to define the attractor within the phase space and it can be estimated from an experimental time series by means of the correlation integrals C(r,m) defined as follows (*Kaplan and Glass, 1995*):

$$C(r,m)=2/N^2 \sum_{i=1}^{N-B} \sum_{j=i+B}^{N} \Theta(r-|V_i-V_j|) \qquad (2)$$

where Θ (u) is the Heaviside function defined as (Θ(u)=1 for u>0 and Θ(u)=0 for u≤ 0), m is the embedding dimension and n is the number of vectors constructed from a time series with N samples, given by the formula n=N-(m-1)τ (Here τ is a delay parameter which is equal to the first zero crossing of the autocorrelation time of the MEG signal). B is a correction factor for spurious influences of autocorrelation (*Theiler and Rapp, 1996*). The correlation integral C(r,m) measures the spatial correlation of the points of the attractor and it is calculated for different values of r in the range from 0 to $r_{max}$ . The $r_{max}$ is equal to $(m)^{1/2}$ $(x_{max}-x_{min})$, (assuming that $x_{max}$ and $x_{min}$ are the maximum and the minimum recorded values in the time series). For a chaotic system the correlation integrals should scale as $C(r,m) \sim r^{D(m)}$ .Thus, the D of the attracting submanifold in the reconstruction phase space is given by :

$$D= \lim_{\substack{r \to 0 \\ m \to \infty}} \partial(\ln C(r,m)) / \partial(\ln(r)) \qquad (3)$$

when we analyze the real data, the scaling region is very often observed to oscillate around some straight line. These oscillations may be either intrinsic sample oscillations caused by the lacunarity of the attractor or finite sample oscillations caused by the limited amount of data (the edge effect). We used a modification proposed by *Dvorak and Klaschka* (*1990*) to compensate for the edge effect:

$$D= \lim_{\substack{r \to 0 \\ m \to \infty}} \partial \ln C(r,m) / \partial \ln(r(2-r)) \qquad (4)$$

In the case of a chaotic signal exhibiting a strange attractor, there is a saturation value, (plateau) in the graph of the slopes D v's ln(r(2-r)). This value remains constant, although the signal is embedded in successively higher-dimensioned phase spaces and gives an estimation of the correlation dimension of the attractor which is estimated by a least-squares method of that linear region. This approach avoids the problem of selecting appropriate reference points on the attractor present in the original algorithm.

For another descriptor of non-linear behavior, LE was calculated. According to this theory, two points close to one another in phase space are chosen and their evolution over time determined. If the system is chaotic, the two trajectories will diverge rapidly reflecting their dependence on initial conditions. The LE is the mean exponential divergences of such trajectories. If the first LE is positive, the system exhibits chaotic behavior (*Frank et al., 1990*) that reflects the tendency of small disturbances to grow exponentially. The basic principle behind most algorithms to compute LE is to consider two or a small number of nearby points on the attractor and to quantify the exponential increase or decrease of the inter vector distances over time. An m-dimensional dynamical system has m LE. The presence of a positive LE indicates chaos. It also quantifies the amount of instability or predictability of the system. A fully deterministic system will have a zero LE since it is fully predictable, whereas a random system will have large positive exponent indicating no predictability (*Keshavana et al., 2004*). Dimensions are static measures of attractors which provide no information on the evolution of trajectories over time. LE can be considered "dynamic" measures of attractor complexity and indicate exponential divergence or convergence of nearby trajectories on the attractor. A system has as many LE as there are directions in state space. The concept of entropy is closely related to that of LE. It is defined as the rate of information loss over time and is equal to the sum of all positive LE (*Stam, 2005*).

## Results

Using the above-described method, the D of the selected MEG time series was estimated for the brain of the 3 study populations. The average values of D and the standard deviations for the epileptic patients are summarized in table 1. It can be seen that epileptic patients had low values of D at the right and left temporal regions whereas the controls have no saturation values. It means that the chaotic activity of MEG in epileptic patients in the temporal areas is lower than that in normal brain. The same occurs for the PD and schizophrenic patients in comparison to controls (tables 2, 3). The D determines the number of independent variables, which are necessary to describe the dynamics of the central nervous system (CNS). The first LE were significantly greater than zero in these groups, which means that the dynamical systems are chaotic. Moreover in epileptic, PD and schizophrenic patients the LE had lower values in compare with controls (tables 1-3).

**Table 1. Mean values of D and LE in the 1st examined group**

| | Right temporal | | Left Temporal | |
|---|---|---|---|---|
| | D | LE | D | LE |
| Epilepsy (10) | 6.7±0.3 | 1.0±0.1 | 6.2±0.6 | 1.1±0.1 |
| Controls (10) | - | 1.2±0.1 | - | 1.3±0.1 |

**Table 2. Mean values of D and LE in the 2nd examined group**

| | Right temporal | | Left Temporal | |
|---|---|---|---|---|
| | D | LE | D | LE |
| Parkinson (10) | 3.7±0.4 | 1.1±0.1 | 4.2±0.5 | 1.0±0.1 |
| Controls (10) | - | 1.2±0.1 | - | 1.3±0.1 |

**Table 3. Mean values of D and LE in the 3rd examined group**

| | Right temporal | | Left Temporal | |
|---|---|---|---|---|
| | D | LE | D | LE |
| Schizophrenia (10) | 8.1±0.5 | 1.1±0.1 | 7.6±0.7 | 1.0±0.1 |
| Controls (10) | - | 1.3±0.1 | - | 1.2±0.1 |

# Conclusion

Functional mapping of the human brain has made tremendous progress in the past years thanks to new technical developments. Single photon emission computer tomography (SPECT), positron emission tomography (PET), fMRI and high-resolution EEG and MEG are currently intensively applied techniques to functional studies, each one having specific properties and disadvantages concerning spatial and temporal resolution. The success of these methods in basic neuroscience research has led to the demand for applying them to clinical questions. Diseases of the central nervous system that lead to brain dysfunction can be ideally explored using these techniques. Of particular importance are those diseases in which a focal neuronal dysfunction is the primary cause and where surgical resection of this focus might be the cure. This is often the case of tumors associated with pathological rhythms development and spread throughout the brain, leading to seizures that severely handicap the patient. Surgical resection of the primary focus is only possible if the focus can be exactly localized and adequately separated from functionally important areas. The only methods that have sufficient temporal resolution to follow neuronal activity in real time are the electrophysiological measures, i.e. the EEG and the MEG.

The importance of the biological time-series analysis, which exhibits typically complex dynamics, has long been recognized in the area of non-linear analysis. Several features of these approaches have been proposed to detect the hidden important dynamical properties of the physiological phenomenon. The analysis of these biological signals is complicated due to its highly irregular and non-stationary property. The nonlinear dynamical techniques are based on the concept of chaos and it has been applied to many areas including the areas of medicine and biology. Efforts have been made in determining non-linear parameters like D for pathological signals and it has been shown that they are useful indicators of pathologies. In analysis of EEG and MEG data, different chaotic measures such as D, LE and entropy are used in recent literature (*Kowalik et al., 2001; Lehnertz, 1999*).

Non-linear analysis offers new tools for the investigation of information processing in the brain by analysis and classification of MEG signals. The recent developments in non-linear dynamics have indicated a new understanding of many biological processes. The hypothesis that the CNS is a dynamical system exhibiting deterministic chaos has offered important tools to investigate the brain function. Identifying families of attractors in phase space analysis can prove valuable in describing a range of behaviors and associated neural activity including sensory and motor repertoires. Additionally, transitions between attractors may serve as useful descriptors for analyzing state changes in neurons and neural ensembles.

Our study revealed the hypotemporality of the complexity in the temporal regions of epileptic, Parkinson diseased and schizophrenic patients. It may be that the abnormal brain has decreased information processing and less flexible neural networks in this area. Our results fit well with previous studies showing that diminished dimensions are found in diseases (*Babloyantz and Destexhe, 1986*), or brain states that can be assumed to be associated with diminished complexity of brain activity (*Babloyantz et al, 1985*). The decreased complex activities in the abnormal brain are consistent with the findings of hypotemporality reported in EEG (*Hughes, 1996*), cerebral blood flow (*Andreasen et al., 1992; Catafau et al.,1994*), MRI (*Barta et al.,1990*), PET (*Buchsbaum et al.,1984*), etc.

While the first LE and D are related (*Peitgen et al., 1992*), the exact nature of the relationship is unproven; it is obvious that both parameters measure different aspects of a system's dynamics. The LE provides a new axis in terms of non-linear systems theory (*Fell et al., 1993*) and estimates the mean exponential divergence or convergence of nearby trajectories in phase space. The calculation of LE expresses sensitive dependence on initial conditions and supports the hypothesis that the investigating system is chaotic. The low values of LE in the temporal hemispheres express a decrease in the information processing and indicate less flexible neural networks in these areas. There have been many publications about the evaluation of the LE of EEG segments in epileptic seizures, electroconvulsive therapy, sleep etc (*Frank et al., 1990; Roschke and Aldenhohh, 1993*). The LE is a non-linear measure of signal chaoticity. It measures the stability of a system and characterizes the signal predictability. Positive LE corresponds to chaotic, negative to the periodic states (*Kowalik et al., 2001; Lehnertz, 1999*).

Loss of neurons in degenerative brain diseases may disrupt anatomical connectivity at the level of functional sources and functional networks. Consequently one might expect that brain dynamics in such disorders, is characterized by a lower level of synchronization of ongoing brain activity, and that this loss of functional connectivity interferes normal information processing. However, at the level of functional sources many studies have reported a loss of dynamical complexity which would suggest increased local levels of synchronization (*Stam, 2005*).

The active neuronal states that sustain cognitive processes are organized through the exchange of excitatory and inhibitory signals, which allow for a balanced oscillation within a functionally integrated CNS. Neurons are coupled to form resonating parallel circuits distributed in diffuse form across the cortex. The activity of these circuits covaries with external input. Therefore, cognitions, emotions, perceptions, and behaviors depend not so much on the activity of isolated neurons as on the interconnections among them. These interconnections are based on a nonlinear chaotic dynamic that is continually interactive with the environment (*Toro et al., 1999*).

New techniques for the visualization of spatiotemporal dynamics in neural ensembles provide opportunities for observing coherent spatial structures of the neural population. New developments in complex systems can be a source of power new analytical tools and insights into the dynamics of neural systems. Particularly the implications of the complexity of the MEG or EEG activities may offer fertile perspectives for understanding the significant features of the pathologic brain.

# References

Aldridge, B; Haller, G; Sorger, P; Lauffenburger D. Direct Lyapunov Exponent Analysis Enables Parametric Study of Transient Signaling Governing Cell Behavior. *Syst. Biol.* 2006; 6:425-432

Andreasen, NC; Rezai, K; Alliger, R; Swayze, VW; Flaum, M; Kirchner, P; Cohen, G; O'Leary, DS. Hypofrontality in neuroleptic-naïve patients and in patients with chronic schizophrenia. *Arch. Gen. Psychiatry.* 1992;49:943-958

Anninos, PA; Tsagas, N; Sandyk, R; Derpapas K. Magnetic stimulation in the treatment of partial seizures. *Int. J. Neurosci.* 1991;60 : 141-171

Anninos, P; Kotini, A; Adamopoulos, A; Tsagas, N. Magnetic stimulation can modulate seizures in epileptic patients. *Brain Topogr.* 2003 ;16:57-64.

Anninos, P; Kotini, A; Tamiolakis, D; Tsagas N. Transcranial magnetic stimulation. A case report and review of the literature. *Acta Neurol. Belg.* 2006 ;106:26-30

Anninos, PA; Adamopoulos, A; Kotini, A; Tsagas, N. Nonlinear Analysis of brain activity in magnetic influenced Parkinson patients. *Brain Topogr*; 2000;13:135-144

Anninos, PA; Tsagas, N; Jacobson, JI; Kotini, A. The biological effects of magnetic stimulation in epileptic patients. *Panminerva Med.* 1999; 41 : 207-215

Babloyantz, A; Salazar, JM; Nicolis, C. Evidence of chaotic dynamics of brain activity during the sleep cycle. *Physics Letters.* 1985;111A:152-156

Baloyantz, A; Destexhe, A. Low dimensional chaos in an instance of epilepsy. *Proc. Natl. Acad. Sci. U S A.* 1986; 83 : 3513-3517

Barta, PE; Pearlson, GD; Powers, RE; Richard, SS; Tune, LE. Auditory hallucinations and smaller superior temporal gyral volume in schizophrenia. *Am. J. Psychiatry.* 1990;147:1457-1462

Buchsbaum, MS; DeLisi, LE; Holcomb, HH; Cappelletti, J; King, AC;Johnson, J et al. Anteroposterior gradients in cerebral glucose use in schizophrenia and affective disorders. *Arch. Gen. Psychiatry.* 1984;41:1159-1166

Catafau, AM; Parellada, E; Lomena, FJ; Bernardo, M; Pavia, J; Ros, D; Setoain, J; Gonzalez-Monclus, E. Prefrontal and temporal blood flow in schizophrenia: Resting and activation technetium-99m-HMPAO SPECT pattern in young neuroleptic naïve patients with acute disease. *J. Nucl. Med.* 1994;35:935-941

Dvorak, I; Klaschka, J. Modification of the Grassberger-Procaccia algorithm for estimating the correlation exponent of chaotic systems with high embedding dimension. *Phys. Lett. A.* 1990; 145:225-231

Elbert, T; Lutzenberger, W; Rochstroh, B; Berg, P; Cohen, R. Physical aspects of the EEG in schizophrenics. *Biol. Psychiatry.* 1992;32:595-606

Fell, J; Roschke, J; Beckmann, P. The calculation of the first positive Lyapunov exponent in sleep EEG data. *Electroencephalogr. Clin. Neurophysiol.* 1993;86:348-352

Frank, GW; Lookman, T; Nerenberg, MAH; Essex, C; Lemieux, J; Blume, W. Chaotic time series analysis of epileptic seizures. *Physica D.* 1990; 46:427-438

Grassberger, P; Procaccia I. Characterization of strange attractors; *Phys. Rev. Lett*; 1983a; 50: 346-349

Grassberger, P; Procaccia I. Measuring the strangeness of strange attractors. *Physica D.* 1983b ;9 : 189-208

Grinvald, A.; Lieke, E; Frostig R.; Gilbert C; Wiesel T. Functional architecture of cortex revealed by optical imaging of intrinsic signals. *Nature.* 1992;324:361-364

Haken, H; Kelso, JAS; Bunz, H. A theoretical model of phase transitions in human hand movements. *Biol. Cybern.* 1985; 51: 347-356

Halgren, E; Dhond, RP; Christensen, N; Van Petten, C; Marinkovic, K; Lewine, J.D. , Dale, AM. N400-like magnetoencephalography responses modulated by semantic context; word frequency; and lexical class in sentences. *Neuroimage.* 2002;17:1101-1116

Hamalainen, M; Hari, R; Ilmoniemi, R; Knuutila, J; Lounasmaa, O. Magnetoencephalography-theory; instrumentation and applications to non-invasive studies of the working human brain. *Rev. Mod. Physics.* 1993; 65:1-93

Hughes, AJ; Daniel, SE; Kilford, L; Lees, AJ. Accuracy of clinical diagnosis of idiopathic Parkinson disease: a clinicopathological study of 100 cases. *J. Neurol. Neurosurg. Psychiatry.* 1992; 55:181-184

Jasper, HH. The ten-twenty electrode system of the International Federation; *Electroencephalogr. Clin. Neurophysiol.* 1958; 10 : 367-380

Kaplan, D; Glass, L. Understanding nonlinear dynamics. New York, Springer, 1995

Keshavana, MS; Cashmerea, JD; Miewalda, J; Yeraganib, VK. Decreased nonlinear complexity and chaos during sleep in first episode schizophrenia: a preliminary report. *Schizophrenia Res.* 2004;71 :263– 272

Kowalik, ZJ; Schnitzler, A; Freund, HJ; Witte, OW. Local Lyapunov exponents detect epileptic zones in spike-less interictal MEG recordings. *Clin. Neurophysiol.* 2001; 112: 60-7

Kristeva-Feige, R; Rossi, S; Feige, B; Mergner, T; Lucking, CH, Rossini P.M. The bereitschafts potential paradigm in investigating voluntary movement organization in humans using magnetoencephalography (MEG). *Brain Res. Protocol.* 1997;1:13-22

Kwong, K; Belliveau, J; Chesler, D; Goldberg, I; Wiskoff, R; Poncelet, B; et al: Dynamic magnetic resonance imaging of human brain activity during sensory stimulation. *Proc. Natl. Acad. Sci. U S A.* 1992; 89: 5675-5679

Lehnertz, K. Non-linear time series analysis of intracranial EEG recordings in patients with epilepsy - an overview. *Int. J. Psychophysiol.* 1999;34: 45-52

Lutzenberger, W; Birbaumer, N; Flor, H; Rockstroh, B; Elbert, T. Dimensional analysis of the human EEG and intelligence. *Neurosci. Lett.* 1992; 143: 10-14

Makela, JP. Neurological application of MEG. *Electroencephalogr. Clin. Neurophysiol. Suppl.* 1996; 47:343-355

Marinkovic, K; Dhond, RP; Dale, AM; Glessner, M; Carr, V; Halgren, E. Spatiotemporal dynamics of modality-specific and supramodal word processing. *Neuron.* 2003 ; 38: 487-497

Mitra, PP, Pesaran B. Analysis of dynamic brain imaging data. *Biophys. J.* 1999; 691-708

Peitgen, HO; Jurgens, H; Saupe, D. Chaos and fractals: New frontiers of science. New York , Springer, 1992

Pijn, JP; Van Neerven, J; Noest, A; Lopes da Silva, FH. Chaos or noise in EEG signals: dependence on state and brain site. *Electroencephalogr. Clin. Neurophysiol.* 1991; 79:371-381

Roschke, J; Aldenhoff, J. Estimation of the dimensionality of sleep-EEG data in schizophrenics. *Eur. Arch. Psychiatry Clin. Neurosci.* 1993;242:191-196

Rosenstein, MT; Collins, JJ; Juca, JD. A practical method for calculation largest Lyapunov exponents from small data sets. *Physica D.* 1993;65:117-134

Stam, CJ. Nonlinear dynamical analysis of EEG and MEG: Review of an emerging field. *Clin. Neurophysiol.* 2005;116:2266-2301

Stam, CJ; Jelles, B; Achtereekte, HAM; Birgelen, JH; van Slaets, JPJ. Diagnostic usefulness of linear and nonlinear quantitative EEG analysis in Alzheimer's disease. *Clin. Electroencephalogr.* 1996;27:69-77

Stam, CJ; Jelles, B; Achtereekte, HAM; Rombouts, SARB; Slaets, JPJ; Keunen RWM. Investigation of EEG nonlinearity in dementia and Parkinson's disease. *Electroencephalogr. Clin. Neurophysiol.* 1995;95:309-317

Takens, F. Detecting strange attractors in the turbulence. *Lect. Notes Math.* 1981; 898: 366-381

Theiler, J; Rapp, PE. Re-xamination of the evidence for low-dimensional nonlinear structure in the human electroencephalogram. *Electroencephalogr. Clin. Neurophysiol.* 1996;98:213-222

Timmermann, L; Gross, J; Dirks, M; Volkmann J; Freund, HJ, Schnitzler, A. The cerebral oscillatory network of Parkinsonian resting tremor. *Brain.* 2003; 126:199-212

Tonoike, M; Yamaguchi, M; Kaetsu, I; Kida, H; Seo, R; Koizuka, I. Ipsilateral dominance of human olfactory activated centres estimated from event-related magnetic fields measured by 122-channel whole head neuromagnetometer using odorant stimuli synchronized with respirations. *Ann. N.Y. Acad. Sci.* 1998; 855:579-590

Toro, MG; Ruiz, JS; Talavera, JA; Blanco, C. Chaos theories and therapeutic commonalities among depression; Parkinson's disease; and cardiac arrhythmias. *Compr. Psychiatry.* 1999 ;40:238-44

Volkmann, J; Joliot, M; Mogilner, A; Ioannides, AA; Lado, F; Fazzini, E; Ribary, U, Llinas, R. Central motor loop oscillations in parkinsonian resting tremor revealed by magnetoencephalography. *Neurology.* 1996; 46:1359-1370

Yambe, T; Asan,o E; Mauyama, S; Shiraishi, Y; Shibata, M; Sekine, K; et al. Chaos analysis of electro encephalography and control of seizure attack of epilepsy patients. *Biomed. Pharmacother*. 2005;59 Suppl 1:S236-8

# Index

## A

## B



## C

## D

## E

## J



## K



## L



## M

## N



## O

## P



## Q



## R

## S

## T



## U

## V



## W



## Y